AGING
Volume 20

The Aging Brain
*Cellular and Molecular Mechanisms of Aging
in the Nervous System*

Aging Series

Aging
Volume 20

The Aging Brain
Cellular and Molecular Mechanisms of Aging in the Nervous System

Editors

Ezio Giacobini, M.D., Ph.D.
Laboratory of Neuropsychopharmacology
Department of Biobehavioral Sciences
The University of Connecticut
Storrs, Connecticut

Guido Filogamo, M.D.
Institute of Human Anatomy
University of Turin Medical School
Turin, Italy

Giacomo Giacobini, M.D.
Institute of Human Anatomy
University of Turin Medical School
Turin, Italy

Antonia Vernadakis, Ph.D.
Departments of Psychiatry
and Pharmacology
University of Colorado School of Medicine
Denver, Colorado

Raven Press ■ New York

Raven Press, 1140 Avenue of the Americas, New York, New York 10036

Made in the United States of America

International Standard Book Number 0-89004-802-9
Library of Congress Catalog Number 81-40542

Great care has been taken to maintain the accuracy of the information contained in the volume. However, Raven Press cannot be held responsible for errors or for any consequences arising from the use of the information contained herein.

Preface

This volume presents current work on the cellular and molecular mechanisms of aging in the nervous system.

The question may arise as to why we are speaking of the mechanisms of aging at a time when early development and differentiation of the nervous system are the topical subjects. The answer is evident if we bear in mind the common impact of both early development and aging upon the population increase "at the two extremes of life." This calls to mind all the implications, socially speaking, of a good physical and psychic state of the population.

The affinity of these two seemingly disparate processes, growth and aging, was explained with authority by Giuseppe Levi, to whom this book is dedicated, in his 1946 monograph *Growth and Aging*. Here he claimed that from investigations based on the structural substrate of development, one may gather much information about the problem of senility. The alterations of the structures of the tissues, from the embryonal stage to that of old age, are inherent in the essential biological properties of organisms and are analogous, constituting one uninterrupted series. Physiological aging is not abstract and devoid of real content, even if it is interwoven with man's actual environment. Much of the substance of this volume documents the legitimacy of the premise of that monograph.

In agreement with Levi, Paul Weiss considered the aging process to be a "corollary of development," and not a "separate and separable encumbrance" superimposed as a contamination of the organism. Therefore, our present task is that of discovering the price we pay for developmental differentiation, the sum of the small errors that each individual accumulates day after day, both in cellular dynamics and in the dynamics of intercellular mutual relationships, slowly altering the neuro-glia unity.

Thus, it is also our task to attempt to combat the deteriorative events from which the decline of efficiency, adaptability, and plasticity derive, so that "if aging is inevitable, we can at least retard its pace."

The Editors

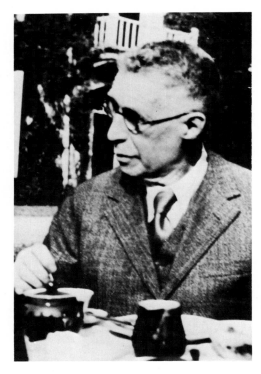

Professor Giuseppe Levi (1872–1965)

Dedication

This volume is dedicated to the great teacher Professor Giuseppe Levi, of the Institute of Normal Human Anatomy of Turin University.

Contents

Aging of Receptor Mechanisms

Human and Clinical Correlates of Brain Aging

General Discussion and Concluding Remarks

Contributors

R. Adolfsson
Umeå Dementia Research Group
Departments of Pathology and Psychiatry
University of Umeå
S-901 87 Umeå, Sweden

M. Aloisi
National Research Council Unit for Muscle
   Biology and Physiopathology
Institute of General Pathology
University of Padova
35100 Padova, Italy

H. H. Althaus
Department of Neurochemistry
Max-Planck Institute for Experimental Medicine
3 Hermann-Rein Street
Gottingen 3400, Federal Republic of Germany

L. Amaducci
Department of Neurology
University of Florence
Via le Morgagni 85
Florence 50134, Italy

Ellen B. Arnold
Departments of Psychiatry and Pharmacology
University of Colorado
School of Medicine and Veterans Administration
   Medical Center
Denver, Colorado 80262

Amico Bignami
West Roxbury Veterans Administration Medical
   Center
Boston, Massachusetts 02132

E. D. Bird
Department of Neurology-Neuropathology
Harvard Medical School
McLean Hospital
Boston, Massachusetts 02178

J. P. Blass
Department of Neurology
Dementia Research Service
Division of Chronic and Degenerative Diseases
Cornell University Medical College
The Burke Rehabilitation Center
785 Mamaroneck Avenue
White Plains, New York 10605

A. Bosio
Department of Pharmacology
University of Brescia
Brescia, Italy

D. M. Bowen
Miriam Marks Department of Neurochemistry
Institute of Neurology
33, John's Mews
London WC1N 2NS, United Kingdom

M. Brunetti
Biochemistry Department
The Medical School
Perugia University
Via del Giochetto
06100 Perugia, Italy

G. Calderini
Department of Biochemistry
Fidia Research Laboratories
Via Ponte della Fabbrica 3/A
35031 Abano Terme, Italy

Richard G. Cutler
Gerontology Research Center
National Institute on Aging
Baltimore City Hospitals
Baltimore, Maryland 21224

Doris Dahl
Department of Neuropathology
Harvard Medical School
Boston, Massachusetts 02115

A. N. Davison
Miriam Marks Department of Neurochemistry
Institute of Neurology
33, John's Mews
London WC1N 2NS, United Kingdom

S. J. Enna
Departments of Pharmacology and of
   Neurobiology and Anatomy
University of Texas Medical School
P.O. Box 20708
Houston, Texas 77025

N. Eshhar
Department of Neurobiology
The Weizmann Institute of Science
Rehovot 76100, Israel

A. Gaiti
Biochemistry Department
The Medical School
Perugia University
Via del Giochetto
06100 Perugia, Italy

Ezio Giacobini
Department of Biobehavioral Sciences
Laboratory of Neuropsychopharmacology
University of Connecticut
Storrs, Connecticut 06268

Gary E. Gibson
Department of Neurology
Cornell University Medical College
Burke Rehabilitation Center
White Plains, New York 10605

S. Govoni
Department of Pharmacology and
    Pharmacognosy
University of Milan
Milan, Italy

Inge Grundke-Iqbal
New York State Institute for Developmental
    Disabilities
1050 Forest Hill Road
Staten Island, New York 10314

James T. Hartford
Department of Psychiatry
University of Cincinnati Medical Center
Cincinnati, Ohio 45267

D. S. Heron
Department of Isotope Research
The Weizmann Institute of Science
76100 Rehovot, Israel

M. Hershkowitz
Department of Isotope Research
The Weizmann Institute of Science
76100 Rehovot, Israel

Antti Hervonen
Department of Biomedical Sciences
University of Tampere
P.O. Box 607
SF 33101 Tampere 10, Finland

Beng T. Ho
Departments of Neurobiology and
    Neurochemistry
Texas Research Institute of Mental Sciences
Houston, Texas 77030

D. W. Hoffman
Laboratory of Neuropsychopharmacology
Department of Biobehavioral Sciences
University of Connecticut
Storrs, Connecticut 06268

D. B. Hudson
Department of Physiology-Anatomy
University of California
Berkeley, California 94720

Khalid Iqbal
New York State Institute for Developmental
    Disabilities
1050 Forest Hill Road
Staten Island, New York 10314

C. Kalcheim
Department of Neurobiology
The Weizmann Institute of Science
Rehovot 76100, Israel

D. A. Kendall
Departments of Pharmacology and of
    Neurobiology and Anatomy
University of Texas Medical School
P.O. Box 20708
Houston, Texas 77025

Patricia M. Kralik
Departments of Neurobiology and
    Neurochemistry
Texas Research Institute of Mental Sciences
Houston, Texas 77030

M. Marchi
Laboratory of Neuropsychopharmacology
Department of Biobehavioral Sciences
University of Connecticut
Storrs, Connecticut 06268

J. Marcusson
Umeå Dementia Research Group
Departments of Pathology and Psychiatry
University of Umeå
S-901 87 Umeå, Sweden

Patricia A. Merz
New York State Institute for Developmental
    Disabilities
1050 Forest Hill Road
Staten Island, New York 10314

C. Miller
Department of Physiology-Anatomy
University of California
Berkeley, California 94720

Y. Mizrachi
Department of Neurobiology
The Weizmann Institute of Science
Rehovot 76100, Israel

I. Mussini
National Research Council Unit for Muscle
*   Biology and Physiopathology*
Institute of General Pathology
University of Padova
35100 Padova, Italy

V. Neuhoff
Department of Neurochemistry
Max-Planck Institute for Experimental Medicine
3 Hermann-Rein Street
Gottingen 3400, Federal Republic of Germany

Y. Nomura
Department of Pharmacology
Institute of Pharmaceutical Sciences
Hiroshima University School of Medicine
Kasumi 1-2-3, Minami-ku
Hiroshima 734, Japan

A. Nordberg
Department of Pharmacology
University of Uppsala
Box 573
S-751 23 Uppsala, Sweden

Michael Norenberg
Departments of Psychiatry and Pharmacology
University of Colorado
School of Medicine and Veterans Administration
*   Medical Center*
Denver, Colorado 80262

K. Oki
Department of Pharmacology
Institute of Pharmaceutical Sciences
Hiroshima University School of Medicine
Kasumi 1-2-3, Minami-ku
Hiroshima 734, Japan

Keith Parker
Departments of Psychiatry and Pharmacology
University of Colorado School of Medicine and
*   Veterans Administration Medical Center*
Denver, Colorado 80262

Matti Partanen
Laboratory of Neurosciences
Gerontology Research Center
National Institute of Aging
Baltimore City Hospitals
Baltimore, Maryland 21224

Christine Peterson
Department of Neurology
Cornell University Medical College
Burke Rehabilitation Center
White Plains, New York 10605

G. Porcellati
Biochemistry Department
The Medical School
Perugia University
Via del Giochetto
06100 Perugia, Italy

Stanley I. Rapoport
Laboratory of Neurosciences
Gerontology Research Center
National Institute of Aging
Baltimore City Hospitals
Baltimore, Maryland 21224

F. Riccardi
Department of Pharmacology and
*   Pharmacognosy*
University of Milan
Milan, Italy

George S. Roth
Endocrinology Section
Clinical Physiology Branch
Gerontology Research Center
National Institute on Aging
National Institutes of Health at Baltimore City
*   Hospitals*
Baltimore, Maryland 21224

T. Samorajski
Departments of Neurobiology and
*   Neurochemistry*
Texas Research Institute of Mental Sciences
Houston, Texas 77030

D. Samuel
Department of Isotope Research
The Weizmann Institute of Science
76100 Rehovot, Israel

H. Schupper
Department of Virology
Section for Electron Microscopy
Israel Institute for Biological Research
P.O. Box 19
Ness-Ziona, Israel

Michal Schwartz
Department of Neurobiology
The Weizmann Institute of Science
Rehovot 76100, Israel

T. Segawa
Department of Pharmacology
Institute of Pharmaceutical Sciences
Hiroshima University School of Medicine
Kasumi 1-2-3, Minami-ku
Hiroshima 734, Japan

A. Shahar
Department of Virology
Section for Electron Microscopy
Israel Institute for Biological Research
P.O. Box 19
Ness-Ziona, Israel

M. Shinitzky
Department of Membrane Research
The Weizmann Institute of Science
76100 Rehovot, Israel

M. L. Simeoni
National Research Council Unit for Muscle
*   Biology and Physiopathology*
Institute of General Pathology
University of Padova
35100 Padova, Italy

N. R. Sims
Miriam Marks Department of Neurochemistry
Institute of Neurology
33, John's Mews
London WC1N 2NS, United Kingdom

Dean O. Smith
Department of Physiology
University of Wisconsin
Madison, Wisconsin 53706

S. Sorbi
Department of Neurology
Dementia Research Service
Division of Chronic and Degenerative Diseases
Cornell University Medical College
The Burke Rehabilitation Center
785 Mamaroneck Avenue
White Plains, New York 10605

P. F. Spano
Department of Pharmacology and
*   Pharmacognosy*
University of Milan
Milan, Italy

R. Strong
Departments of Pharmacology and of
*   Neurobiology and Anatomy*
University of Texas Medical School
P.O. Box 20708
Houston, Texas 77025

P. S. Timiras
Department of Physiology-Anatomy
University of California
Berkeley, California 94720

G. Toffano
Department of Biochemistry
Fidia Research Laboratories
Via Ponte della Fabbrica 3/A
35031 Abano Terme, Italy

M. Trabucchi
Department of Pharmacology
University of Brescia
Brescia, Italy

M. R. Ven Murthy
Department of Biochemistry
Faculty of Medicine
Laval University
G1K 7P4 Québec, Canada

Antonia Vernadakis
Departments of Psychiatry and Pharmacology
University of Colorado
School of Medicine and Veterans Administration
*   Medical Center*
Denver, Colorado 80262

Z. Vogel
Department of Neurobiology
The Weizmann Institute of Science
Rehovot 76100, Israel

B. Winblad
Umeå Dementia Research Group
Departments of Pathology and Psychiatry
University of Umeå
S-901 87 Umeå, Sweden

Henryk M. Wisniewski
New York State Institute for Developmental
*   Disabilities*
1050 Forest Hill Road
Staten Island, New York 10314

I. Yorsumoto
Department of Pharmacology
Institute of Pharmaceutical Sciences
Hiroshima University School of Medicine
Kasumi 1-2-3, Minami-ku
Hiroshima 734, Japan

L. Yurkewicz
Laboratory of Neuropsychopharmacology
Department of Biobehavioral Sciences
University of Connecticut
Storrs, Connecticut 06268

*The Aging Brain: Cellular and Molecular
Mechanisms of Aging in the Nervous System,*
edited by E. Giacobini et al., Raven Press, New
York © 1982.

The Dysdifferentiative Hypothesis of Mammalian Aging and Longevity

Richard G. Cutler

Gerontology Research Center, National Institute on Aging, Baltimore City Hospitals, Baltimore, Maryland 21224

What to Expect from Gerontological Research?
Science editorial, Sept. 5, 1980, Vol. 209.
  "Medical care, one might say, remains in its infancy as long as it
  cannot forestall intrinsic pathogenesis as effectively as that
  originating in the environment. To overcome this limitation is
  the true aim of gerontological research. In initiating the revo-
  lutionary step from an environmentally oriented health care to one
  centered on man himself, it becomes the very foundation of future
  scientific medicine."
  --Frederic C. Ludwig, Dept. of Pathology, College of Medicine,
    University of California, Irvine.

Biological aging is manifested by a progressive uniform loss of optimum health and vigor. The biology of aging is clearly complex. Most
physiological functions are involved in aging and decline at approxima-
tively the same rate. Thus, the problem of separating out cause and
effect is extremely difficult.
    Over the past ten years my interest in gerontology has been aimed at
gaining an understanding of the biology of general health maintenance
rather than the biology of general health loss governing aging rate. It
was hoped that by this approach some of the complexities of aging could
be avoided and an understanding of processes governing aging rate at the
mechanistic level would be more readily gained.
    The fundamental assumption of this research approach is that the
biology of general health maintenance is indeed somewhat less complex
than the biology of the whole organism. It was therefore important to
determine if a special set of health maintenance processes do exist
which act to govern aging rate and, if so, what are they, how do they
function, and what might their genetic complexity be? In this paper I
have reviewed some of the major points of the working hypothesis formed
over the course of this research effort which was designed to answer
these questions and some of our recent findings.

THE WORKING HYPOTHESIS OF MAMMALIAN AGING AND LONGEVITY

    Much of the theoretical basis of the working hypothesis that has been
used to guide my research program has been of an evolutionary nature.
A summary of the rationale and major concepts developed from this evolutionary viewpoint which forms the basis of the working hypothesis
follows.

1. The existance of living systems (life forms) and their evolution are suggested to be based fundamentally on the preservation of information which can preserve this same information (11,12,15). By necessity, this information is encoded in a physical structure having a finite life span, and thus a key feature of all living systems is the protection and repair of this physical structure. Any time-dependent alteration in the physical structure which contains this information leading towards an increased probability of its loss is considered, in a broad sense, to be an aging process. All processes acting to preserve this information, such as repair and protective mechanisms, are considered in a broad sense to be anti-aging processes. DNA is an example of a physical structure where such information is stored, and DNA replication an example of one of the most primitive and essential information preservational processes which have evolved (11). The information set of an organism can theoretically be preserved indefinitely (immortality) in a mortal physical setting.

2. Throughout the evolution of all living systems the opposition of anti-aging vs aging forces has prevailed (16,19). The biological makeup of all life forms consequently reflects the interplay and trade-offs moulded by the actions and counteractions of these two forces, which are reflected in every characteristic of life. The longevity of an individual of a given life form is only one of many different types of strategies that have evolved to ensure continued preservation of its characteristic set of information. Thus, since the origin of life, longevity processes have evolved, not senescent or aging processes, although the primary source of the senescent processes in life forms is the result of endogenously produced pleiotropic by-products of their information preservational processes, such as energy metabolism, differentiation and development.

3. On studying the evolution of longevity in mammalian species, it is found that, in general, longevity of the individual has steadily increased (13,14,17). Also, few if any individuals in their natural ecological niche are able to live much beyond a chronological age where the aging process seriously decreases their health status or physiological functions. This evidence opposes the postulated existance of specific aging genes or hormones that are necessary to age an individual for the good of its species. It also supports the concept that senescence did not evolve nor is it a result of a special evolutionary selected genetic program. Instead, it is predicted that longevity has evolved in mammalian species as a result of an evolutionary positive pressure.

4. The characteristic lifespan of an individual of a given mammalian species can be explained as an evolutionary adaptation to ensure optimum health and physical vigor throughout its normal life span, as determined by the environmental hazards of its ecological niche (15). This life span is where the probability of death due to these environmental hazards reaches a point where further longevity has little benefit for the preservation of the information which defines the species. In primates and other mammalian species there is a good correlation between the longevity of an individual and its dependence for its evolutionary success on "learned behavior", as opposed to "instinctive behavior". The amount of "learned behavior" a species is capable of and expresses in turn plays an important role in determining the resultant intensity of the hazards of the species' ecological niche (15,16,19).

5. The remarkable similarities of the primate species in terms of morphology, physiology, biochemistry and genetic-encoded information

suggest that their evolutionary developmental beginnings from a common ancestor 65 million years ago were accomplished mainly through changes in regulatory genes which affected the timing and degree of expression of a common unchanging set of structural genes (13,14,17). The high evolutionary rate of increase in longevity of primates along the hominid ancestral-descendant sequence indicates a similar genetic mechanism of evolution for the increase in longevity. Only a few mutations in these regulatory genes or chromosomal sequence rearrangements relative to the structural genes they control appear to have been necessary to account for the observed increase in longevity. It is estimated that a maximum of about 0.6% of the total cellular genetic information in a cell was involved in the recent evolutionary history of man, which includes all aspects of recent hominid evolutionary changes in addition to longevity (13,14).

6. The above results were used to postulate the existance of a specific set of structural genes whose role is to govern the duration of time that general health and vigor of an organism is to be maintained. The functions these genes code for are called "longevity determinant processes" (LDPs). All mammalian species are predicted to have the same set of LDPs and the species' characteristic duration of good health or longevity is a result of their timing during development and the intensity of their expression (12,15,16). This timing and extent of expression are postulated to be governed by a specific set of regulatory genes. It is these regulatory genes governing the levels of LDPs which have evolved during the evolution of longevity in the primate species.

7. The primary causes of aging are predicted to be of a pleiotropic nature; that is, they are by-products of normally beneficial metabolic and developmental processes (17). Two basic types are postulated: (a) "continuously-acting biosenescent processes" (CABPs) and (b) "developmentally-linked biosenescent processes" (DLBPs). Evolution of longevity depended on the coordinated reduction of these two causes of aging (72). Examples of CAPBs are the by-products of oxygen metabolism, such as the superoxide radical $O_2^{-\cdot}$, the hydroxyl radical $\cdot OH$, and hydrogen peroxide H_2O_2. Their corresponding LDPs are superoxide dismutase, glutathione peroxidase, and catalase. Examples of DLBPs are the hormones associated with sexual maturation, and their corresponding LDP is the postponement of their appearance by the general decrease in rate of development.

8. The CAPBs and DLBPs are postulated to act largely by epigenetic/ mutational-like processes slowly destabilizing the proper differentiated state of cells (18). Thus, aging of an individual is considered to be largely a result of a time-dependent disorderly, dysdifferentiative process--the opposite of the orderly differentiation and developmental processes which initially created the individual. The longevity of a species is determined then on the species' innate ability to maintain the proper differentiated state of its cells over a given time period. The time-dependent stability of a differentiated cell is the result of the level of perturbation a cell's genetic apparatus receives. This is equal to the difference of the CABPs and DLBPs' levels and the counteracting levels of LDPs (28,59).

9. This hypothesis suggests (a) a new interpretation of the forces involved in the origin of life and the evolution of species, which are predicted to be reflected in many of the morphological, physiological, cellular and biochemical features of all forms of life and whose presence could not otherwise be explained, (b) a new experimental approach in

aging research investigating the biochemical and non-systemic processes governing the general maintenance of health by the comparison of genetically closely-related species having substantial differences in innate aging rates, and (c) the existance of a specific set of genes called the LDPs, which determine the time-dependent stability of cells capable of maintaining their proper state of differentiation and thus govern a species' duration of good health and resultant life span (22).

10. Recent experimental evidence suggests that some LDPs may be genetically linked and/or under control of a common regulatory gene element in prokaryotic and eukaryotic single-cell organisms, as well as in multicell organisms. Some of these common regulatory gene elements appear to be located in or near the histocompatibility loci in mouse and human (particularly the major histocompatibility complex), and mutations in these loci appear to govern tissue levels of DNA repair, superoxide dismutase, catalase and cAMP, as well as lifespan of H-2 congenic strain mice. These results, plus the effects of the human major histocompatibility complex on onset frequency of a number of diseases, suggest that the major and minor histocompatibility gene clusters in mammalian species may represent superstructural and regulatory gene loci for LDPs. These LDPs would then appear to have a common basis for their mechanism of action, which is the maintenance of proper self through self- and non-self recognition processes (20,21).

EXPERIMENTAL APPROACH TO TESTING THE WORKING HYPOTHESIS

As previously stated, pleiotropic by-products of metabolism and development are predicted to be the primary causes of aging and are of two types or sets. In terms of metabolism, one set of aging processes is called "continuously-acting biosenescent processes" (CABP). Examples are the various energy- or heat-producing reactions producing free radicals, such as during oxygen metabolism. These are the superoxide free radical $O_2^{-\cdot}$, the hydroxyl radical $\cdot OH$, and hydrogen peroxide H_2O_2. Corresponding longevity determinant processes (LDPs) would be superoxide dismutase, glutathione peroxidase and catalase. The second set of aging processes is associated with development and is called "developmentally-linked biosenescent processes" (DLBP). Examples are the hormones and growth factors involved in the control of growth and sexual maturation (44,45). A corresponding LDP to the DLBPs would be the postponement of their expression in terms of chronological time by slowing down the rate of development.

These two types of aging processes produce their aging effects by destabilizing the differentiated state of cells by way of epigenetic/mutational interaction with the genetic processes determining a cell's state of differentiation. Thus, the phenotypic expression of aging is predicted to be largely the result of cellular dysdifferentiation processes and not necessarily only the result of cellular intrinsic impairments. The LDPs act to stabilize the differentiated state of cells in all mammalian species. The longer the stability of the cells is maintained, the longer is the period of good health, vigor and longevity. Thus, the problem of determining what governs aging rate is that of determining what stabilizes the differentiated state of cells. It is predicted that LDPs are the key stabilizing forces of the differentiated state of mammalian cells. The probability of a cell suffering a change leading to a dysdifferentiative type of change is directly proportional to its steady-state equilibrium load of epigenetic and mutational

alterations in the genome. This load does not necessarily have to increase with age and is governed by the resultant intensity of harmful
agents which reach and damage the genome and the intensity of repair
processes which remove the damage. The following diagram illustrates
this concept.

Dysdifferentiational Model of Cellular Aging

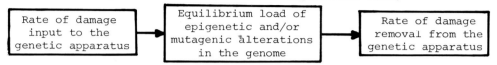

The rate of damage input to the genetic apparatus is determined by the
primary generation rate of damage (being proportional to specific metabolic rate in many cases) and the intracellular levels of protection. The
rate of output damage removed from the genetic apparatus is determined
by the levels of DNA repair and the chromatin turnover rate. The genetic
apparatus will show a continuous turnover of alterations scattered along
the genome, some areas being more intense than others, which do not
necessarily build up with age. Old cells will be largely free of damage
and normal in all respects with regard to viable processes. The equilibrium load (similar to mutational load) is defined by the level of input
of **damage and** the level of output of damage. Longer-lived species are
predicted to have a characteristic lower equilibrium load of epigenetic/
mutational alterations in their cells throughout their lifespan than
shorter-lived species and thus a lower probability of drifting towards
different differentiated states.

According to this model, an equation can be derived that relates
longevity (MLP) to the degree of protection and repair of the genetic
apparatus in cells. This equation is:

$$MLP = K \cdot \frac{(protection)(repair)}{(specific\ metabolic\ rate)}$$

where K is a constant and protection might be the tissue level of superoxide dismutase and repair the level of UV DNA repair. Thus, this model
can be tested by determining if MLP does vary with repair, protection,
and specific metabolic rate according to the above functions.

DYSDIFFERENTIATIVE NATURE OF MAMMALIAN AGING PROCESSES

The mammalian aging process is usually thought to be a result of a
time-dependent increase of impairment of vital functions occurring at the
cellular level which, if allowed to continue long enough, would eventually result in cell death (10,35,50,55,67,70,71). In contrast to this
view, a hypothesis has been described pointing out that most dysfunctions
associated with aging could be accounted for by a small accumulative age-
depedent drift of cells from their proper state of differentiation, where
vital cellular functions would not necessarily become impaired (16,59).
Specific age-dependent diseases such as autoimmune diseases (48) or
cancer (27,46,77), the age-dependent appearance of abnormal proteins (78)
or abnormal cell morphology (64), the loss of specific proteins such as
hormone receptors (63), and the appearance of specific types of cells in

the wrong tissues (metaplasias)(36) support the dysdifferentiative
hypothesis of aging. The dysdifferentiative process is proposed to be
a result of an age-dependent accumulation of genetic changes due to the
natural instability of DNA (26) (such as in transposon element migration)
and the long-term interaction of the genetic apparatus with endogenously-
produced hormones, growth factors, or toxic by-products of metabolism
(28,59). Thus, the differentiated state of cells is considered to be
innately unstable, requiring positive functions for its maintenance.

The general effect of the proposed dysdifferentiation process is a
slow but increasing inability of tissues to carry out functions at an
optimum efficiency. The same type of accumulative change in cells is
also predicted to lead to specific types of dysfunctions such as cancer
(8,60), where in this case the specific change (the loss of proper cell
growth restriction) results in an amplification of the dysdifferentiated
cell by increased cell number (59).

Thus, the biological aspects of longevity and aging are viewed as a
problem in the maintenance of the proper state of cell differentiation
after sexual maturity has been reached. Accordingly, cells from longer-
lived species are predicted to have evolved means (intrinsically and/or
through extracellular means) to ensure a longer time-dependent state of
proper differentiation. Evidence that intracellular levels of superoxide
dismutase may be such a stabilizing agent of differentiation has been
reported (72).

The dysdifferentiated model of mammalian aging and longevity is
summarized in outline form as follows.

A. Hypothesis
   1. Aging rate of an organism is directly related to the innate
      ability of the cells making up that organism to maintain their
      proper state of differentiation as a function of time.
   2. Differentiated cells are inherently unstable, and their rate of
      drift away from their proper state of differentiation is
      governed by the level of expression of LDPs.

B. Prediction of hypothesis
   1. A time-dependent increase in improper gene expression will be
      found, resulting in an altered differentiated state of cells.
   2. The rate of dysdifferentiation will be found to be inversely
      related to longevity or maximum lifespan potential of an
      organism.

C. Supportive data from other laboratories
   1. Many aspects of cancer cells reflect a dysdifferentiative state.
      The age-dependent increase in onset frequency of cancer is an
      expression of a specific case of the dysdifferentiative process,
      a case where proper regulation of cell division is lost (60).
   2. Many aspects of the age-dependent autoimmune diseases can be
      explained as the result of the derepression of cellular proteins
      that were repressed before immunocompetence developed (60).
   3. The age-dependent expression of endogenous viruses (slow
      viruses) could represent dysdifferentiation (30).
   4. Appearance of foreign-like proteins associated with senile
      dementia diseases (neurofibrillary tangles)(78).
   5. Changes in cell morphology (64), enzyme induction (1), loss of
      hormone receptors (63), and general decrease in ability to
      carry out specific functions (66).
   6. Lack of detection of any serious cellular impairment in cells

taken from old animals that could account for the types of dysfunctions associated with aging (62).

D. Supportive data from our laboratory
  1. We have investigated if there is an age-dependent increase in the presence of a gene product in a given differentiated type of cell in tissue where this gene is thought to be normally repressed. The experimental method uses radioactive cDNA probes of specific genes to detect the presence of a complementary RNA sequence in an RNA preparation from tissues of different-aged mice.
  2. Experimental results
     a. Structural genes. Age-dependent derepression of globin and casein genes were studied in liver and brain tissues of C57BL/6J male mice. Results show a two-fold increase in globin in nuclei and cytoplasm of brain and liver over an age range of 6-24 months (59). No changes were found for casein genes (24).
     b. Endogenous virus genes. Age-dependent derepression of mouse leukemia virus (MuLV) and mouse mammary tumor virus (MMTV) were studied in liver and brain tissues of C57BL/6J male mice. Results show a four-fold qualitative increase in gene expression of the viral genome in the nuclei but no change in the cytoplasm (28,59). These results suggest that stabilization of nuclear membrane integrity and selective transcription processes are essential in maintaining differentiated stability of cells. Understanding the mechanism of selective transport of RNA to the cytoplasm may lead to important insight to understanding (a) the stabilization of differentiation and (b) a regulatory gene dysfunction which occurs with increasing age.

Our present general approach for determining if aging is related to dysdifferentiational processes is to continue along these lines, as follows:

A. Look for the derepression of specific genes using cDNA probes
  1. Structural proteins where cDNA probes are available
     a. α and β -hemoglobin (mouse and human)
     b. casein (mouse)
     c. α-fetoprotein (mouse)
     d. insulin (mouse and human)
     e. growth hormone (mouse and human)
     f. albumin (rat)
  2. Endogenous viruses where cDNA probes are available
     a. mouse leukemia viruses (MuLV)
     b. mouse mammary tumor viruses (MMTV)
     c. adenoviruses (primates)
     d. retroviruses (primates)

B. Search for possible changes in distribution of isoenzymes. Over 20 isoenzymes have shown changes in their isoelectric PAGE profile as a function of different states of differentiation and/or normal vs cancerous tissue (77).

C. Search for possible anatomical cellular changes (36,37)
  1. metaplasias (tissues appearing in the wrong organs)
  2. Dysfunctional tissues (as carcinomas)

3. Increased frequency of nodules, benign foci or lesions, precursor lesions appearing in normal tissue

THE SEARCH FOR LONGEVITY DETERMINANT PROCESSES

Superoxide Dismutase

We are presently studying potential LDPs acting against the by-products of metabolism that are not developmentally-linked. We have focused on LDPs that would act against free radicals, namely the superoxide radical $O_2^{-\bullet}$. Its corresponding LDPs are superoxide dismutase (SOD), glutathione peroxidase and catalase. The experimental approach has been to see if a correlation exists between the maximum life span potentials of primate species and their life-long constitutive levels of these protective enzymes. The following figure shows a typical result found for superoxide dismutase levels in different primate species (72).

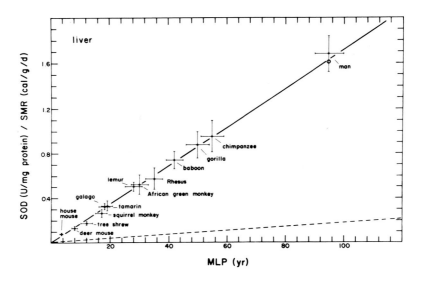

FIG. 1. Correlation between maximum lifespan potential (MLP) and the ratio of superoxide dismutase (SOD) specific activity to specific metabolic rate (SMR) for liver. Data represent mean $\pm$ SD. Taken from (72).

Similar results were found for brain and heart tissues, and these results can be described by the following function:

SOD = K (MLP)(SMR) = K (MCC)

where: SOD = specific activity of superoxide dismutase
       MLP = maximum lifespan potential
       SMR = specific metabolic rate of the particular tissue
       MCC = maximum lifespan potential calorie consumption

Uric Acid

Recently Bruce Ames and coworkers have found that uric acid (a normal constituent of plasma) is an excellent free radical scavenger (personal communication). They have proposed that uric acid may be an important protective agent against membrane lipid peroxidation and, because of its higher levels in man than in other species, it may therefore be an important longevity determinant process. We have looked for such a correlation in the primate species using literature values for plasma uric acid concentration and have found that in general a good correlation does exist. This data is shown in the following figure.

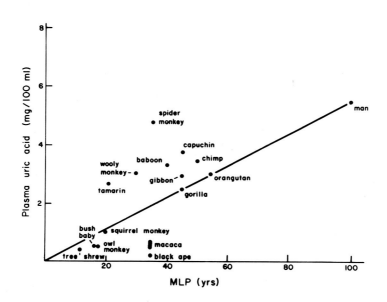

FIG.2 Blood plasma concentration of uric acid as a function of maximum lifespan potential (MLP) in primates. Uric acid values are taken from (7,52).

Guanylate Cyclase

The activity of guanylate cyclase can be increased by its direct interaction with free radicals and a number of mutagenic agents (25,51). We were therefore interested to see if this enzyme might play an important role in the detection and gene regulation of LDPs in a cell. Our initial investigations were to determine if the activity of soluble guanylate cyclase correlated with the maximum lifespan potential of primate species. We found a good inverse correlation, the opposite of what was found for SOD. Typical results for guanylate cyclase activity in brain are shown in the following figure.

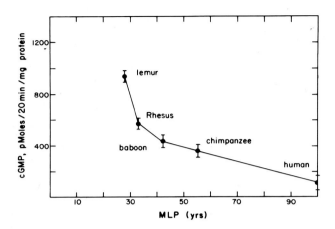

FIG. 3. Guanylate cyclase as a function of maximum life span
potential (MLP) in brain tissues of primates.

These guanylate cyclase results are consistent with the following
function:

SOD = K_1 (MLP)(SMR)

(GC)(SOD) = constant = K_1 (GC)(MLP)(SMR), giving

$$(GC) = \frac{K_2}{(SMR)(MLP)}$$

From these results it is suggested that guanylate cyclase may act
importantly as a free radical detector and thus as a regulatory enzyme
governing the intracellular redictive/oxidative potential by regulating
the levels of a number of antioxidants. A simple model for this control
is shown in the diagram below.

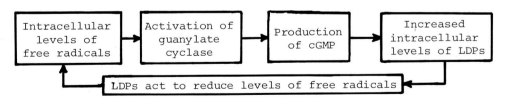

Sensitivity of the feedback loop is predicted to determine the constitutive intracellular levels of free radicals. An increased sensitivity
of the feedback loop would be predicted for longer-lived primate species,
resulting in higher levels of LDPs and lower levels of free radicals.
An age-dependent increase of guanylate cyclase activity, and consequently
cGMP, would be consistent with an increased level of mutagens and free
radicals in the cell, which might reflect excess damage within the cell.

General Classes of Potential Longevity Determinant Processes

The correlation of superoxide dismutase, guanylate cyclase and urate activity levels in tissues with MLP supports their role as possible longevity determinant processes. A general list of potential longevity determinant processes which can be tested by this comparative approach by seeking a correlation with MLP is as follows.

A. Immunological system
   1. Sensitivity and specificity of immunological reactions
   2. Inducibility of immunological reactions

B. Interferon
   1. Sensitivity and specificity of the various types of interferons
   2. Inducibility of interferon production

C. Intracellular mechanisms stabilizing the differentiated state of cells
   1. Protection and repair of critical regulatory components
   2. Redundancy of control-regulatory processes
   3. Cyclic genetic reprogramming during cell division
   4. Independent-acting gene regulatory processes (no operons)

D. Detoxification processes (40)
   1. Mixed function oxidases
   2. Oxidation-reduction enzymes
   3. Conjugation and hydralic enzymes
   4. Peptide bond and mercapturic acid reactions

E. DNA repair processes
   1. X-ray
   2. Ultraviolet light
   3. Endogenous chemical mutagens
   4. Depurination

F. Free radical scavengers
   1. Superoxide dismutase
   2. Glutathione peroxidase
   3. Catalase
   4. Glutathione
   5. Cysteine
   6. Vitamin C
   7. Vitamin E
   8. Unsaturated fatty acids
   9. Polyamines
   10. Urate and related derivatives
   11. Retinoids and related derivatives

G. Cellular renewal processes
   1. Non-selective protein and lipid degradation
   2. Selective protein (abnormal) degradation
   3. Organelle turnover (mitochondria, peroxisomes, lysosomes)
   4. Cell replacement (turnover)
   5. Chromatin protein turnover

H. Redundancy processes
   1. Molecular level
      a. Information storage (redundant structural genes)
      b. Information control (redundant regulatory genes)

2. Cellular level
   a. Cellular structure and organelles
   b. Cell number per tissue
3. Organ level
   a. Overlap function of organs and tissues
   b. Number of separate organs of same function

I. Reduction of specific metabolic rate
  1. Body size increase
  2. Decreased ratio of heat energy/kinetic energy production
  3. Decreased body temperature

J. Decrease in the rate of development and differentiation
  1. Postponement in the appearance of growth inhibitors
  2. Postponement in the appearance of steroids and hormones asscciated with sexual maturation processes
  3. Possible protective role of dehydroepiandrosterone (DHEA) against the long-term harmful effects of hormones and growth factors related to development

K. Increase in precision of homeostasis control
  1. Intracellular processes
  2. Extracellular processes

L. Shifts in the relative levels of enzymes in metabolic pathways, resulting in less toxic by-product production
  1. Change in the ratio of the isoenzymes of lactate dehydrogenase
  2. Alteration in the amount of the various mixed function oxidase enzymes

M. Shifts in the relative levels of structural components of a cell
  1. Change in the ratio of unsaturated/saturated fatty acids
  2. Change in the amino acid content in proteins. Decrease in methionine and other amino acids subject to high oxidation/racemization rates

MAJOR HISTOCOMPATIBILITY COMPLEX: A NEW PROPOSAL FOR ITS BIOLOGICAL ROLE

Mutations occurring within the H-2 loci of mice have been reported by other laboratories to change the levels of (a) DNA repair in response to ultraviolet light and bleomycin in lymphocytes (75), (b) tenth decile of longevity of H-2 congenic mouse strains (68), (c) superoxide dismutase levels in liver (58), (d) catalase levels in kidney (39), and (e) cAMP levels in liver (49). On integrating these difference sources of data, we found a positive correlation of the levels of DNA repair, superoxide dismutase, catalase and cAMP with the tenth decile longevity of these H-2 congenic mouse strains (20,21). These data, shown in Table 1, suggested to us that the H-2 region might act importantly in governing a wide spectrum of LDPs, in addition to its involvement in the immune system.

A summary of other evidence suggesting a role for the MHC as a cluster of LDP regulatory genes is given.

1. Mutations in the H-2 loci of mice coordinately change the levels of SOD, catalase, DNA repair, cAMP and life span of the mice in the expected direction; that is, higher levels result in greater life span.

2. Similar coordinated effects produced by a single mutation have been found in other organisms:

E. coli   - catalase, glutathione peroxidase, SOD (38)
Neurospora - catalase, glutathione peroxidase, SOD, life span (53,54)

TABLE 1. Correlation between expression of potential longevity determinants and major histocompatibility genes in congenic mouse strains

Mouse strain	H-2 allele	Life span[a]	SOD[b]	cAMP[c]	Ultraviolet DNA repair[d]	Bleomycin DNA repair[d]
B10Br/Sg	k	149 ± 1.1	23 ± 2	0.95 ± 0.2	2.0 ± 0.18	72
C57BL/10	b	155 ± 4.0	46 ± 2	1.29 ± 0.18	3.7 ± 0.28	120
B10A/2R	h2	-	46 ± 2	1.76 ± 0.32	-	-
B10A/4R	h4	-	48 ±	1.76 ± 0.32	-	-
A.BY	b	114 ± 3.5	45 ± 1	1.39 ± 0.16	-	-
A.CA	f	127 ± 3.0	48 ± 2	1.48 ± 0.13	-	-
C3H/HeDi	k	138 ± 0.7	18 ± 1	0.99 ± 0.28	1.7 ± 0.15	90
C3H.SW	b	150 ± 1.2	58 ± 1	1.25 ± 0.37	2.1 ± 0.23	125

[a] Tenth decile, male (68).

[b] Units SOD/mg protein in liver (58).

[c] Picomoles cAMP/mg liver, wet weight (43).

[d] Expressed as amount of unscheduled DNA replication in treated lymphocytes at a given dose divided by amount of DNA replication of untreated cells (75).

<u>Drosophila</u> - SOD, DNA repair, sensitivity to chemical mutagens,
          life span (3,5)
     3. Age-dependent derepression of endogenous viruses is affected by
H-2 loci.
     4. Lower than normal levels of LDPs have been found in a number of
human inherited diseases, some of which are also known to be associated
with specific HLA alleles. A few examples are:
     a. systemic lupus erythematosus: MHC-linked and low level of
        DNA repair (6)
     b. rheumatoid arthritis: MHC-linked and low level of SOD (61)
     c. diabetes mellitus: MHC-linked, low level of SOD, altered levels
        of cyclic nucleotides similar to those found in older patients
        (76)
     d. Down's syndrome: high levels of Cu/Zn SOD and interferon
        receptor and low level of Mn SOD (4)
     e. Parkinson's disease: low levels of glutathione peroxidase and
        catalase (2)
     f. Fanconi's anemia: low level of SOD (41)
     g. granulomatous disease: low level of glutathione peroxidase (65)
     5. Aryl hydrocarbon hydroxylase (Ah) levels appear to be correlated
with life span in some mouse strains and may be regulated by genes on the
same chromosome as the H-2 loci (56,57,80).

     To summarize our interest in the major histocompatibility complex, the
following points are made.
     1. The function of the immune system is the maintenance of proper self
through self- and non-self recognition processes acting at the cellular
level against abnormal cells or organisms coming from the external environment.
     2. The function of the LDPs is also the maintenance of proper self, a
number of which are through self- and non-self recognition processes such
as DNA repair and selective protein degradation, but acting at the
molecular level against intrinsic types of pathology. In this regard,
the role of scavengers like SOD and glutathione peroxidase is also the
maintenance of proper self, such as through the protection of cell membranes. This is necessary for maintaining proper hormone receptor levels
and cell-cell interactions, among other things, which are essential for
the cell to be able to maintain its state of differentiation.
     3. We have proposed that the immune system may be part of the LDPs,
with a common purpose and acting through a common mechanism. Another
system which may also be part of the LDPs and is related in function to
the immune system is interferon.
     4. It appears that all of these LDPs have a long and common evolutio-
nary history, some of which emerged from common ancestral genes. The
discovery that regulatory genes governing the levels of molecular as well
as cellular LDPs might be clustered together in a few common gene loci
such as the MHC might therefore be expected. The coordinate control of
the LDPs by a few supergenes would provide certain adaptive advantages
for the control of aging processes, as well as to enable a rapid rate of
coordinate evolution of longevity (23).
     5. The proposed mechanism of how MHC gene loci control LDPs is by the
governing of the sensitivity of certain membrane receptors of cells to
specific humoral factors; that is, LDP levels within a cell are not an
independent intrinsic cellular property but are instead determined at
least in part by the presence of specific cell membrane receptors and
humoral factors. It is the sensitivity of these receptors and the

effectiveness of the humoral factor(s) which play(s) a role in determining a cells LDP level and in turn the longevity of the animal. Perhaps the receptor involves guanylate cyclase, which in turn is involved
in determining intracellular levels of cGMP and cAMP (9,47).

MEMBRANE SURFACE AND HUMORAL HORMONE-LIKE FACTORS GOVERNING INTRACELLULAR LEVELS OF LONGEVITY DETERMINANT PROCESSES

An important assumption made concerning our efforts to understand the
mechanism(s) controlling intracellular levels of longevity determinant
processes (LDPs) and how these levels might be enhanced is that the
levels of LDPs are controlled by some type of intracellular mechanism(s).
For example, the higher levels of SOD and DNA repair found in the cells
of longer-lived species were thought to be entirely due to intracellular
gene-control mechanisms and independent of extracellular influences.
Most of the scientific community appears to have assumed this concept to
be true, and to my knowledge no one has seriously questioned it. In
fact, this assumption underlies much of the past and present work using
tissue culture techniques, where cells have been examined for their
innate properties of DNA repair and sensitivity to various mutagens and
carcinogens. The extracellular environment of cells grown in tissue
culture is the tissue culture growth media, which usually consists of
essential salts and minerals plus serum (usually from calf). The possible effects this growth media has or the possibility that there might be
specific extracellular regulatory factors of a humoral nature that might
act to govern intracellular levels of DNA repair and other protective
processes apparently has never been considered in these studies.

However, there are now reasons to suggest that LDPs in all the cells
of the organism might be largely controlled by the concentration of
specific types of hormone-like factors in the blood. Evidence for this
suggestion comes from work concerning the major histocompatibility complex. A brief outline of the rationale leading to this suggestion is as
follows.

1. It is known that H-2 congenic strain mice (strains that are genetically different only in alleles at the H-2 genetic locus) have different
organ levels of DNA repair (75), SOD (58), and cAMP (43).

2. In these H-2 congenic mouse strains, the levels of DNA repair, SOD,
and cAMP increase together, and high levels correlate with longer life
span (mean and 10th decile)(68).

3. The H-2 genetic locus is known to affect the composition of the
membranes of all cells of an organism. In particular, a number of
specific types of H-2-determined proteins have been described, which are
glycoproteins and are located on the surface of the membrane, as well as
being found in the plasma (32,69).

4. A research group at the Johns Hopkins University, Drs. D. Meruelo,
W. Lafuse and M. Edidin, has found that the H-2 locus controls the level
of cAMP in tissues by modifying the binding affinity of receptor proteins
to hormones known to modify intracellular concentrations of cAMP. Using
crude liver plasma membranes prepared from H-2 congenic strain mice,
these workers found that basal, NaF and GMP-DNP-stimulated adenylate
cyclase activity was identical in all strains. However, differences
were found in the K_m for glucagon stimulation that correlated with the
cAMP levels. Thus, the cAMP correlation with the H-2 locus is not a
result of a difference in levels of enzymes synthesizing or degrading
cAMP but rather a result of the different sensitivities of the hormone

receptors on the membrane to stimulation by hormones such as glucagon (43).

5. Because intracellular levels of cAMP appear to be controlled by H-2-determined membrane/humoral factors and because cAMP levels are also correlated with DNA repair/SOD levels and longevity for the same H-2 strains, then these membrane-humoral factors might also govern the intracellular levels of DNA repair and SOD, as well as other LDPs.

6. These concepts are further supported by experiments showing that cAMP injected into mice enhances their resistance to x-rays (47, and non-published data from our laboratory). There are a number of other data suggesting that DNA repair and SOD, as well as other LDPs, might be governed by membrane/humoral factors. For example, skin fibroblasts grown in tissue culture media undergo a progressive decrease in DNA repair level with increasing passage number, but at the same time the cells are known to lose their histocompatibility antigens (33,34). Primate fibroblast skin cells taken from species having different life spans have similar DNA repair levels when grown in tissue culture media with calf serum (24,42,79). A correlation might have been found with life span if the cells were grown in homologous serum: human cells in human serum--not human cells in calf serum. When fresh lymphocytes were tested, a good correlation of DNA repair with longevity was found.

This concept can be tested in the following ways.

1. Determining the sensitivity of mouse and human cells grown in tissue culture to various mutagens (UV light and a few chemical mutagens) when grown in calf serum as compared to when grown in homologous serum and serum taken from species having different life span potentials.

2. Determining the levels of SOD, cAMP and DNA repair in parabiotic mouse pairs using strains having different individual levels of SOD, cAMP and DNA repair.

3. Studying the effects of UV light and chemical mutagens on cells grown with various hormone/growth factors added to the tissue culture media.

It may be that each type of cell has a characteristic sensitivity to the common circulating humoral factor(s) which determine(s) each cells unique level of LDPs and in turn the life span of the organism. Thus, a simple increase in concentration of the humoral factor(s) may effect a uniform and coordinated increase in LDPs throughout the entire organism.

CORRELATION OF THE LATENT PERIOD BETWEEN INITIATION AND APPEARANCE OF CANCER WITH SPECIES' INNATE AGING RATE

There is a substantial amount of pathology data in the literature indicating that human aging is a result of an accumulation of dysdifferentiation-like processes (36). One example is intestinal metaplasia (37). In this regard, the most common effect of many carcinogens is not the production of cancer but the dysdifferentiation of cells to an accelerated "aged" state. Also, the role nitrates and nitrites have in gastrointestinal aging and cancer and how glutathione, polyamines and specific types of gastric and intestinal micins (polypeptides having a high percentage of cysteinyl residues) may be important as anti-aging and anti-cancer agents (37).

One mechanism of how cancer might be produced is by a multistep process involving initiation and promotion. The initiation step is usually thought to be a mutation and the promotion step to be an epigenetic-like effect. The time period between the initiating event and the appearance of a cancer is called the latent period (73). It appears that, for a number of mutagens, the duration of this latent period is proportional to the longevity or maximum life span potential of a species. For example, for a given mutagen, the latent period is found to be 20 years in man and about 4-6 months in mouse. How good this correlation might be for a large number of different mammalian species is not known but is currently being investigated.

These data suggest that the rate of accumulation of promotion steps is determined by LDPs and is therefore related to the aging rate of an organism. Also, these data support the idea that many types of cancer are products of the same processes causing aging. The sensitivity of a cell to become initiated by a mutagen and its time-dependent progress from the initiated state to a cancer would be related to the endogenous levels of the LDPs; that is, the stability of a cell towards dysdifferentiation not only determines an organism's aging rate but also its rate of progress towards the cancerous state after it has been initiated by a mutagenic event. In this regard, it would be predicted that promoter agents such as the phorbal esters should accelerate aging.

REFERENCES

1. Adelman, R.C. (1979): Fed. Proc., 38:1968-1971.
2. Ambani, L.M., Van Woert, M.H., and Murphy, S. (1975): Arch. Neurol., 32:114-118.
3. Baker, G.T. (1975): Gerontologia, 21:203-210.
4. Baret, A., Baeteman, M.A., Mattie, J.F., Michel, P., Broussolle, B., and Giraud, F. (1981): Biochem. Biop. Res. Comm., 98:1035-1043.
5. Bartosz, G., Leyko, W., and Fried, R. (1979): Experientia, 35:1193.
6. Beighlie, D.J. and Teplitz, R.L. (1975): J. Rheumatol., 2:149-160.
7. Benirschke, K., Garner, F.M., and Jones, T.C., editors (1978): Pathology of Laboratory Animals, Vol. II. Springer-Verlag, New York.
8. Burnet, F.M. (1974): Intrinsic Mutagenesis: A Genetic Approach to Ageing. J. Wiley and Sons, New York.
9. Chirkov, Yu. Yu., Chesnokova, L.P., Sobolev, A.S., and Lomonosov, M.V. (1979): Biull. Eksper. Biol. Medit., 87:230-232.
10. Comfort, A. (1979): The Biology of Senescence. Elsevier, New York.
11. Cutler, R.G. (1972): In: Adv. in Geront. Res., Vol. 4, edited by B.L. Strehler, pp. 219-321. Academic Press, New York.
12. Cutler, R.G. (1974): Mech. Ageing. Develop., 2:381-408.
13. Cutler, R.G. (1975): Proc. Natl. Acad. Sci. U.S.A., 72:4664-4668.
14. Cutler, R.G. (1976): J. Human Evol., 5:169-204.
15. Cutler, R.G. (1976): In: Interdiscipl. Topics Geront., Vol. 9, edited by R.G. Cutler, pp. 83-133. Karger, Basel.
16. Cutler, R.G. (1978): In: The Biology of Aging, edited by J.A. Behnke, C.E. Finch, and G.B. Moment, pp. 311-360. Plenum Press, New York.
17. Cutler, R.G. (1979): Gerontology, 25:69-86.
18. Cutler, R.G. (1979): Mech. Ageing. Develop., 9:337-354.
19. Cutler, R.G. (1980): In: Adv. in Pathobiol., Vol. 7. Aging, Cancer and Cell Membranes, edited by C. Borek, C.M. Fenoglio, and D.W. King, pp. 43-79. Thieme-Stratton, New York.
20. Cutler, R.G. (1980): The Gerontologist, 20:88a.
21. Cutler, R.G. (1981): XII Intern. Congr. Gerontol., Hamburg, pg. 272a.
22. Cutler, R.G. (1981): In: Aging: Biology and Behavior, edited by J.L. McGaugh and S.B. Kiesler, pp. 31-76. Academic Press, New York.
23. Dausset, J. and Contu, L. (1980): Human Immunol. 1:5-17.

24. Dean, R.G., Socher, S.H., and Cutler, R.G. submitted for publication.
25. DeRubertis, F.R. and Craven, P.A. (1980): Adv. Cyclic Nucleotide Res. 12:97-109.
26. Fahmy, M.J. and Fahmy, O.G. (1980): Cancer Res. 40:3374-3382.
27. Fishman, W.H. and Sell, S., editors (1976): Onco-Developmental Gene Expression. Academic Press, New York.
28. Florine, D.L., Ono, T., Cutler, R.G., and Getz, M.J. (1980) Cancer Res. 40:519-523.
29. Francis, A.A., Lee, W.H., and Regan, J.D. (1981): Mech. Ageing and Develop. 16:181-189.
30. Gajdusek, D. (1972): In: Adv. in Geront. Res., Vol. 4, edited by B.L. Strehler, pp. 201-218. Academic Press, New York.
31. Getz, M.J. and Florine, D.L. (1980): In: Biological Mechanisms in Aging Conference, National Institute on Aging, Bethesda.
32. Gill, T.J. (1980): Arch. Pathol. Lab. Med., 104:559-562.
33. Goldstein, S. and Singal, D.P. (1972): Exp. Cell Res., 75:278-282.
34. Goldstein, S. and Singal, D.P. (1973): J. Clin. Invest., 52:2259.
35. Harley, C.B., Pollard, J.W., Chamberlain, J.W., Stanners, C.P., and Goldstein, S. (1980): Proc. Natl. Acad. Sci. U.S.A., 77:1885-1889.
36. Hartman, P. (1979): Genetics, 91:s45.
37. Hartman, P. (1981): In: Chemical Mutagens. Principles and Methods for Their Detection, Vol. 7, edited by F.J. deSerres and A. Hollaender, in press.
38. Hassan, H.M. and Fridovich, I. (1977): J. Bact., 129:1574-1583.
39. Hoffman, H.A. and Grieshaber, C.K. (1976): Biochem. Genet., 14:59-66.
40. Jakoby, W.B., editor (1980): Enzymatic Basis of Detoxication, Vols. I and II, Academic Press, New York.
41. Joenje, H., Eriksson, A.W., Frants, R.R., Arwert, F., and Houwen, B. (1978): The Lancet, January 28, I:204.
42. Kato, H., Harada, M., Tsuchiya, K., and Moriwaki, K. (1980): Japan. J. Genet., 55:99-108.
43. Lafuse, W., Meruelo, D., and Edidin, M. (1979): Immunogenet., 9:57-65.
44. Landfield, P.W. (1978): In: Parkinson's Disease II. Aging and Neuro-endocrine Relationships, edited by C.E. Finch, D.E. Potter, and A.D. Kenney, pp. 179-199. Plenum Press, New York.
45. Landfield, P.W., Sundberg, D.K., Smith, M.S., Eldridge, J.C., and Morris, M. (1980): Peptides, 1:185-196.
46. Lehmann, F.G., editor (1979): Carcino-Embryonic Protein, Elsevier/North Holland Biomedical Press, New York.
47. Lehnert, S. (1979): Rad. Res. 78:1-12.
48. Meredith, P.J. and Walford, R.L. (1979): Mech. Ageing Develop., 9:61-77.
49. Meruelo, D. and Edidin, M. (1980): In: Contemp. Topics Immunobiol., Vol. 9, edited by J.J. Marchalonis and N. Cohen, pp. 231-253, Plenum Press, New York.
50. Miquel, J., Economos, A.C., Fleming, J., and Johnson, J.E. (1980): Exp. Gerontol., 15:575-592.
51. Mittal, C.K. and Murad, F. (1977): J. Cyclic Nucleotide Res., 3:381-391.
52. Morrow, A.C. and Terry, M.W. (1972): Urea Nitrogen, Uric Acid and Creatinine in the Blood of Nonhuman Primates. A Tabulation of the Literature. Primate Information Center.
53. Munkres, K.D., Furtek, C., and Goldstein, E. (1981) Age, abstr., in press.

54. Munkres, K.D. and Rana, R.S. (1981): Age, abstr., in press.
55. Murray, V. and Holliday, R. (1981): J. Molec. Biol. 146:55-76.
56. Nebert, D.W. (1979): Molec. & Cell. Biochem., 27:27-46.
57. Nebert, D.W. and Jensen, N.M. (1979): Crit. Rev. Biochem., 6:401-437.
58. Novak, R., Bosze, Z., Matkovics, B., and Fachet, J. (1980): Science, 207, 86-87.
59. Ono, T. and Cutler, R.G. (1978): Proc. Natl. Acad. Sci. U.S.A., 75:4431-4435.
60. Peto, R. (1977): In: Origins of Human Cancer, Book C, edited by H.H. Hiatt, J.D. Watson, and J.A. Winsten, pp. 1403-1428, Cold Spring Harbor, New York.
61. Rister, M., Bauermeister, K., Gravert, U., and Gladtke, E. (1978): The Lancet, May, 20, I:1094.
62. Rosen, R. (1978): Intern. Rev. Cytol., 54:161-191.
63. Roth, G.S. (1979): Fed. Proc. 38,1910-1914.
64. Scheibel, M.E., Lindsay, R.D., Tomiyasu, O., and Scheibel, A.B. (1975): Exp. Neurol. 47:392-403.
65. Serfass, R.E. and Ganther, H.E. (1975): Nature, 255:640-641.
66. Shock, N.W. (1970): J. Amer. Diet. Assoc., 56:491-496.
67. Sinex, F.M. (1975): In: Handbook of the Biology of Aging, edited by C.E. Finch and L. Hayflick, pp. 37-62. Academic Press, New York.
68. Smith, G.S. and Walford, R.L. (1977): Nature, 270:727-729.
69. Snell, G.D. (1981): Science, 213:172-178.
70. Sohal, R.S. and Buchan, P.B. (1981): Exp. Gerontol., 16:157-162.
71. Strehler, B.L. (1978): Time, Cells, and Aging. Academic Press, New York.
72. Tolmasoff, J.M., Ono, T., and Cutler, R.G. (1980): Proc. Natl. Acad. Sci. U.S.A., 77:2777-2781.
73. Trosko, J.E. and Chang, C. (1980): Med. Hypothesis, 6:455-468.
74. Walford, R.L. (1974): Fed. Proc., 33:2020-2027.
75. Walford, R.L. and Bergmann, K. (1979): Tissue Antigens, 14:336-342.
76. Walford, R.L., Weindruch, R.H., Gottesman, S.R.S., and Tam, C.F. (1981): In: Ann. Rev. Geront. & Geriat., Vol. 2, edited by C. Eisdorfer, B. Starr, and V. Cristofalo, in press. Springer-Verlag, New York.
77. Weinhouse, S. and Ono, T., editors (1972): Isozymes and Enzyme Regulation in Cancer, University Park Press, Baltimore.
78. Wiśniewski, H.M. and Terry, R.D. (1976):In: Neurobiology of Aging, edited by R.D. Terry and S. Gershon, pp. 265-280. Raven Press, New York.
79. Woodhead, A.D., Setlow, R.B., and Grist, E. (1980): Exp. Gerontol. 15:301-304.
80. Yamasaki, H., Huberman, E., and Sachs, L. (1975): J. Biol. Chem., 250:7766-7770.

The Aging Brain: Cellular and Molecular
Mechanisms of Aging in the Nervous System,
edited by E. Giacobini et al., Raven Press, New
York © 1982.

Biological Activity and Sequence Complexity of Membrane-Bound and Free Polysomal Messenger RNAs of Young and Old Rat Brains

M. R. Ven Murthy

Department of Biochemistry, Faculty of Medicine, Laval University, Québec, Québec, Canada G1K 7P4

Structural characteristics and biological activity of mRNAs from membrane-bound and free polysomes of young (20 days) and old (1 year) rat brains were examined. The results showed that the S-100 protein and neuron specific enolase (NSE) were predominantly synthesized by free polysomes whereas tubulin was synthesized by both types of polysomes. The young brain polysomes were more active in tubulin synthesis whereas the old brain polysomes exhibited a higher activity for synthesis of S-100 and NSE proteins. The average nucleotide lengths of mRNAs and of poly-A tracts also showed differences depending on the types of polysomes and the age of animals from which they were isolated. Saturation hybridization of rat DNA with excess mRNA showed that mRNAs from free and membrane-bound polysomes contained a majority of overlapping sequences. However, there was also a significant portion of nonoverlapping sequences indicating that the different cellular locations of these polysomes may be a reflection of functional specificity.

INTRODUCTION

All mammalian cells examined so far contain two types of cytoplasmic ribosomes distinguishable by their existence as free particles (free ribosomes : refered to hereafter as F-ribosomes) or as constituents of the rough endoplasmic reticulum (membrane-bound ribosomes : refered to hereafter as B-ribosomes). Tissues such as liver and pancreas which synthesize protein for secretion are found to be particularly rich in B-ribosomes whereas cells from tissues such as brain and muscle and HeLa cells which manufacture proteins primarily for intracellular use have a greater proportion of F-ribosomes (24). Although the early view that B-ribosomes may be exclusively involved in export has been revised by more recent findings, there exists extensive evidence showing that a number of secretory proteins are synthesized predominantly by B-ribosomes whereas many intracellular proteins are made by F-ribosomes (39).

Using homologous as well as heterologous translation systems containing intact polysomes or ribosomal subunits and brain mRNA, it has been shown that brain specific proteins S-100, neuron specific enolase (NSE) and myelin basic proteins are synthesized mainly by F-ribosomes (4, 7). No brain specific protein has so far been reported to be formed exclusively by B-ribosomes, although indirect evidence using antibody fluorescence technique has suggested that proteolipid protein and glycoprotein of myelin may be products of B-ribosomes (40).

21

Earlier work from our laboratory revealed that the structural and functional characteristics of F- and B-ribosomes of rat brain underwent significant changes as a result of maturation, aging and sensory deprivation (30-32). Brain maturation was accompanied by a decrease in the proportion of B-ribosomes and an increase in F-ribosomes (29). Deprivation of light stimulation during the neonatal and postnatal periods reduced protein and RNA synthesis predominantly in the visual cortex. B-ribosomes were more severely affected by this treatment than F-ribosomes indicating that the former could have a special role in the utilization or processing of sensory information (34). Translation of mRNA in reconstituted brain in vitro systems containing ribosomal subunits from young and old cerebral cortices, in homologous or hybrid combinations, showed that both the 40S and 60S subunits of the aged brain were inferior to those of the young in the synthesis of brain proteins (33).

The above results suggested that factors that influence the functioning of brain such as aging or changes in sensory input could produce changes in the distribution and protein synthetic activities of F- and B-ribosomes in the brain cell by affecting the integrity of the membrane and the ribosomes and the nature of the mRNAs attached to them. The studies reported in this communication were undertaken with the following objectives : a) to find whether the mRNAs isolated from the two types of polysomes were different in structural properties such as molecular weight and size of the poly (A) segment; b) to determine what proportions of these two mRNAs were made up of common sequences or of unique nonoverlapping sequences, by using the technique of saturation hybridization with homologous DNA and c) to verify whether the young and the old rat brains differed from each other in regard to any of the above characteristics.

EXPERIMENTAL PROCEDURES

Cytoplasmic Free and Membrane-bound Polysomes :

Male, Sprague-Dawley rats, 20 days (young) or 12 months (old) of age were used in these studies. F- and B-ribosomes were prepared by a modification of the method of Ramsey and Steele (37). The modifications were as follows : a) use of high levels (200 mM) of K^+ ions in all homogenization and fractionation buffers in the form of potassium acetate instead of KCl since chloride ions at such concentrations have been shown to inhibit mRNA activity and depress the efficient utilization of K^+ ions (42); b) raising the concentration of Mg^{2+} ions to 10 mM in all solutions since high levels of Mg^{2+} have been reported to stabilize polysomal structure during isolation (44); c) use of rat liver ribonuclease inhibitor (20 µg/ml) throughout the preparation of the ribosomes and the use of a second inhibitor, heparin (1 mg/ml) during the fractionation of ribosomes from the postnuclear supernatant; d) avoidance of the use of the ionic detergent sodium deoxycholate in favor of a higher concentration of the nonionic detergent Triton X-100 (2 %) for releasing the B-ribosomes from the nuclear pellet.

Polysomal mRNAs :

Total RNA was extracted from the polysomes according to Palmiter (35). mRNAs of F- and B-polysomes (refered to hereafter by the abbreviations P_f-mRNA and P_b-mRNA respectively) were isolated by oligo (dT) cellulose chromatography of corresponding total polysomal RNA by the procedure of Bantle et al. (2) except that washing of the column with 0.1 M NaCl was omitted. mRNA was purified by two successive cycles of adsorption and elution on oligo(dT) cellulose.

Translation of Brain mRNA in Reticulocyte Lysate System :

Reticulocyte lysate was prepared and pretreated with micrococcal nuclease as described by Pelham and Jackson (36). Reaction mixture for protein synthesis consisted of the following ingredients whose concentrations were previously optimized for translation of rat brain mRNA : 20 mM HEPES buffer (pH 7.4), 2 mM dithiothreitol. 1 mM ATP, 0.2 mM GTP 15 mM creatine phosphate, 150 µg per ml of creatine phosphokinase, 30 µM of each of 19 non-radioactive protein amino acids excepting L-leucine, 400 µCi per ml of [^{3}H] leucine (180 Ci/mmol; Amersham), 1 mM magnesium acetate, 80 µM spermine, 120 mM K$^+$ (35 mM as chloride and other anions and the rest as acetate), 30 µM hemin, 80 µg per ml of brain tRNA, 40 µg per ml of appropriate mRNA and sufficient reticulocyte lysate to give 6.5 A$_{260}$ units of ribosomes per ml. Incubation was at 30°C for 1 hr. S-100 and NSE proteins synthesized in vitro were determined by immunoprecipitation of the reaction mixtures and SDS-poly-acrylamide gel electrophoresis of the immunoprecipitates according to the procedure of Mahony et al. (22). Synthesis of tubulin was estimated by the method of Gozes et al. (16) by vinglastine precipitation of tubulin from the soluble fraction of the reaction mixture followed by gel electrophoresis.

Size Distribution of mRNA and of Poly(A) Tracts :

The molecular size of mRNA was determined by sucrose-formamide density gradient centrifugation (10) followed by hybridization of mRNA fractions from the gradient with excess [^{3}H] Poly(U) (38). The number average nucleotide lengths of mRNA were estimated according to Bantle et al. (1). Poly(A) tracts were isolated from mRNA by treatment with a mixture of RNase A and RNase T$_1$. They were then subjected to polyacrylamide gel electrophoresis and the amounts of poly(A) in successive sections of the gel were determined by hybridization with [^{3}H] Poly(U) (1). Lengths of the poly(A) tracts in each fraction were estimated according to Kaufman and Gross (20) by using plots of log molecular weight against electrophoretic migrations of poly(A) standards of known length.

Preparation and [^{3}H] Labeling of Single Copy DNA :

Nuclei were prepared from livers of 4 week old rats by the method of Widnell and Tata (43). DNA was extracted according to a method described by Gaubatz and Cutler (14). DNA was dissolved in 0.12 M phosphate buffer (pH 6.8) and was fragmented by shearing in a French pressure cell. Heavy metal ions and any residual polypeptide materials were removed by passing the solution over a column of AG50/-X2 (BioRad) overlaid on Chelex-100. Single copy DNA was isolated from these fragments by three cycles of reassociation at Cot = 250 and hydroxylapatite chromatography. Sedimentation on alkaline sucrose density gradients (41) or electrophoresis in alkaline agarose gels (23) was used for determining the average size of DNA fragments which was found to be approximately 500 nucleotides for the above preparation. The single copy DNA which was reassociated to Cot = 60 000 was used as template for the synthesis in vitro of [^{3}H] labeled DNA (13, 19) using E. coli DNA polymerase 1. The [^{3}H] DNA prepared in this manner reassociated to a maximum of 90% when mixed with freshly denatured driver DNA$_5$ from rat liver and incubated at equivalent Cot values of upto 1×10^5. The DNA-RNA hybridization values were corrected for the presence of this fraction (10%) which was apparently not accessible for interaction with complementary DNA, and presumably not with complementary RNA also, under experimental conditions used in these studies.

[^{3}H] DNA-mRNA Hybridization :

Mixtures containing single copy [^{3}H] DNA and polysomal mRNA in 0.41 M phosphate buffer - 0.1% sodium dodecyl sulphate (1) were distributed in small aliquots into 5 µl capillary tubes and sealed. The tubes were immersed in boiling water for 5 mins to denature the DNA and then incubated at 70°C for various periods of time to obtain the desired Rot values for hybridization. At the end of reaction, the tubes were quick frozen in dry ice-acetone when necessary for storage. The samples were thawed and expelled into 1 ml of 50 mM phosphate buffer and passed through a column of Sephadex G-100 equilibrated with the same buffer. The exclusion peak in the eluate was collected and fractionated in a 1 ml column of hydroxylapatite at 60°C according to Bantle and Hahn (1). The extent of DNA-mRNA hybrids formed was estimated as the difference between the total radioactive DNA bound following treatment of the sample with RNase A and RNase T$_1$ (12). Equivalent Rot values of reaction mixtures were obtained by correcting to 0.12 M buffer salt concentration (6).

RESULTS

Fractionation of F- and B-Ribosomes :

Biochemical and metabolic studies on F- and B-ribosomes using isolated preparations of these organelles are often open to question on the ground that the particles obtained by a given procedure may not represent qualitatively or quantitatively the two classes of ribosomes existing in vivo. Avoidance of differential losses or cross contamination of the two classes of ribosomes in the course of isolation is particularly crucial to experiments whose objective is to discover the existence of differences between them. However, investigations carried out during the last few years by a number of workers have greatly clarified the nature of specific interactions that bind the ribosomes to the endoplasmic reticulum and the susceptibility of this binding to various physicochemical and enzymatic situations generally encountered in cell fractionations (24). Based on this knowledge, several methods have been devised for a satisfactory separation of the two classes of ribosomes from a variety of tissues including brain. We used a modified method based on that of Ramsey and Steele (37) who estimated a recovery of 95% of polysomes of both categories from the brain homogenate. There was less than 10% contamination of B-ribosomes with F-ribosomes and less than 2% of reverse contamination.

Some characteristics of F- and B-Ribosomes :

It it seen from Table 1 that the yields of both F- and B-ribosomes from the old rat brain were considerably diminished. The decrease was particularly marked for B-ribosomes which were a third less than the amount recovered from the young brain. This represented a relatively higher concentration of free ribosomes (F/B ratio) in the old tissue as compared to the young.

TABLE I. <u>Some characteristics of free and membrane-bound ribosomes of rat brain</u>

	Young brain ribosomes		Old brain ribosomes	
	Free (F)	Membrane-bound (B)	Free (F)	Membrane-bound (B)
Total yield (μg RNA/gm tissue)	718 ± 25	532 ± 20	621 ± 18	361 ± 15
Polysome ratio (F/B)	1.35		1.72	
Polysome ratio[a] (Heavy/light)	4.2 ± 0.6	4.8 ± 0.5	2.8 ± 0.5	3.1 ± 0.4
Protein Synthesis (%)[b]	100	145 ± 22	92 ± 11 (100)	62 ± 15 (75)
Poly-phe/Protein ratio in the presence of Poly-U[c]	4.9 ± 1.0	4.5 ± 0.8	6.3 ± 1.2	7.2 ± 1.5
Inhibition of protein Synthesis by aurine tricarboxylic acid (ATA) (%)	73	75	62	48

a Following sucrose density gradient centrifugation of polysomes, the optical density peaks consisting of upto four ribosomes were collected and arbitrarily designated as light polysomes and those consisting of five or more ribosomes as heavy polysomes. b Incorporation of L-[14C] leucine into protein *in vitro* by ribosomes. The activity of free ribosomes from young rat brain is taken as 100. The numbers in parenthesis compare membrane-bound ribosomes of old rat brain with free ribosomes in the same tissue. c Ratios of L-[14C] phenylalanine radioactivity incorporated into polyphenylalanine and into protein respectively in the presence and in the absence of added polyuridylic acid to the reaction mixture synthesizing protein *in vitro* (28). The values in the table represent averages of 15-20 different analyses carried out at different times.

When analyzed by sucrose density gradient centrifugation, the proportions of heavy agregates were also found to be lower in both classes of ribosomes from the old brain. The capacity of these ribosomes to synthesize protein *in vitro* was tested by incubating them with a radioactive amino acid under conditions optimum for this reaction. Synthesis of protein directed by endogenous mRNA was lower for the ribosomes of old brain as compared to the young tissue. On the other hand, old brain ribosomes produced a higher proportion of polyphenylalanine when [14C]-phenylalanine and poly(U) were added to the reaction mixture, indicating the presence of a larger number of inactive monomers. The ability of isolated ribosomes to initiate protein synthesis was examined by the addition of aurine tricarboxylic acid which is known to inhibit the initiation step specifically when used in low concentrations. This substance caused a lower inhibition of amino acid incorporation in the old brain ribosomal system indicating that the polypeptides formed by these ribosomes contained fewer newly initiated chains as compared to the young brain ribosomes. The lowered efficiency of protein synthesis for the old brain reflected in the above results was found, in all cases, to be more pronounced for the membrane-bound ribosomes than for the free ribosomes, although both classes of ribosomes were affected to a significant degree in the old animal.

Synthesis of S-100 Protein, Neuron Specific Enolase (NSE) and Tubulin :

In order to examine the presence of functionally intact mRNAs in the two classes of ribosomes, mRNAs were isolated and translated in the reticulocyte lysate system. Syntheses of two brain specific proteins S-100 and NSE and of tubulin were measured. The first two proteins were very largely synthesized by P_f-mRNA (Table 2).

TABLE 2. Synthesis of proteins in reticulocyte lysate system programmed by rat brain mRNA[a]

Age of rat	Source of mRNA	Incorporation (CPM)/ml of reaction					
		S-100 protein	%	NSE	%	Tubulin	%
Young	F-ribosomes	1025	100	614	100	2160	100
	B-ribosomes	190	18.6	178	29.0	1710	79.2
Old	F-ribosomes	1450	100 (142)	950	100 (155)	1470	100 (68.2)
	B-ribosomes	328	22.3 (170)	270	28.5 (152)	772	52.4 (45.2)

a Preparation of reticulocyte lysate, conditions employed for protein synthesis and procedure for determination of S-100 protein, NSE and tubulin synthesized in vitro were as described in EXPERIMENTAL PROCEDURES. The percentage values of incorporation given in parenthesis compare the free and bound polysomal mRNAs of old brain with corresponding preparations from the young brain taken as 100.

These results are in conformity with previous data showing the predominant role played by F-ribosomes in the synthesis of these two brain specific proteins in homologous translation systems (45). Synthesis of these proteins by both P_f- and P_b-mRNAs was higher in the old as compared to the young rat brain. This is probably a reflection of the fact that the concentrations of these two proteins increase in brain as a function of age (4).

In contrast to the mRNAs coding for S-100 protein and NSE, tubulin mRNAs were present in F- and B-ribosomes in a more balanced proportion. For example, tubulin mRNA activity in the B-ribosomes of young brain was nearly 80% of that measured using the mRNA of F-ribosomes (Table 2). This was in conformity with earlier in vitro translation experiments, using intact polysomes or isolated mRNA, which had shown that both F- and B-ribosomes in brains of young animals had the ability to synthesize tubulin (11, 8). Our results showed, in addition, that there was a marked reduction in tubulin mRNA in both F- and B-ribosomes of old rat brain. This reduction was more pronounced for the B-ribosomes than for F-ribosomes with the result that the P_b-mRNA of old rat brain contained only half of tubulin synthesizing capacity of the P_f mRNA from the same tissue.

Tubulin, is believed to have an important role in the development of neuronal processes and in maintaining axoplasmic flow (11) and hence its synthesis by membrane-bound ribosomes could have special significance for the structural and functional development of brain. The fall in the proportion of tubulin mRNA in membrane-bound ribosomes suggests the possibility that the interaction between the membranes of the endoplasmic reticulum and the ribosomes may be damaged in the old rat brain. A number of studies have suggested a deterioration in the structure and function of cell membranes in parallel with aging (46). Aging of rat brain may be accompanied by a redistribution of tubulin mRNA between the B- and F-ribosomes due, at least in part, to a reduced or faulty interaction between the ribosomes and the endoplasmic reticulum. In view of the subunit structure and microheterogeneity of tubulin and the reported existence of multiple forms of mRNA for coding different isotubulins (15), it is possible that further investigations will reveal functional and structural differences between the tubulins synthesized on F- and B-ribosomes and their role in the aging of brain.

Size Distribution of mRNA and of Poly(A) Tracts :

The mRNAs from F- and B-ribosomes of both young and old rat brains exhibited an optical density profile ranging from approximately 4S to 30 S with a maximum at about 18 S. The average nucleotide lengths of rat

TABLE 3. Some characteristics of rat brain polysomal mRNAs[a]

	Young rat brain		Old rat brain	
	P_b–mRNA	P_f–mRNA	P_b–mRNA	P_f–mRNA
Average nucleotide length of mRNA	1712	1675	1680	1615
Average nucleotide length of poly(A) tracts	98	87	72	61
Average Poly(A) content (%)	5.8	5.2	4.2	3.7

a The average nucleotide lengths of mRNA and of poly(A) tracts were calculated from sedimentation data and polyacrylamide gel electrophoretic migrations, as described in EXPERIMENTAL PROCEDURES. Poly(A) content was estimated as the percentage of total mRNA nucleotides. The values represent an average of 5-6 determinations.

brain mRNAs (Table 3) were in the size range reported for poly(A) mRNAs from rodent brains and brain cells in culture (10, 1) and ranged between 1600 to 1700 nucleotides. There were no striking differences in the sizes of P_f- or P_b-mRNAs or those isolated from young or old rat brains, although the old brain mRNAs in general and P_f-mRNAs in particular tended to be shorter than the young brain mRNAs and P_b-mRNAs. This was apparently not due to shorter coding regions in the P_f-mRNAs, but rather to lower poly(A) contents of P_f-mRNAs as compared to P_b-mRNAs. Poly(A) content and the number average nucleotide lengths of poly(A) showed much greater differences between the P_f- and P_b-mRNAs and between the mRNAs of young and old rat brains than did the mRNA size. The following observarions were made : a) both the P_f- and P_b-mRNAs of old rat brain had, on the average, shorter poly(A) tracts and smaller poly(A) contents than the corresponding mRNAs from young rat brain; b) P_b-mRNAs in both young and old rat brain had, on the average, longer poly(A) tracts and higher poly(A) contents than P_f-mRNAs.

In certain mammalian cells, such as the HeLa (27), the poly(A) segment of P_b-mRNA is reported to be directly attached to the membrane indicating that poly(A) may be involved in the specificity of the membrane-polysome interaction. It is conceivable that the longer poly(A) tracts of P_b-mRNAs in the young as well as old rat brain may confer an advantage or a means for interaction with the membrane. On the other hand, the lower poly(A) content of P_f-mRNA could indicate the presence in this mRNA of molecules originally attached to membrane and later released from this site because of poly(A) shortening as part of the process of mRNA turnover (44).

Complexities and Sequence Homology of P_f- and P_b-mRNAs :

In order to verify the degree of homology between P_f- and P_b-mRNAs, two types of experiments were performed. In one, the tracer [^{3}H] DNA was first saturated with P_f-mRNA; P_b-mRNA was then added to the reaction mixture and incubation was continued to sufficiently high Rot values until a second saturation was attained. In the second type of experiment, [^{3}H] DNA was first saturated with P_b-mRNA and incubation was then continued in the presence of added P_f-mRNA until the latter was annealed to the maximum extent. If no common sequences existed between the two mRNAs, the degree of hybridization by the two mRNAs together should be the sum of the values obtained with each mRNA alone. If, in the other extreme case, there was a complete overlapping of sequences between the two mRNAs, then addition of one or other of the mRNAs to a system already saturated with one of the mRNAs should lead to no further hybridization and should, therefore, show no elevation in the saturation point.

P_f-mRNAs from young and old rat brains hybridized to saturation with single copy [^{3}H] DNA at approximately 3.5% and 4.3% respectively (Figure 1) indicating that the F-ribosomes of old rat brain possessed a higher complexity of mRNA than the young F-ribosomes. The difference in the levels of saturation of P_b-mRNAs of young and old rat brains was not as striking as for P_f-mRNAs, although, even in this case, the old rat brain exhibited a slightly higher complexity (3.2% saturation) as compared to the young brain (2.9% saturation) (Figure 2).

Addition of P_b-mRNA to [^{3}H] DNA already saturated with P_f-mRNA resulted in a further hybridization finally reaching a new saturation plateau (Figure 1) which was less than additive for either young or old rat brain (Table 4). Similarly addition of P_f-mRNA to [^{3}H] DNA previously annealed with P_b-mRNA raised the saturation to a level which was also less than additive (Figure 2 and Table 4). The saturation plateaus reached by both types of hybridization experiments were the same (approximately 4.1% for young brain and 4.5% for old brain) indicating that whatever the order of addition of mRNAs, the [^{3}H] DNA was independently accessible to both mRNAs without mutual interference. Calculations based on the hybridization data revealed the following points : a) Approximately 35% of the P_f-mRNA and 21% of the P_b-mRNA of young rat brain constituted sequences unique to these classes of mRNA; in the old brain, the unique sequences of P_f-mRNA comprised the same proportion as in the young brain, but the proportion of unique sequences in the P_b-mRNA fell to only 8%. b) Total cytoplasmic polysomal mRNA of young rat brain was made up of 55% of sequences which were present in both P_f- and P_b-mRNAs, 30% which was present only in P_f-mRNA and 15% that was only in P_b-mRNA. In the old rat brain, the proportion of total mRNA sequences unique to the free poly-

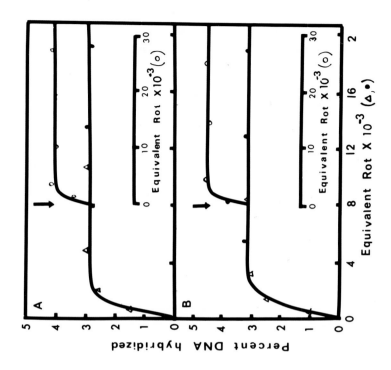

FIG. 1. Hybridization of single copy [^{3}H] DNA with P_f-mRNA and then with P_b-mRNA. (A) Young rat brain : P_f-mRNA only ($\triangle$,$\bullet$); P_f-mRNA + P_b-mRNA (o). (B) Old rat brain : P_f-mRNA only ($\triangle$,$\bullet$); P_f-mRNA + P_b-mRNA (o)

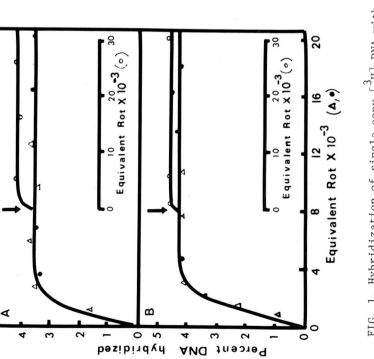

FIG. 2. Hybridization of single copy [^{3}H]DNA with P_b-mRNA and then with P_f-mRNA. (A) Young rat brain : P_b-mRNA only ($\triangle$,$\bullet$); P_b-mRNA + P_f-mRNA (o). (B) Old rat brain : P_b-mRNA only ($\triangle$,$\bullet$); P_b-mRNA + P_f-mRNA (o)

TABLE 4.   Complexities of Polysomal mRNAs of young and old rat brains

mRNA	Young rat brain				Old rat brain			
	Saturation Hybridn. corr. (%)[a]	Relative Proportion (%)	Complexity[b] Ntx10^8	Complexity[b] No. aver. Molecules X 10^-3	Saturation Hybridn. corr. (%)[a]	Relative Proportion (%)	Complexity[b] Ntx10^8	Complexity[b] No. aver. MoleculesX10^-3
P_f-mRNA only[c]	3.50	85	1.85	112	4.27	94	2.25	136
P_b-mRNA only[d]	2.89	70	1.53	93	3.15	70	1.66	101
P_f-mRNA+P_b-mRNA (sum)	6.39	–	3.38	205	7.42	–	3.91	237
P_f-mRNA+P_b-mRNA[c] (obs)	4.12	100	2.18	132	4.52	100	2.39	145
P_b-mRNA+P_f-mRNA[d] (obs)	4.12	100	2.18	132	4.52	100	2.39	145
Overlapping sequences in P_f-mRNA	2.27 (65%)[e]	55	1.20	73	2.90 (68%)[e]	64	1.53	93
Unique sequences in P_f-mRNA	1.23 (35%)[e]	30	0.65	39	1.37 (32%)[e]	30	0.72	44
Overlapping sequences in P_b-mRNA	2.27 (79%)[e]	55	1.20	73	2.90 (92%)[e]	64	1.53	93
Unique sequences in P_b-mRNA	0.62 (21%)[e]	15	0.33	20	0.25 (8%)[e]	6	0.13	8

[a]The mRNA hybridization values were corrected for "non available DNA" (see EXPERIMENTAL PROCEDURES).
[b]The complexities of mRNAs were calculated assuming a total rat genome single copy DNA complexity of 2.64×10^9 nucleotide pairs (19), and that RNA annealed to only one of the two strands of DNA because of assymetric transcription. For calculation of complexity as number average mRNA molecules, the number average nucleotide length for brain mRNAs was taken to be 1650 nucleotides (Table 3). [c,d]Saturation hybridization values for P_f- and P_b-mRNAs were based on results represented in Figures 1 and 2 respectively. "P_f-mRNA + P_b-mRNA" refers to experiments where P_b-mRNA was added to the hybridization reaction after the tracer DNA had already been saturated with P_f-mRNA (Figure 1). In the experiment "P_b-mRNA + P_f-mRNA" the order of addition of mRNA for hybridization was reversed (Figure 2). [e]Percentages in parenthesis indicate the proportion of overlapping and unique mRNA sequences based on each class of polysomal mRNA separately as 100. Nt = nucleotides. The values in the table represent averages from 4–6 different experiments.

somes was similar to that in the young tissue (30%), but those uniquely present in bound polysomes were reduced to 6%. The sequences common to the two classes of polysomes were elevated to 64%.

DISCUSSION

The very high complexity of brain polysomal mRNAs that we observed in the present work was in agreement with previous studies demonstrating that the number of different species of mRNA molecules present in brain was several fold greater than that found in any other mammalian tissue so far examined (1, 19). It has been suggested that this has to do with the functional diversity of the different types of cells composing the nervous system and with the capacity of this tissue to respond to a variety of endogenous and environmental stimuli.

Our results also showed that both P_f- and P_b-mRNAs contained sequences, parts of which were common to both and parts which were unique to each class of molecules (Table 4). This raises a number of questions about both the unique and common mRNAs, in regard to the compartmentation itself and in regard to the nature of proteins synthesized by these mRNAs. For example, what mechanisms exist to segregate the unique mRNAs into either F- or B-ribosomal compartments? Are the mRNAs common to both F- and B-ribosomes identical in their structure and if so, what enables them to circumvent the restrictions imposed on the unique mRNAs and move from one compartment to the other? Alternatively, do the common mRNAs possess identical structure in the message region, but different structural features in other parts of the molecules which would permit some of them to bind to the membrane and some others to exist as free polysomes? Do these different classes of mRNAs synthesize proteins that fulfill different functions in the tissue? Some of these questions have, atleast in part, been answered for secretory cells. A number of observations have indicated that, in such cells, the interaction between the ribosome and the membrane was specially adapted to permit the synthesis and transport of proteins to certain intracellular or extracellular locations using the cisternal spaces of the endoplasmic reticulum. The ribosomes appear to bind to specific sites on the membrane through the 60S subunit with a stable linkage provided by ionic bonds and the nascent polypeptide chain (5). B-ribosomes have been found to contain extra proteins not present in free ribosomes and which may be implicated in specific attachment to the membrane (5). The mRNAs translated by B-ribosomes are shown to possess a region that codes for a hydrophobic N-terminal polypeptide sequence in the translation product (3). It is suggested that this sequence called the "signal peptide" serves to anchor the ribosome to the membrane and to assist the entry of the nascent protein into the cisternal space for eventual transportation elsewhere.

Neither the nature of membrane-ribosome interaction nor the role of proteins synthesized by the different classes of polysomes is clear for tissues such as brain which do not manufacture large quantities of proteins for export like liver and pancreas. In this connection, it is interesting to note that the membrane-bound ribosomes of brain contained a large portion of total cytoplasmic mRNAs and out of this, a significant proportion was unique to this compartment (15% in the young and 6% in the old brain). In contrast, Mechler & Rabbitts (26) have recently reported that in the highly secretory mouse myeloma cells, the membrane-bound ribosomes contained unique mRNA sequences which constituted only 2.5% of the number of unique sequences present in the free ribosomes. Mechler

(25) also found that the attachment of polysomes to membrane was determined by the N-terminal amino acid sequence of the nascent polypeptide chain suggesting that these proteins were those that were destined for eventual export. Although such specialized protein synthesis is not a general property of brain cells, the fact that there is a heavy traffic of materials from the neuronal perikariya, over comparatively long distances, to the cell peripheries by axoplasmic flow (18) suggests that synthesis and transport of certain proteins may be synchronized and facilitated by the membrane net work to which the ribosomes are attached. It is possible that the mechanism of interaction of polysomes with the membrane and the density of attachment in such a situation could be different from that found in the case of cells where newly synthesized proteins are transferred to external locations. In Hela cells, for example, mRNA has been shown to be attached directly to the endoplasmic reticular membrane by means of the Poly(A) fragment (27).

The P_f- and P_b-mRNAs of old rat brain showed a number of structural and functional differences as compared to corresponding young brain mRNAs. To summarize, (1) the poly(A) contents and the average lengths of poly(A) tracts of both P_f- and P_b-mRNAs of old rat brain were smaller as compared to those of postnatal rat brain (Table 3); (2) the proportions of unique and overlapping sequences in the P_f- and P_b-mRNAs underwent striking changes in the old rat brain as compared to the young brain (Table 4) and (3) there was evidence by in vitro translation, for atleast a quantitative redistribution of certain specific mRNAs, for example, the ones coding for tubulin, between the free and membrane-bound polysomes. These results can be interpreted to signify an orderly adjustment in the spectrum of mRNAs in the two ribosomal populations as a function of age and to reflect the need for a changing pattern of protein synthesis. On the other hand, the general decline in the protein synthetic activity of old brain polysomes, particularly of those attached to the membrane (Table 1), would suggest that the redistribution of mRNAs in the two compartments may, atleast partly, be a result of damage caused to the membrane structure due to aging and to a consequent haphazard release of degradative enzymes affecting polysomal integrity and function.

An interesting result of the hybridization studies was the observation that the complexity of P_f-mRNA and, to a lesser extent, even of P_b-mRNA was higher in the old as compared to the young brain. Colman et al. (9), in a recent communication, reported that they found no differences in either the yield or the complexity of total polysomal poly(A) RNA of brains of rats aged from 2 to 32 months, which led them to conclude that there were no global alterations of genomic function in most brain cells during the rodent life span. The discrepancy between our results and those of the above authors could be related to the procedures used for the preparation of polysomes and the ages of the rats which were compared. Colman et al. (9) isolated polysomes from a 14,500 g postmitochondrial supernatant which is known to result in the sedimentation of different proportions of free and bound ribosomes in the nuclear-mitochondrial fraction (29, 30, 37). These differential losses were probably aggravated by the low concentration of K^+ in the homogenization medium (25 mM), since Ramsey and Steele (37) have shown that concentrations of K^+ lower than 250 mM led to reduced recovery of free ribosomes due to their entrapment in the membrane fraction and in the nuclear pellet. The yield of ribosomes (measured as μg polysomal RNA per gm brain) using postmitochondrial supernatant, by Coleman et al. (9) was 1/5th of that obtained by Ramsey and Steele (37) and 1/3 to 1/5th of our values (Table 1) using the total brain homogenate. On the other hand, as a result of procedures used in our study, our preparations of bound and free ribosomes included small amounts of ribosomes contributed by mitochondria and by RNP particles respectively. In addition, our results refer to comparison between brains of a sexually immature rats with adult rats of fairly advanced age whereas the youngest animals in the studies of Coleman et al. (9) were 2 months old. Our results are more consistent with the observations of Grouse et al. (17) that the portion of genome transcribed in mouse brain increased strikingly with age both before birth and between the young and the adult animal. The increase of complexity of brain mRNA during a period when the capacity for total protein synthesis declines (Table 1) suggests that the old brain may produce a greater diversity of proteins in smaller amounts as compared to the younger brain and many of these proteins could be meant for use primarly in functional and maintenance roles. In the young brain on the other hand, higher protein synthetic activity with lower diversity may reflect a preferential need for proteins which could serve as building blocks for elaboration of new cellular structures.

ACKNOWLEDGMENTS

This work was supported by grants from the Medical Research Council of Canada and the Commission de la Recherche Scientifique, Ministère de l'Education, Gouvernement du Québec. My grateful thanks are due to Professor B. Dastugue of Faculty of Medicine, Clermont-Ferrand for facilities accorded to me for some parts of this work and to J.L. Couderc and F. Gachon for assistance and helpful discussions.

REFERENCES

1. Bantle, J.A. and Hahn, W.E. (1976) Cell 8, 139-150
2. Bantle, J.A., Maxwell, J.A. and Hahn, W.E. (1976) Anal. Biochem. 72, 413-423
3. Blobel, G. (1978) in FEBS Symposium, vol. 43, pp. 99-108, Pergamon, Oxford
4. Bock, E. (1978) J. Neurochem. 30, 7-14
5. Borgese, D., Blobel, G. & Sabatini, D.D. (1973) J. Mol. Biol. 74, 415-438
6. Britten, R.J., Graham, D.E. and Neufeld, K. (1974) Methods in Enzymol. vol. 29, Eds L. Grossman and K. Moldave, pp. 363-418, Academic Press, N.Y.
7. Campagnoni, A.T., Carey, G.D. and Yu, Y.T. (1980) J. Neurochem. 34, 677-686
8. Cleveland, D.W., Kirschner, M.W. and Cowan, N.J. (1978) Cell 15, 1021-1031
9. Colman, P.D., Kaplan, B.B., Osterburg, H.H. and Finch, C.E. (1980) J. Neurochem. 34, 335-345
10. Felsani, A., Berthelot, F., Gros, F. and Croizat, B. (1978) Eur. J. Biochem. 92, 569-577
11. Floor, E.R., Gilbert, J.M. and Nowak, T.S. Jr. (1976) Biochim. Biophys. Acta 442, 285-296
12. Galau, G.H., Britten, R.J. and Davidson, E.H. (1974) Cell 2, 9-21
13. Galau, G.A., Klein, W.H., Davis, M.M., Wold, B.J., Britten, R.J. and Davidson, E.H. (1976) Cell 7, 487-505
14. Gaubatz, J.W. and Cutler, R.G. (1978) Gerontology 24, 179-207

15. Gozes, I., De Baetselier, A. and Littauer, U.Z. (1980) Eur. J. Biochem. 103, 13-20
16. Gozes, I., Schmitt, H. and Littauer, U.Z. (1975) Proc. Nat. Acad. Sci. U.S.A. 72, 701-705
17. Grouse, L., Chilton, M.-D., and McCarthy, M.D. (1972) Biochemistry 11, 798-805
18. Jeffery, P.L. and Austin, L. (1973) Progress in Neurobiol. 2, 207-245
19. Kaplan, B.B., Schachter, B.S., Osterburg, H.H., de Vellis, J.S. and Finch, C.E. (1978) Biochemistry 17, 5516-5524
20. Kaufman, S.J. and Gross, K.W. (1974) Biochim. Biophys. Acta 353, 133-145
21. Kreibich, G., Czako-Graham, M., Grebenau, R., Mok, W., Rodriguez-Boulan, E. and Sabatini, D.D. (1978) J. Supramol. Struct. 8, 279-302
22. Mahony, J., Brown, I., Labourdette, G. and Marks, A. (1976) Eur. J. Biochem. 67, 203-208
23. McDonnell, M.W., Simon, M.N. and Studier, F.W. (1977) J. Mol. Biol. 110, 119-146
24. McIntosh, P.R. and O'Toole, K. (1976) Biochim. Biophys. Acta 457, 171-212
25. Mechler, B. (1981) J. Cell. Biol. 88, 42-50
26. Mechler, B. and Rabbitts, T.H. (1981) J. Cell. Biol. 88, 29-36
27. Milcarek, C. and Penman, S. (1974) J. Mol. Biol. 89, 327-338
28. Murthy, M.R.V. (1966) Biochim. Biophys. Acta 119, 599-613
29. Murthy, M.R.V. (1970) in Protein metabolism of the nervous system, Lajtha, A., Ed., pp. 109-127, Plenum Press, New York
30. Murthy, M.R.V. (1972) J. Biol. Chem. 247, 1936-1943
31. Murthy, M.R.V. (1972) J. Biol. Chem. 247, 1944-1950
32. Murthy, M.R.V. (1980) in Biochemistry of Brain, Kumar, S., Ed., pp. 505-521, Pergamon Press
33. Murthy, M.R.V., Bharucha, A.D., Charbonneau, R. and Chaudhary, K.D. (1977) in Mechanisms, regulation and special functions of protein synthesis in brain, Roberts, S., Lajtha, A. and Gipsen, W.H., Eds, pp. 21-28, Elsevier Press, New York
34. Murthy, M.R.V., Roux, H., Bharucha, A.D. and Charbonneau, R. (1977) in Behavioural Neurochemistry, Delgado, J.M.R. and DeFeudis, F.V. Eds., pp. 192-216, Spectrum Press
35. Palmiter, R.D. (1974) Biochemistry 13, 3606-3615
36. Pelham, H.R.B. and Jackson, R.J. (1976) Eur. J. Biochem. 67, 247-256
37. Ramsey, J.C. and Steele, W.J. (1977) J. Neurochem. 28, 517-527
38. Robash, M. and Ford, P.J. (1974) J. Mol. Biol. 85, 87-101
39. Rolleston, F.S. (1974) Sub-Cell. Biochem. 3, 91-117
40. Sternberger, N.H., Itoyama, Y., Kies, M.W. and Webster, D. de F. (1978) J. Neurocytol. 7, 251-263
41. Studier, F.W. (1965) J. Mol. Biol. 11, 373-390
42. Weber, L.A., Hickey, E., Maroney, P.A., and Baglioni, C. (1977) J. Biol. Chem. 252, 4007-4010
43. Widnell, C.C. and Tata, J.R. (1964) Biochem. J. 92, 313-317
44. Wilson, M.C., Sawicki, S.G., White, P.A. and Darnell, J.E. (1978) J. Mol. Biol. 126, 26-36
45. Zomzely-Neurath, C., York, C. and Moore, B.W. (1973) Arch. Biochem. Biophys. 155, 58-69
46. Zs-Nagy, I. (1979) Mech. Ageing Dev. 9, 237-246

The Aging Brain: Cellular and Molecular Mechanisms of Aging in the Nervous System, edited by E. Giacobini et al., Raven Press, New York © 1982.

"Aging" in Cerebral and Motor Neurons of Fetal and Adult Origin in Long-Term Cultures

A. Shahar, H. Schupper, *H. H. Althaus, and *V. Neuhoff

*Department of Virology, Section for Electron Microscopy, Israel Institute for Biological Research, Ness-Ziona, Israel; *Department of Neurochemistry, Max-Planck Institute for Experimental Medicine, Gottingen 3400, Federal Republic of Germany*

Neurons, being post-mitotic cells which can not regenerate through cell division, are known to undergo sequential degenerative changes during their lives (8,11). Some of these changes might be due to vascular alterations, others are part of the dynamic process of aging. Morphological changes in the brain seem to correlate with a decline in intellectual and other behavioural capacities (13). It is doubtful, therefore, whether the term "aging" can be legitimately used in the case of neuronal cultures. This is also because cultured nerve cells represent only a fraction of the total nervous system. Cultured for a short period of time, they have a different pattern of growth and differentiation according to their fetal or adult origin. However, during cultivation, nerve cells may reach a state of maturation that mimics their natural development in animals. Furthermore, degenerative morphological changes such as accumulation of lipofuscin and osmophilic dense bodies, membrane whorls, etc., which appear in nerve cells of aged animals, are also found in neurons grown in long-term culture (14,15). So, in a way, neuronal cultures may provide a useful model for the study of morphological changes which occur at the cellular level during and after cell maturation.

In the present paper, the growth pattern and morphological events which occur in single neurons of fetal origin are compared with neurons of adult origin, during their long-term cultivation. In addition, we describe here further differentiation and myelination in dissociated fetal central nervous system (CNS) cultures, as a result of the addition of new fresh fetal CNS cells.

MATERIALS AND METHODS

Fetal CNS neurons were dissociated from the brain and spinal cord of rat fetuses, at 16 and 14 days, respectively. Cells were mechanically dissociated using the trituration method by Pasteur pipet (5,6,10). $1X10^6$ cells were seeded in 35 mm plastic dishes either directly or on round coverglasses, previously coated with 0.1% polylysin (17). Cultures for brain cells were incubated at $37^{\circ}C$ in a CO_2 incubator. The nutrient medium for brain cells consisted of 63.5% Eagle's Basal Medium, 20% heat inactivated fetal calf serum, and 10% egg ultra-filtrate, supplemented by 1% L-Glutamin (2 mM), 3% gentamicin in a concentration of 1.6 gamma/ml; 2.5% of a 20% dextrose solution provide a final concentration of 600 mg %. For dissociated spinal cord cultures the nutrient medium consisted of 74.5% Eagle's Basal Medium, 20% inactivated horse serum, 3% gentamicin and 2.5% dextrose (as above). 1.5 g/liter of $NaHCO_3$ was added to the Eagle's medium to increase buffering capacity. Nutrient media were replaced once a week at which time freshly dissociated cells ($1X10^6$/dish) were added to ongoing cultures. New cells were added either once or repeatedly, 2 or 3 times at one week intervals.

Adult CNS neurons were obtained by bulk separation (1,7) from the cerebral cortex and from the spinal cord (motor neurons) of Sprague-Dawley male rats. Animals weighing 120-180 grams were anaesthetized by IP injection of sodium pentobarbital solution (Nembutal Abbot 60 mg/ml) and perfused through the carotid arteries with 100 ml of an enzymatic mixture composed as follows: 0.1% collagenase (Worthington), 0.1% W/v hyaluronidase (Sigma) and 1.5 mM $caCl_2$ (Merk). The enzymes were dissolved in a hyperosmotic medium containing 280 mM glucose (Merk), 280 mM fructose (Merk) and 1% ficoll70 (Pharmacia). The perfusion medium was adjusted to a pH of 7.4 and oxygenated for 20 minutes before being perfused at $37^{\circ}C$ at a steady flow rate of 4 ml/minute. After perfusion the brain and the cervical part of the spinal cord were removed, chopped separately with a razor blade and homogenized in a loose glass homogenizer (Brown-Melsungen). Cell suspension was layered on a metrizamide step gradient as shown in Fig. 1.

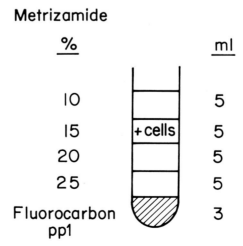

FIG. 1

After centrifugation for 15 minutes at 7500 rpm, approximately 10^7 neurons were collected from the interface of metrizamide and the fluorocarbon. The majority of the neurons retain the proximal part of their processes. Optimal culture conditions for cerebral neurons were: cultivation in a CO_2 incubator in 35 mm petri dishes coated with poly-L lysin and a nutrient medium consisting of 77% Eagle's MEM, 15% fetal calf serum, 3% chick embryonic extract, and 1% L-glutamin (2 mM). The medium was suppplemented with 2.5% of a 20% dextrose solution to give a final concentration of 600 mg%; 1% of insulin 5 gamma/ml and 0.5% of penicillin and streptomycin. Motor neurons were cultured in the same medium but their support was reconstituted rat tail collagen substrate (4). Adult cerebral neurons were added to fetal dissociated brain cultures after about one week in culture. Fetal dissociated brain cells were added to ongoing cultures of adult cerebral neurons after 3 weeks in culture. Cultures were observed daily under a phase contrast microscope. Samples were selected at different stages of cultivation and processed for histology, Cresyl Echt violet stain, histochemical reaction for cholinesterase (ChE) according to Karnovsky (9), transmission and scanning electron microscopy. For TEM all the following steps were carried out directly in plastic dish. Cultures were fixed in 2.5% glutaraldhyde for 30 minutes. After 3 rinses in 0.1 M phosphate buffer (pH 7), the material was post-fixed in 1% osmium tetroxide and dehydrated in graded alcohols. Embedding was carried out in a mixture of epon and methacrylate (the latter was used instead of the usual propylene oxide in order to avoid melting of the plastic dish) and replaced by a 5 mm thick layer of epon for 24 hours, first at $37^{\circ}C$ and then at $80^{\circ}C$ for 48 hours. This method enables the removal of the hardened epon with the cells as a whole mount. Selected areas were punched out with a leather puncher and glued on to epon stubs for sectioning. Sections were cut with a OMU-2 Reichert ultra-microtome, stained with uranyl acetate and lead citrate and observed in a JEM 100B electron microscope. For SEM the fixation and dehydration procedures were the same. The final dehydration step was done in acetone. The material was critical point dried with liquid CO_2, vacuum coated with a 100-200 $\overset{\circ}{A}$ layer of gold paladium (Polaron sputter unit) and observed in a JSM 35 C scanning electron microscope at 15-30 Kv.

RESULTS

<u>Dissociated fetal brain and spinal cord neurons</u> (Fig. 2) have a well known growth patttern in culture (16,17). It consists of an initial period of 2-3 days which is mainly characterized by nerve fiber regeneration along with cellular division of glial and meningeal elements. Neurons appear at this stage as dark cells on phase contrast microscopy and their structure is not yet clearly defined. During the following 2 weeks, these dark cells become flattened, the nucleus and nucleolus are clearly visible, the perikaryon has enlarged, the fibers have increased in length and diameter and they have established synapses. The non neuronal elements have divided intensively to form a monolayer of "flat" cells. Around the 3rd week of cultivation and onward the cells undergo a series of changes, which consist of a decrease in the number of neurons, a marked increase in the amount of macrophages and in the appearance of numerous giant astrocytes. The remaining neurons show a drop in

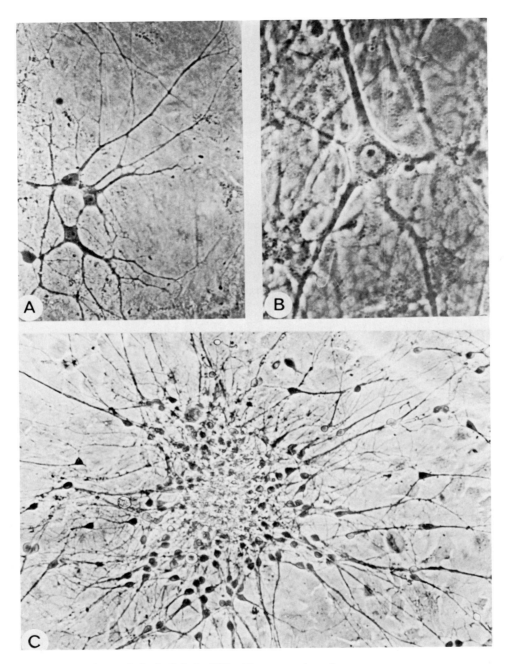

FIG. 2. - Dissociated fetal CNS. Phase contrast
A,C - Cerebral neurons
A - 3 weeks in culture, X 298 and C - 48 hours in vitro, X 230
B - Motor neuron, 21 days in culture, X 595

cholinesterase activity, and degenerative morphological alterations evidenced by the appearance of refractile granulation, frequency of dense bodies, and vacuoles containing myelin figures, observed along the membrane of fibers and the perikarya (Fig. 3). The addition of newly dissociated cells to ongoing fetal CNS cultures induced further differentiation and the onset of myelination (Fig. 4A-C). The cultures which have received new cells, unlike control cultures, preserved most of their "old" neuronal population (recognized by their large size in comparison to the size of the added neurons) even after 3 months in culture. These neurons showed abundant Nissl substance and had well-developed axons which became visibly ensheathed by myelin over long portions. Many of the nerve cells gave also a positive reaction to ChE.

Adult cerebral neurons (Fig. 5) have usually a triangular or pyramidal shape, are 10-30 microns in length and retain most of the proximal part of their processes after the gradient separation procedure. During the first week in culture, the neurons undergo a slow process of recovery. In phase contrast microscopy, a glow, indicative of cell survival, is visible around a great number of cells. The round swollen nucleus, whose outline was obscured by cytoplasmic granules, becomes slightly more irregular in shape and its outline clearer. A prominent nucleolus is visible. The Nissl substance becomes densely packed and evenly distributed throughout the cytoplasm. In some cells a few vacuoles are visible. In SEM (Fig. 5C,D) the neuron soma and its processes have a rough membrane surface with numerous spherical varicosities, except for one thin elongated process, which always has a smooth surface all along its length. This process emerges usually on the opposite side of the apical dendrite and is identified as the nerve cell axon. From the time the neuron has attached to the substrate in culture, the tips of the apical dendrite and other preserved processes appear as sturdy truncated "stumps". During the first week of adjustment in culture these "stumps" remain in a stationary state and do not undergo any changes in diameter or in length. After approximately one week in vitro, the first signs of neuritic regeneration become apparent. They are expressed by the formation of new, thin processes, emerging from the perikarya of the larger or medium size neurons. These newly formed processes end with a growth cone consisting of a membranous expansion with ruffled edges and often dotted with vesicles, probably pinocytic vesicles. In addition to the regeneration of processes originating from the perikaryon, a thin outgrowth zone can be identified at the tips of some pre-existing processes as well. This outgrowth consists of a growth cone with many extended protoplasmatic microspikes. The addition of glial conditioned medium to the cultures (12) enhanced not only the formation of growth cones in a greater number of neuronal processes, but also bifurcation of their tips and collateral sprouting along the processes. Positive staining for cholinesterase activity was found in many of the large neurons. Medium and small size neurons did not stain at all or showed different degrees of faint staining. After the addition of adult cerebral neurons to dissociated fetal brain cultues, morphological changes appeared in the adult neurons after 24-48 hours. These cells became rounded, granulated and refracticle; some of them floated in the medium, others adhered to the support and assumed the form of motile macrophages. In the fetal brain cultures many glial- like elements appeared with intensive membrane activity consisting of elongation and retraction of their pro-

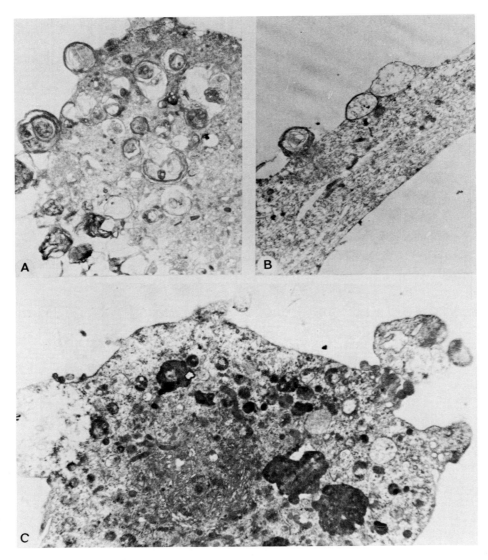

FIG. 3. – TEM of fetal cerebral neurons
A,C – nerve cells, X 3230, X 8160
B – Part of a nerve fiber. Note: presence of many vacuoles containing
myelin figures and osmophylic dense bodies. X 5695

cesses (Fig. 4D-F). In contrast, the addition of dissociated fetal
brain cells to cultured adult cerebral neurons did not induce any significant morphological changes in adult nerve cells, but the fetal brain
cells aggregated and degenerated.

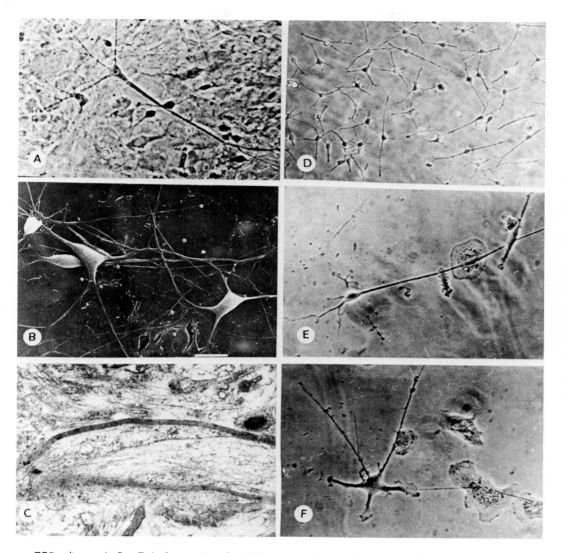

FIG. 4. - A-C. Fetal cerebral cultures after addition of newly dissociated cells.
A - An "old" neuron, 71 days in vitro (DIV) with several dark neurons
added after one week. X 270.
B - SEM preparation of neurons from culture 37 DIV on which newly dissociated neurons were added after 30 DIV. Bar: 10 microns
C - TEM section of a myelinated axon in a 91 DIV culture which received
cerebral neurons after 51 DIV. X 11200
D-F - Phase contrast microscopy of a 12 day fetal brain culture, 3 days
after addition of neurons from adult rat. Note: glial-like elements
with long processes and macrophages. D, X 150; E,F, X 270.

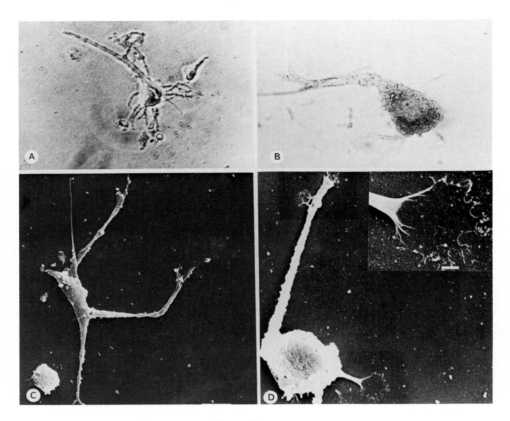

FIG. 5. - Adult brain neurons in culture.
A - Phase contrast micrograph of a pyramidal neuron, 18 DIV. Note: the "stump"-like shape of the tip of an apical dendrite. X 340.
B - A cerebral neuron 48 hours in culture stained for cholinesterase. X 1913.
C,D - SEM of neurons 20 and 10 DIV respectively. The thin smooth elongated process in C is probably the axon. D, note regeneration of a process with a growth cone from the perikaryon and a growth cone at the tip of the apical dendrite. Bars, 10 microns; inset, 1 micron

In phase contrast microscopy (Fig. 6A) adult motor neurons are multipolar and have a characteristic polygonal shaped perikaryon 30-50 microns in diameter, with a centrally positioned nucleus and a prominent nucleolus. The dendrites emerge from the perikaryon with a stout base, tapering and branching distally. Most of the motor neurons show a positive histochemical reaction of varying intensity to ChE (Fig. 6B). The stain is mainly localized in the perikaryon and to a lesser degree in the processes. A few small cells (probably interneurons) remain unstained. In SEM (Fig. 6C) motor neurons have, for the most part, the same morphological features as those described for cerebral neurons. However, unlike cerebral neurons, formation of growth cones or new processes have been observed in only a few cells even after several months

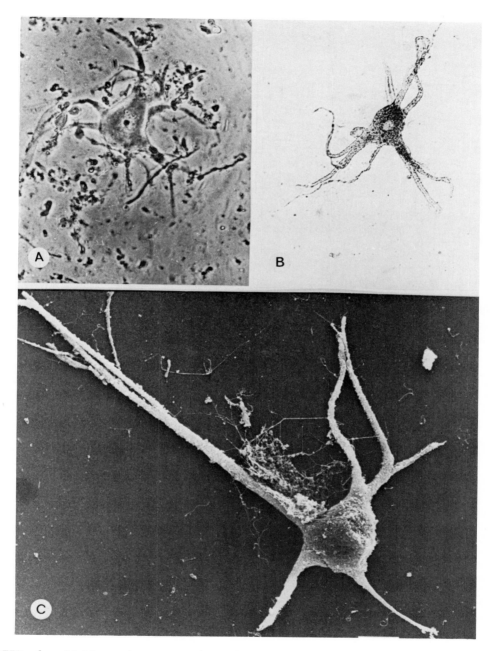

FIG. 6.- Adult cord neurons in culture with preserved processes and a
positive reaction to cholinesterase.
A - 24 hours in culture, phase contrast, X 595
B - 8 DIV, bright field, X 383
C - 10 DIV, SEM. Bar: 10 microns

in culture. Such newly formed processes were regenerated from pre-existing processes rather than from the perikaryon.

DISCUSSION

"Aging" in fetal CNS cultures can be defined at the cellular level as
a continuous process of morphological and physiological changes occuring
in neuronal and glial elements in the course of time. Such changes may
depend, on one hand, upon intrinsic genetic cellular factors causing
wear and tear of certain organelles due to their active or defective
metabolism; or on the other hand, may be induced by the external environment and express the effects of malnutrition, electrolyte imbalance,
depletion of hormonal factors or toxicity. Since morphological changes
appearing after long term cultivation in dissociated fetal CNS are basi-
cally of the same type as those observed in neurons exhibiting cytotoxic
effects _in vitro_, we can assume that they result from the combination of
both extrinsic and intrinsic factors and that the relative contribution
of one factor or another will determine the intensity of the changes in
cellular morphology.

The addition of new _fetal CNS_ cells to ongoing dissociated _fetal CNS_
cultures favors further differentiation and myelination in long-term
cultures which otherwise show degenerative morphological changes and
loss of neurons. It is difficult to estimate whether the enhanced differentiation and onset of myelination are induced by the added cells or
by some other factors. However, the observation that the new neuronal
and glial elements, added to older cultures, interact with the "aged"
cells to form new organotypic-like structures suggest the active
involvement of these added cells in the process of differentiation and
myelination. Thus the introduction of new oligodendroglia to an already
established fascicular network of nerve fibers might create suitable
conditions for myelin formation. Addition of new nerve cells might
induce an increase of synapse formation, as to improve neuronal function.

Adult dissociated CNS neurons were successfully cultivated provided
that they were isolated in fairly good morphological condition by the
bulk separation technique (1,2,7). Unlike fetal CNS nerve cells, adult
CNS neurons regenerate very slowly only a few thin processes, mainly
from the perikarya or from pre-existing processes, and do not form
interconnections among them during cultivation. The slowing rate of
regeneration in adult neurons after injury is attributed to age-related
changes in their intrinsic properties, such as axonal flow as well as to
changes in extrinsic factors (3). The fact that diffusible factors such
as glia factors can promote regeneration of adult neurons in culture
supports the assumption that slow regenerative capacity of these cells
depends upon extrinsic rather than intrinsic factors.

In contrast to the growth promoting and differentiation effects of
fetal CNS cells added to ongoing fetal CNS cultures, the fate of cultures in which fetal cells are added to cultures made of adult cells, or
vice versa, depends on which of these cells grew first, and which were
added later. The reason for this apparent incompatibility between adult
and fetal cells is not yet clear.

We have demonstrated for the first time that adult motor neurons can be isolated and maintained in long term cultures. In contrast to adult cerebral neurons, the growth of motor neurons in culture is not affected by glial factor(s). Experiments are now being conducted on co-cultures of adult motor neurons and fetal muscle cells.

REFERENCES

1. Althaus, H.H., Huttner, W.B., and Neuhoff, V. (1977): Hoppe-Seyler's Z. Physiol. Chem., 358:1155-1159.

2. Althaus, H.H., Neuhoff, V., Huttner, W.B., Monzain, R., and Shahar, A. (1978): Hoppe-Seyler's Z. Physiol. Chem., 359:773-775.

3. Black, M.M. and Lasek, R.J. (1979): Exp. Neurol., 63:108-119.

4. Bornstein, M.B. (1958): Lab. Invest., 7:134-137.

5. Burry, R.W. and Lasher, R.S. (1978): Brain Res., 147:1-15.

6. Dichter, M.A. (1978): Brain Res., 149:279-293.

7. Huttner, W.B., Meyermann, R., Neuhoff, V., and Althaus, H.H. (1979): Brain Res., 171:225-137.

8. Johnson, J.E., Jr. & Miquel, J. (1974): In: Mechanisms of Aging and Development, edited by B.L. Strehler, pp. 203-224. Elsevier Sequoia, S.A. Lausanne.

9. Karnovsky, M.J. and Roots, L. (1964): J. Histochem. Cytochem., 12:219-221.

10. Peacock, J.H., Nelson, P.G., and Goldstone, M. (1973): Develop. Biol., 30:137-152.

11. Shahar, A. and Edery, H. (1976): In: Electron Microscopy, 1976. Volume II: Biological Sciences, edited by Y. Ben-Shaul, pp. 614-615. Tal International Publishing Co., Jerusalem.

12. Shahar, A., Schupper, H., Mizrachi, Y., and Schwartz, M. (1981): Submitted to Develop. Brain Res.,

13. Shewin, I. and Seltzer, B. (1977): In: Senile and Pre-senile Dementia: a Clinical Overview, edited by Nandy and I. Sherwin, pp. 285-297. Plenum Press, New York.

14. Spoerri, P.E. and Glees, P. (1973): Exp. Geront., 8:259-263.

15. Spoerri, P.E. and Glees, P. (1974): In: Mechanism of Aging and Development, edited by B.L. Streher, pp. 131-155. Elsevier Sequoia, S.A. Lausanne.

16. Yavin, E. & Menkes, J.H. (1973): J. Cell. Biol., 57:232-237.

17. Yavin, E. and Yavin, Z. (1974): J. Cell Biol., 62:540-546.

*The Aging Brain: Cellular and Molecular
Mechanisms of Aging in the Nervous System,*
edited by E. Giacobini et al., Raven Press, New
York © 1982.

Target-Derived Trophic Factors for the Adult Goldfish Regenerating Retina

Michal Schwartz, N. Eshhar, C. Kalcheim, Y. Mizrachi, and Z. Vogel

Department of Neurobiology, The Weizmann Institute of Science, Rehovot 76100, Israel

ABSTRACT

Functional recovery of a damaged nerve depends on axonal growth, guidance and formation of new synapses. The ability of a central nervous
system neuron to support regeneration is decreased during development
and aging. In contrast, low vertebrates exhibit functional recovery of
damaged neurons throughout their entire lifespan. The goldfish visual
system provides a good model system for the study of central nervous
system regeneration. Investigation of the involvement of a diffusible
factor(s) originating in the target towards which the regenerative
fibers grow is the subject of this report.

An extract from the goldfish brain induces and supports neuritic outgrowth from the regenerating retina. The effect is mediated by molecules distinct from nerve growth factor. In addition to growth promoting
activity, goldfish brain extract can induce aggregation of acetylcholine
receptor molecules on cultured rat myotubes. The process of aggregation
of acetylcholine receptor molecules has been associated with synapse
formation at the neuromuscular junction. It is very likely that two
distinct molecules are responsible for the two functions. Further analysis and purification of these molecules should help in the understanding of their mode of action and their relevance to adult CNS plasticity.

INTRODUCTION

It has been hypothesized and supported by experimental evidence that
mammals lose their capability to regenerate damaged axons in the central
nervous system (CNS) upon maturation (review,33). Thus for example,
Ramon y Cajal's observations of axon sprouting, especially in the tran-
sected or hemisected spinal cord of young kittens, supports this notion.
The low regenerative capacity of the CNS of mature mammals represents a
major problem for the neurologist and neurobiologist.

For many years damage to a mammalian CNS neuron has been considered
as irreversible. Only recently it has begun to appear that a damaged
CNS neuron is intrisically capable of supporting regeneration, and that
the failure to regenerate might therefore result from environmental factors rather than from genetically determined properties of the cell
body. This issue can be investigated using two approaches: (1) Discovering the changes which occur upon maturation in the environment of CNS
neurons which makes them different from mammalian peripheral nervous

47

system. (2) Establishing the role of various diffusible factors in nerve regenerating systems in those instances in which functional recovery of a nerve is taking place. This type of study should help in determining whether CNS neurons in adult mammals experience the lack of permissive factors or the existence of inhibitory factors in their environment.

One of the systems which is well suited for studying the mechanism of adult CNS regeneration is the goldfish visual system (1,2,10,11,14,29), with the reservation that this model can serve effectively provided that there are no genetic differences between higher and lower vertebrate CNS neurons. Due to the plasticity in growth and their reproductive capacity, fish provide a unique model for a wide range of experimental manipulations (34). It should be mentioned that in mammals, the periods of growth and aging are more defined, in fish the aging is a consequence of growth cessation which is characterized by an increase in mortality (34).

The goldfish visual system has been thoroughly investigated for the last 10 years, both in vitro and in vivo (1). Following traumatic damage to the goldfish optic nerve the retinal ganglia cell body undergoes several biochemical and morphological changes, which facilitate the subsequent functional recovery of the nerve (6-9,11,13,14). The new fibers which make up the optic nerve emerge from the retinal ganglia and eventually reach the contralateral tectum. The process of nerve regeneration comprises three major stages: axonal growth, guidance and synapse formation (10). The nature of the signal which initiates the response to the injury as well as the mechanisms of the guidance and the formation of new synapses have not been discovered.

Indications for the involvement of humoral factor(s) in the process of the optic nerve regeneration have emerged from studying the association between polyamine synthesis and regeneration (15,25). The involvement of target-derived factors in various stages of the regenerating process have been investigated in the present study, in vitro.

In vitro model for regeneration.

It has been demonstrated by Landreth and Agranoff (16,17) that the regenerative capacity of the goldfish retina is expressed in vitro by the extensive outgrowth from explanted retina in medium supplemented with 10% fetal calf serum, provided that the ipsilateral optic nerve has been crushed several days (10-14) prior to the in vitro explantation (11,16,17) (Fig. 1).

This in vitro model system for regeneration is very useful for investigating the possible involvement of neurotrophic factor(s) in the regeneration process, at least at the stage of growth induction and elongation. For this purpose, the regenerating retinal explants were kept in suboptimal condition, namely, in medium containing a limiting amount of fetal calf serum (FCS). Under these conditions poor neuritic outgrowth from the regenerating retinal explants could be observed, and thus, enhancement induced by growth promoting factors added to the medium could be detected.

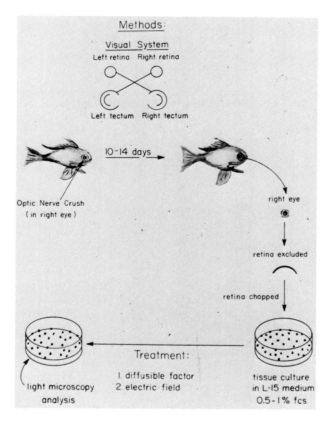

FIG. 1. Schematic presentation of the explantation procedure.

Retinas removed from the fish, from the eye ipsilateral to the crushed nerve, were chopped into pieces of 500 um square and placed on poly-L-lysine coated dishes (12) in L-15 (Leibovitz) medium supplemented with HEPES (20 mM, N-2-hydroxyethyl-piperazine-N'-2-ehtanesulfonic acid, pH 7.2), gentamicine sulfate (0.1 mg/ml), 5'-FudR (0.1 mM, 5'-fluorodeoxyuridine) and uridine (0.2 mM).

The addition of goldfish brain extract (high speed supernatant of homogenized goldfish brain) to the nutrient medium promotes the extent of outgrowth from the goldfish regenerating retina (26) (Fig. 2). The effect was noticeable even in the presence of high concentrations of FCS, but was far more pronounced when only 1% FCS was present. It has been reported that the goldfish brain has an appreciable amount of nerve growth factor (NGF) like activity (4), however, the effect on the outgrowth appears to be mediated by distinct molecules (26). The goldfish brain factor(s) represent an example for target-derived factor(s) involved in a process of regeneration. Similar factor(s) derived from the target have been described (18,review 32). Other factors derived from brain affecting outgrowth from neuronal cells have been described recently (20). These molecules, like the goldfish brain factor(s) described here, are distinct from NGF.

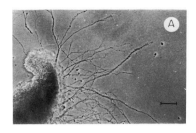

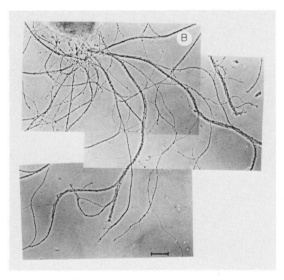

FIG. 2. Phase micrographs of explanted regenerating retinas. (a) Explants which were kept in poly-L-lysine coated dishes in L-15 medium containing only 1% FCS. (b) Explants which were kept in medium containing 1% FCS supplemented with high speed supernatant from homogenized brain (0.5 mg protein/ml).

In the course of the studies we were able to demonstrate that the factor(s) within the goldfish brain affecting the neuritic outgrowth from the explanted regenerating retina are composed of several molecular species. It is possible that the high molecular weight component is an aggregation or the precursor of the low molecular weight species (Fig. 3). It is also possible that the various components are completely unrelated and that the mode of their actions are different in spite of the fact that they are limiting to a similar phenomenon. Thus far we have studied the effect of the brain factor(s) on the neuritic growth indices. As this parameter is a result of a complex process which includes the attachment of the explant to the substrate, sprouting and elongation, it is possible that each of the various molecular species affects a different stage, even though it does not appear different in the net growth effect.

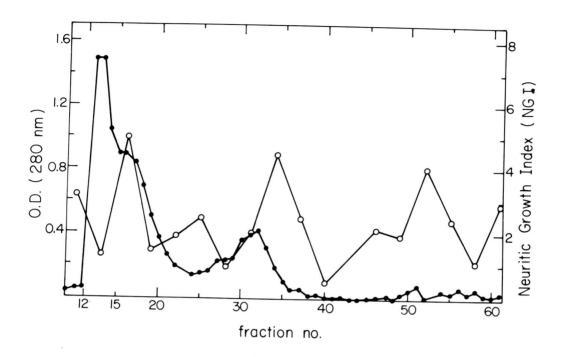

FIG. 3. Fractionation of goldfish brain extract on gel filtration column. Goldfish brain extract (5 mg protein) was applied to Sephadex G-100 column in phosphate buffer (10 mM9. Fractions of 1 ml were collected, protein content was determined by optical density in 280 um and each fraction was assayed for biological activity using goldfish retinal explants. Fractions were diluted 1:40 in L-15 media supplemented with 1% FCS. •—• optic density and o—o NGI.

So far we have been able to demonstrate that extract from tectum derived from uncrushed fish exhibit also trophic effect on the outgrowth from the regenerating retina. At this stage no information has been accumulated regarding the effect of the optic nerve lesion on the specific activity of the tectal or the brain neuritic outgrowth inducing factor(s).

Factor(s) derived from goldfish brain induce aggregation of acetylcholine receptor molecules.

Functional recovery of a nerve requires the growth of the new fibers toward the appropriate target and the formation of new synapses. The various steps of regeneration, including guidance and synapse formation, are probably regulated by different mechanisms in which it seems likely that several factors are involved. So far data regarding synapse formation have been accumulated only from investigations of the neuromuscular junction (9). There are certain basic physiological similarities

between the neuromuscular junction and central neural synapses. Studies
on the neuromuscular junction have provided hypotheses that are suitable
for testing on neural synapses. In the latter it has been shown that
neuronal tissue or factors derived from them can induce redistribution
of acetylcholine receptor molecules on muscle, and thereby cause aggregation of these receptor molecules.

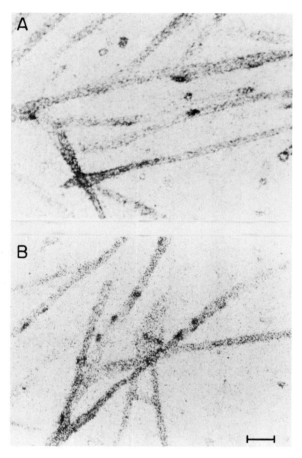

FIG. 4. Autoradiographic micrographs of rat embryonic cultured myotubes
labeled with ^{125}I-α-Butx. A. Control. B. Goldfish brain extract
treated culture (0.2 mg protein/ml).
Space bar = 100 um.

The neuromuscular junctions are disrupted by the degeneration of the
myofibers and the nerves that supply them (5,7,22). It has been established that synapses are formed in the regenerated muscle of amphibian,
and mammals almost always at the site of the original endplate (19).
Aggregation of acetylcholine receptor molecules has been hypothesized to
associate with this type of synapse formation. The effect of denervation on synapse formation has been studied by autoradiography using
^{125}I-α-Butx to examine the distribution of acetylcholine receptor in
endplates. The density and distribution of AChR within newly formed

endplates were not significantly different from those of innervated and uninjured muscle.

Recently, α-bungarotoxin binding sites have been found in goldfish optic nerve fibers and tecta (23,24). Some of the contralateral tectum α-Butx sites are lost following optic nerve axotomy. Since recovery of the visual function following the optic nerve crush is associated with formation of new synapses we have tested whether this process is accompanied by enhanced activity of AChR aggregation inducing factors.

Primary cultures of muscle provide a suitable bioassay for measuring the effect of various factors on AChR distribution (2,3). The cultured rat myotubes were prepared according to Nelson et al. (21). Five to 7 day old cultures were treated for 16 hours with serum free medium containing the appropriate amount of the high speed supernatant of the homogenized goldfish brain. Following the treatment, cultures were labeled for 1 hour at 37°C with 5 x 10^{-9} M ^{125}I-α-Butx. Following the labeling the cultures were fixed with 2% glutaraldehyde and autoradiographed with Ilford K-5 emulsion.

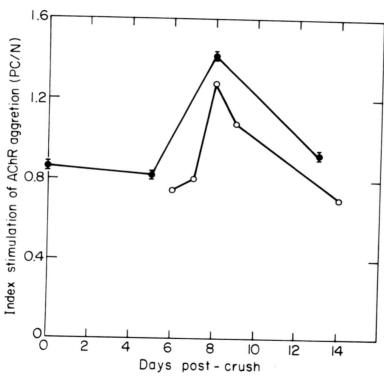

FIG. 5. Effect of optic nerve crush on goldfish brain aggregation activity. High speed supernatants were prepared from goldfish brains at different time points following the crush and assayed for aggregation activity (0.3 mg/ml protein) as described in the legend to Figure 4. The curves represent two separate experiments. The first time point after the crush represents the aggregation activity of an extract prepared 2 hours following the operation. PC/N represent the ratio between the values obtained from post-crush and normal fish respectively.

The extent of aggregation was determined by light microscopic count-ing of AChR aggregates, taking into account only the large aggregates with dimensions of 10-25 um. The results of the present study indicate that a high speed supernatant of homogenized goldfish brain (GSF) induces the formation of AChR aggregates on rat muscle fibers in primary culture. Figure 4 is an autoradiograph representing the distribution of AChR molecules (labeled with ^{125}I-α-Butx) in control and goldfish brain extract treated cultured myotubes. Spontaneous aggregates are seen also in the lack of any neuronal effect; however, in the presence of the brain supernatant, a higher frequency of AChR aggregates is detected. The degree of aggregation is concentration-dependent and saturable. Maximal activity is achieved at 0.3mg/ml of brain protein.

Since the same extract demonstrates both neurite inducing factor and aggregative activity, it is not possible to resolve whether they are exerted by the same molecules. The activity of the aggregation-inducing factors is increased following the optic nerve lesion (Fig. 5), a pheno-menon which suggests that some of the plasticity of the adult goldfish CNS is regained by these changes. At the present stage it is hard to resolve whether the enhanced activity is restricted to the tectum or occurs in other parts of the brain. One should also keep in mind that the aggregation inducing activity within the brain has been examined on rat myotubes, it is still to be studied in the original target. Furth-ermore, its relation to the synapse formed during the regeneration should be investigated.

Since goldfish brain, in contrast to brain of other species, contains high amounts of NGF-like molecules (4) and exhibits good CNS plasticity it has been hypothesized that NGF contributes to the goldfish CNS visual plasticity.

Based on the present findings it appears that NGF-like molecules are not involved in the process of growth and synapse formation. Turner et al. (30,31) have shown that NGF contributes to the goldfish regenerating capacity. The different results suggest that NGF is probably involved in other stages than those examined in the present work.

Other neuronal sources such as glioma cells have also demonstrated recently as growth promoters of neurites from the regenerating retina (27). At the moment it is not clear whether normal glial cells or nor-mal brain cells can release in situ these factors and how relevant they are to the process of regeneration.

It is possible that the molecules within the brain extract contribut-ing to the neuritic outgrowth and to the redistribution of AChR molec-ules are of a distinct nature and are completely unrelated to each other. Each component can contribute to the CNS plasticity of the gold-fish via a completely different mechanism and the presence of one does not necessarily imply the presence of the others. It is also possible that upon aging, the mammalian CNS deficiency is expressed only on the level of one stage and not the two of them. The last statement might be true mainly in view of the known observations that the initial sprouting occurs even from adult mammalian neurons while the aggregation inducing activity of neuronal extracts is decreasing upon aging.

ACKNOWLEDGMENTS

This work was supported by grants from the Jewish Agency and MDA to M.S. M.S. is an incumbent of the Helena Rubinstein Career Development Chair.

REFERENCES

1. Agranoff, B.W., Feldman, E., Heacock, A.M., and Schwartz, M. (1980): Neurochem., 1:487-500.
2. Anderson, M.J., Cohen, M.W., Zorychta, E. (1977): J. of Physiol., 268:731-756.
3. Anderson, M.J., and Cohen, M.W. (1977): J. of Physiol., 268:757-773.
4. Benowitz, L.I., and Greene, L.A. (1979): Brain Res., 162:167-172.
5. Burden, S.J., Sergent, P.B., and McMahan, U.J. (1979): J. Cell. Biol., 82:412-425.
6. Burrell, H.R., Heacock, A.M., Water, R.D., and Agranoff, B.W. (1979): Brain Res., 168:628-634.
7. Burrell, H.R., Doka, L.A., and Agranoff, B.W. (1978): J. Neurochem., 31:289-295.
8. Carlson, B.M., Wagner, K.R., and Max, S.R. (1979): Muscle Nerve, 2:304-307.
9. Fambrough, D.M. (1977): Physiol. Rev., 59(1):165-227.
10. Goldberg, S. (1976): Surv. Ophthalmol. 20:261-272.
11. Grafstein, B. (1977): In: Neuronal Plasticity, edited by C.N. Cotman, pp. 155-195. Raven Press, N.Y.
12. Heacock, A.M., and Agranoff, B.W. (1978): Science, 198:6466-6469.
13. Heacock, A.M., and Agranoff, B.W. (1976): Proc. Natl. Acad. Sci. USA, 73:828.
14. Jacobson, M., editor (1970): Dev. Neurobiology, Holt, New York.
15. Kohsaka, S., Schwartz, M., and Agranoff, B.W. (1981): Dev. Brain Res., 1:391-401.
16. Landreth, G.E., and Agranoff, B.W. (1976): Brain Res., 118:299-303.
17. Landreth, G.E., and Agranoff, B.W. (1979): Brain Res., 161:39-52.
18. Manthorpe, M., Skaper, S., Adler, R., Landa, K., and Varon, S. (1980): J. of Neurochem., 34:69-75.
19. Marshall, L.M., Saves, J.R., and McMahan, U.J. (1977): Proc. Nat. Acad. Sci. USA, 74:3073-3077.
20. Monard, D., Stockal, K., Goodman, R., and Thoenen, H. (1975): Nature (Lond.), 258:445-446.
21. Nelson, P., Christian, C., and Nirenberg, M. (1976): Proc. Natl. Acad. Sci. USA, 73:127-131.
22. Sanes, J.R., Marshall, L.M., and McMahan, U.J. (1978): J. Cell Biol., 78:176-198.
23. Schechter, N., Francis, A., Deutsch, D.G., and Gassaniga, M.S. (1975): Brain Res., 166:57-64.
24. Schwartz, M., Axelrod, D., Feldman, E.L., and Agranoff, B.W. (1980): Brain Res., 194:171-176.
25. Schwartz, M., Kohsaka, S., and Agranoff, B.W. (1981): Dev. Brain Res., 1:403-413.
26. Schwartz, M., Mizrachi, Y., and Eshhar, N. (1981): Dev. Brain Res., (in press).
27. Schwartz, M., Mizrachi, Y., and Kimhi, Y. (1981): Dev. Brain Res., (in press).
28. Singer, M., Nordlander, R.H., and Egar, M. (1979): J. Comp. Neuronal., 185:1-22.
29. Sperry, R.W. (1966): In: Nuerosciences Research Symposium

Summaries, Vol. 1, edited by F.O. Schmitt and T. Melnechink, pp. 213-219. M.I.T. Press, Cambridge.

30. Turner, J.E., Delaney, R.K., and Johnson, J.E. (1980): Brain Res., 197:319-330.
31. Turner, J.E., Delaney, R.Y., and Johnson, J.E. (1981): Brain Res., 204:283-294.
32. Varon, S., and Adler, R. (1981): Adv. Cell. Neurobiol. 2:115-165.
33. Puchala, E., and Windle, W.F. (1977): Exp. Neurol., 55:1-42.
34. Woodhead, A.D. (1977): Exp. Geront., 13:125-140.

The Aging Brain: Cellular and Molecular Mechanisms of Aging in the Nervous System, edited by E. Giacobini et al., Raven Press, New York © 1982.

Role of Glial Cells in CNS Aging

Antonia Vernadakis, Keith Parker, Ellen B. Arnold, and Michael Norenberg

Departments of Psychiatry and Pharmacology, University of Colorado, School of Medicine and Veterans Administration Medical Center, Denver, Colorado 80262

Although the differentiated neuron is not capable of mitosis, there is considerable neuronal plasticity possible in the mature neuron (see reviews 30, 31). Epigenetic factors involved in regulation of neuronal plasticity may be closely associated with glial cell function, a major regulator of the neuronal microenvironment.

It has been accepted that glial cells continue to proliferate throughout their life span. However, there is no definite evidence whether all types of glial cells proliferate. The accepted view is that astrocytes may be the predominant cell type proliferating in aging brain. Recently morphological changes in number and volume of astroglial cells have been reported in the various brain areas in the aging rat brain (8, 14, 15). Using Cajal's gold stain for astrocytes and light microscopic analysis Landfield et al. (14) and Lindsey et al. (15) found astrocytic reactivity (hyperthrophy), increased numbers of thickened processes in the hippocampus, caudate nucleus, and neocortex. Moreover, an increase in the volume of hippocampus occupied by astroglial fibers was observed with aging. We and others have proposed that changes in glial cells activity including proliferation with aging may be compensatory mechanisms to the adaptation of neuronal function decline (31).

Extensive evidence about possible glial cell properties and function has accumulated during the last decade from studies using glioma cells and more recently from primary glial cells in culture (see several reviews in 27; review 35). These culture studies provide support for two basic phenomena regarding glial cells: (1) glial cells may change functional characteristics with age and (2) glial cells may differ among brain areas.

In this paper we will discuss some of our findings on glial cell properties using a glioma cell line (C-6 glial cells) in culture. We propose morphological and biochemical differentiation in culture induced either by hormones or cell passage in culture may reflect aging in glial cells.

MORPHOLOGICAL AND BIOCHEMICAL DIFFERENTIATION: CELL DENSITY AND CELL PASSAGE FUNCTIONS

Using glioma cells (C-6 glial cells, 2B clone, courtesy of Dr. Jean de Vellis) we have performed several studies to characterize these cells in culture. In early studies we and others found that glioma cells, which appear as very primitive glioblasts, when exposed to analogs of cyclic AMP such as dibutryrl cyclic AMP (DBcAMP) differentiate into astrocytic-like cells (36). Since these cells were originally derived from a rat astrocytoma it appears that exposure to DBcAMP stimulates these cells to express their programmed function. This differentiating function of glial cells from glioblastic to astrocytic can also be expressed in primary glial cells cultured from rat or mouse brain (see reviews 10, 21). The questions that have been proposed are: are these cells that differentiate into astrocytes precursors of astrocytes; are oligodenrocytes transdifferentiating into astrocytes; or are the glial cells a multipotential cell capable of expressing several functions in response to neuronal demand and change in the microenvironment.

Responses of cells to cell density has been interpreted by many investigators to reflect the ability of the cells to respond to cell-cell contact, and thus growth patterns in vitro frequently reflect influences of cell contact. We have found that in C-6 glial cells the amounts of RNA and protein per cell are high at low density (50-100 cells per mm²) and progressively decrease with increasing cell density. Another important finding is that DNA content per cell is high at low cell densities (50 to 100 cells per mm²). We have interpreted these findings to mean that cells at low cell density are relatively more active, metabolically, in attempting to make cell-cell contacts (Figs. 1, 2, 3) (36).

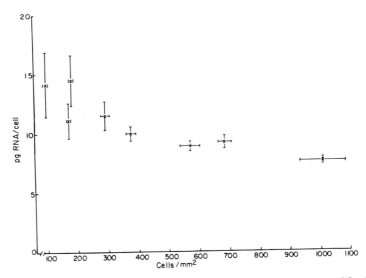

FIG. 1. Changes in RNA content of D-6 glial cells with cell density. Points with bracketed lines represent means ± S. E. of 6-8. {From Vernadakis and Nidess, (36)}

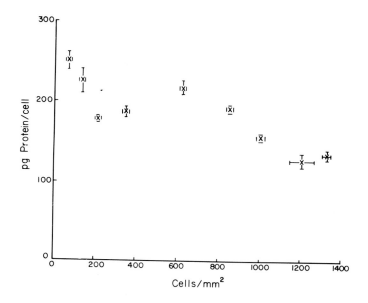

FIG. 2.   Change in protein content of C-6 glial cells with cell density. Points with bracketed lines represent ± S. E. of 6-8 cultures. {From Vernadakis and Nidess, (36)}

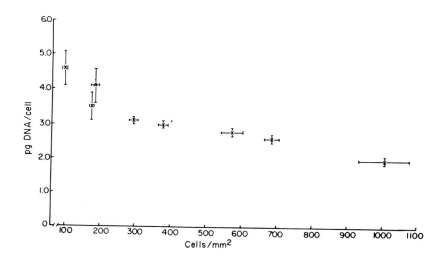

FIG. 3.   Change in DNA content of C-6 glial cells with cell density. Points with bracketed lines represent means ± S. E. of 6-8 cultures. {From Vernadakis and Nidess, (36)}

Several studies using cell culture as a model have been exploring cell changes with aging. More specifically, using somatic cells as a model changes with cell passage in culture have been interpreted as changes with aging (29). Thus we have been using early passage (20-25) and late passage (50-90) C-6 glial cells as a model to study changes in glial cells with aging in culture. We compared the doubling time in young (25 passage) and old (54 passage) C-6 glial cells plated at low density (1-1.5 x 10^5 cells/flask, 25 cm^2) or high density (1-1.5 x 10^6 cells/flask). Young passage cells plated at low cell density appear to proliferate at similar rate to that of old passage cells (Figs. 4 and 5). However, when cells are plated in high cell density old passage cells have a doubling time of approximately 12 to 16 hrs. whereas young passage cells show a doubling time of over 24 hrs. The rapid proliferation of the old passage cell is reflected in the higher protein and RNA content per cell in general (Figs. 6 and 7). This biochemical difference between young and old passage cells was also reflected in the cell, size, the old passage cells being larger (19).

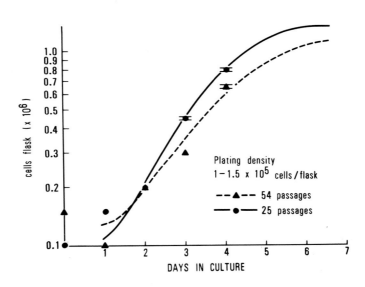

FIG. 4. Cell cycle of C-6 glial cells, cell passage 25 (solid line) and 54 (broken lines plated at 1-1.5 x 10^6 cells/flask. Point represent means $\pm$ S. E. of 10-12 cultures.

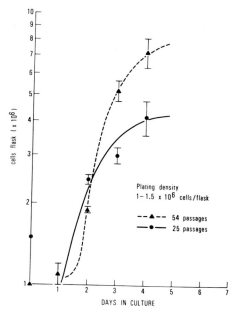

FIG. 5. As in FIG. 4 except that cells were plated at 1-1.5 x 10⁶ cells/flask.

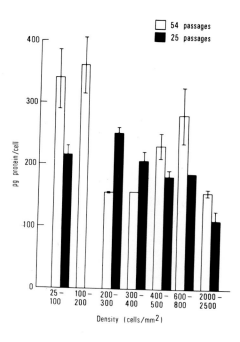

FIG. 6. Changes in protein content per cell in C-6 glial cells of 25 cell passage (filled bar) and 54 cell passage (empty bar). Points with bracketed lines represent means ± S. E. of 6-8 cultures.

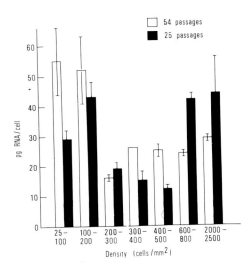

FIG. 7. Changes RNA content per cell. Points as in Fig. 6.

Using the enzyme markers 2', 3' cyclic nucleotide 3' phosphohydrolase (CNP) for oligodendrocytes (20) and glutamine synthetase (GS) for astrocytes (18) we examined changes in the activity of these enzymes in C-6 glial cells with cell passage (19, 38). For the CNP studies cells of either 21 or 82 passages were used. The activity of CNP was markedly higher in cells of young passage as compared to old passage of confluency (10 days in culture); enzyme activity was similar in both cell passage at logarithmic growth (Fig. 8). Moreover, CNP activity increases in the young passage cells with days in culture perhaps reflecting the increase in synthesis of this enzyme protein. That CNP activity did not change and in fact decreased in the old passage cells with days in culture suggests a basic cellular change occuring in these cells with cell passage. That this is the case is substantiated by the results in GS activity (Fig. 9). In contrast to the CNP activity, GS activity was markedly high in the old passage cells and low in the young passage cells. Moreover, the change in GS activity with days in culture was more marked in the old passage cells. Thus young passage cells express predominantly oligodendrocytic properties and old passage cells are predominantly astrocytic.

We have proposed that with aging in culture glial cells transdifferentiate. That oligodendrocytes may differentiate into astrocytes is further suggested by observations in primary cultures. In measuring the maturational profile of CNP and GS in dissociated brain cell cultures from chick embryos, we found that CNP activity is high during early culture then plateaus, whereas GS activity continuously increases in culture (38). These studies also showed the continuous proliferation of astroglia in culture and further support the observations of continuous gliogenesis with age. In an early study we found that the activity of acetycholinesterase (AChE), an ectoenzyme present in both neurons and glial cells markedly increases in the cerebral hemispheres and cerebellum of chickens with age (32). Since the enzyme choline

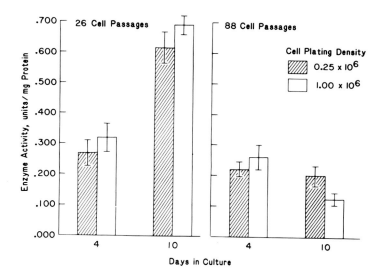

FIG. 8. Changes in 2', 3' cyclic nucleotide 3' phosphohydrolase activity in C-6 glial cells of different cell passage. Cell plating densities were 0.25 x 10⁶ cells (empty bars). Activity is expressed per mg protein. Units of activity represent μmoles phosphate produced per minute derived from a standard curve phosphate produced from 2' adenosine monophosphate. Points were bracketed lines represent mean ± S. E. {From Vernadakis et al., (38)}

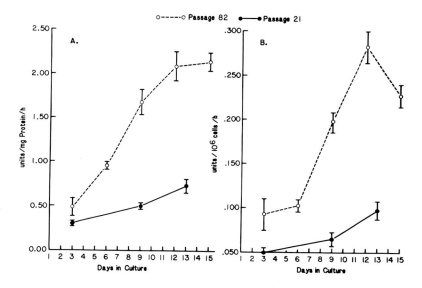

FIG. 9. Changes in glutamine synthetase activity in C-6 glial cells of different cell passages. (A) Activity expressed per mg protein. (B) Activity expressed per 10⁶cells. Units of activity represent μmoles of γ-glutamylhydroxamic acid formed. Points with bracketed lines represent means ± S. E. {From Parker et al., (19)}

acetyltransferase, a marker for cholinergic neurons is markedly low in
the aging chicken brain, the high AChE activity is interpreted to
reflect proliferation of glial cells. We further propose that these
glial cells represent predominantly astrocytes. Recently Raju et al.
(22) reported that aging included a dramatic increase in the number of
glial fibrillary acidic protein (GFA), another astrocytic marker.
Autoradiographic studies of young animals have suggested the possibility
that astrocytes and oligodendrocytes may have a common origin and that
one cell type can be transformed into another (28).

RESPONSES OF GLIAL CELLS TO HORMONES IN CULTURE

We and others have shown that hormones markedly influence glial cells
in culture. For example, we have found that cortisol, 1×10^{-9}M,
enhances proliferation of glial cells in cerebellar explants in culture
(33). More recently we have found that early treatment of chick embryos
with cortisol (0.25 µg/egg) enhances glial differentiation, as shown
by increased activity of glutamine synthetase in the cerebral hemispheres (1). Cortisol treatment, 1×10^{-5}M, increase protein synthesis
in undifferentiated glioblastic C-6 glial cells but not in DBcAMP-
differentiated astrocytic C-6 glial cells (36, 37). Numerous studies
by de Vellis and associates have shown induction of glycerol phosphate
dehydrogenase in early passage glial cells by cortisol (6, 7). In
addition glutamine synthetase is induced by cortisol in chick retina
(17) and this effect represent Muller cells, the glial cells of the
retina. More recently Juurlink et al. (12) reported induction of
glutamine synthetase in mouse primary astrocyte cultures.
In a preliminary study we examined the response of young and old
passage C-6 glial cells to cortisol or DBcAMP (Figs. 10, 11, 12, 13, 14).

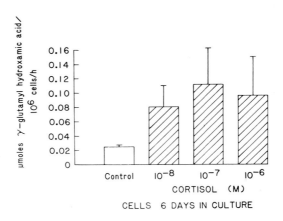

FIG. 10. Effects of cortisol on glutamine synthetase activity in C-6
glial cells of 19 cell passage. Cells were exposed to treated
cortisol for three days before the day of harvesting in the medium.
Points with bracketed lines represent means + S. E. of 4-6 cultures.

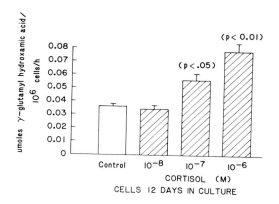

FIG. 11. As in FIG 10 except for days in culture before harvesting.

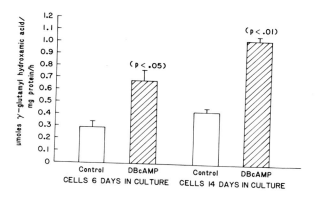

FIG. 12. As in FIGS 10 and 11 except that cultures were treated with DBcAMP.

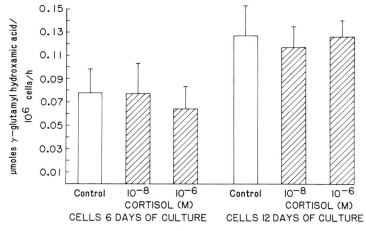

FIG. 13. As in FIGS. 10 and 11 except that cells were of 79 cell passage.

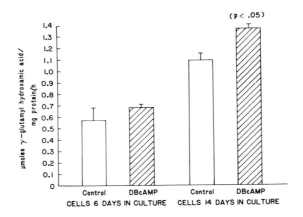

FIG. 14. As in FIG. 12 except that cells are passage 84 and treated with DBcAMP.

Cells were exposed to either cortisol or DBcAMP for three days prior to harvesting at either 6 days (logarithmic) or 12 days (confluency) of subculturing. Glutaminesynthetase activity was increased in the young passage glial cells after cortisol or DBcAMP treatment relative to controls; in contrast, GS activity in the old passage cells was increased only after DBcAMP treatment. The lack of response to cortisol of the old cells we interpret to reflect either changes in uptake of cortisol due to cell surface changes with age and/or a decrease in hormone receptors. Cortisol receptors in C-6 glial cells have been reported (2, 11, 16, 37). Moreover cortisol has been shown to produce changes in the morphology of glial cells reflecting cell surface changes (3, 4). In addition changes in cell surface have been associated with glucocorticoid receptors. For example, McGinnis and de Vellis (16) found that exposure of C-6 glial cells, normal astrocytes, and oligo-dendrocytes to Con A results in the loss of more than 90% of the gluco-corticoid receptor activity. The authors suggest that the response to glucocorticoids of oligodendrocytes and astrocytes can be regulated in vivo by cell surface contact with endogenous lectins, neighboring cells, or both. A decrease in glucocorticoid receptors with aging has been reported in many rat tissues and cells (23, 24, 25, 26).

GENERAL CONCLUSIONS

Several roles have been attributed to glial cells in CNS function and include myelination (5), modulation of extraneuronal microenvironment (13, 39), neurotransmitter concentration in the synaptic cleft (9, 34). Changes therefore in glial cells with aging will influence the function of the neuron and may contribute to its malfunction and ultimate degeneration. The findings disucssed here in cultured glial cells demonstrate that glial cells change their expression with age and that their response to intrinsic substances such as hormones and nucleotides is altered with age. Thus, although neuronal degeneration is not a primary finding in CNS aging, the decreased response of the neuron to its microenvironment with age may be a function of the glial cell a major regulator of the neuronal microenvironment.

ACKNOWLEDGEMENTS

The original work in this paper was supported by a USPHS Training Grant T32 HD 07072 and a Developmental Psychobiology Research Group Endowment and the Medical Research Service of the Veteran Administration. Dr. Norenberg is a Clinical Investigator at the Veterans Administration.

REFERENCES

1. Bau, D. and Vernadakis, A. (1981): The Pharmacologist. 23: 218.
2. Bennett, K., McGinnis, J. and de Vellis, J. (1977): J. Cell Physiol. 93: 247-260.
3. Berliner, J. A., Bennett, K. and de Vellis, J. (1978): J. Cell Physiol. 94: 321-334.
4. Berliner, J. A. and Gerschenson, L. E. (1975): J. Cell Physiol. 86: 523-532.
5. Bunge, R. O. (1968): Physiol. Rev. 48: 197-215.
6. De Vellis, J., Inglish, D., Cole, R. and Molson, J. (1971): In: Influence of Hormones on the Nervous System, edited by D. Ford, pp. 25-39. S. Karger, Basel.
7. de Vellis, J. and Kukes, G. (1973): Texas Reports on Biology and Medicine. 31: 271-273.
8. Geinisman, P., Bondareff, W. and Dodge, J. T. (1978): Am J. Anat. 153: 537-544.
9. Henn, F. A. and Hamberger, A. (1971): Proc. Natl. Acad. Sci. USA. 68: 2686-2690.
10. Hertz, L. (1977): In: Cell, Tissue and Organ Cultures in Neuro-biology, edited by S. Fedoroff and L. Hertz, pp. 39-47, Academic Press, New York.
11. Holbrook, N., Grasso, R. J. and Hackney, J. F. (1981): J. Neurosci. 6: 75-88.
12. Juurlink, B. H. J., Schousboe, A., Jorgensen, O. S. and Hertz, L. (1981): J. Neurochem. 36: 136-142.
13. Kuffler, S. W. (1967): Proc. R. Soc. 168: 1-21.
14. Landfield, P. W., Rose, G., Sundles, L., Wohostadter, T. C. and Lynch, G. (1977): J. Gerontol. 32: 3-12.
15. Lindsey, J. D., Landfield, P. W., Lynch, G. (1979): J. Gerontol. 34: 661-671.
16. McGinnis, J. F. and de Vellis, J. (1981): Proc. Natl. Acad. Sci. USA. 78: 1288-1292.
17. Moscona, A. A. and Piddington, R. (1966): Biochem. Biophys. Acta. 121: 409-411.
18. Norenberg, M. D. and Martinez-Hernandez, A. (1979): Brain Res. 161: 303-310.
19. Parker, K., Norenberg, M. and Vernadakis, A. (1980): Science. 208: 179-181.
20. Poduslo, S. E. and Norton, W. T. (1972): J. Neurochem. 19: 727-736.
21. Prasad, K. N. (1975): Biol. Rev. 50: 129-265.
22. Raju, T. K., Bignami, A. and Dahl, D. (1980): Brain Res. 200: 225-230.
23. Roth, G. S. (1974): Endocrinology. 94: 82-90.
24. Roth, G. S. (1975): Fed. Proc. 34: 183-185.
25. Roth, G. S. (1979a). Mech. Aging Devel. 9: 497-514.

26. Roth, G. S. (1979b): Fed. Proc. 38: 1910-1914.
27. Schoffeniels, E., Frank, G., Hertz, L. and Tower, D. B. Eds. (1978). Dynamic Properties of Glial Cells. Pergamon Press, Oxford.
28. Smart, J. and Leblond, C. P. (1961): J. Comp. Neurol. 116: 346-367.
29. Strehler, B. L. (1977): Time, Cells and Aging. Academic Press.
30. Szekely, G. (1979): Trends in Neurosci. 2: 245-249.
31. Timiras, P. S. and Vernadakis, A. In: Developmental Physiology and Aging, editor and author P. S. Timiras, PP. 502-526, The MacMillan Company, New York, 1972.
32. Vernadakis, A. (1973): Prog. Brain Res. 40: 231-243.
33. Vernadakis, A. (1971): In: Influence of Hormones on the Nervous System, edited by D. Ford, pp. 42-55. S. Karger, Basel.
34. Vernadakis, A. (1974): In: Proceeding of the Mie Conference of the International Society for Psychoneuroendocrinology, edited by N. Hatotain, pp. 251-258. S. Karger, Basel.
35. Vernadakis, A. and Culver, B. (1980): In: Neural Tissue Culture: A Biochemical Tool, edited by S. Kumar, pp. 407-477. Pergamon Press, Oxford.
36. Vernadakis, A. and Nidess, R. (1976). Neurochem. Res. 1: 385-402.
37. Vernadakis, A., Culver, B. and Nidess, R. (1978): Psychoneuro-endocrinology. 3: 47-64.
38. Vernadakis, A., Parker, K. and Norenberg, M. (1980): In: Tissue Culture in Neurobiology, edited by E. Giacobini, A. Vernadakis and A. Shahar, pp. 411-426. Raven Press, New York.
39. Vernadakis, A., Nidess, R., Culver, B. and Arnold, E. B. (1979): Mech. Aging Devel. 9: 553-566.

The Aging Brain: Cellular and Molecular Mechanisms of Aging in the Nervous System, edited by E. Giacobini et al., Raven Press, New York © 1982.

Age-Related Modifications in Chick Iris Muscle

I. Mussini, M. L. Simeoni, and M. Aloisi

National Research Council Unit for Muscle Biology and Physiopathology, Institute of General Pathology, University of Padova, 35100 Padova, Italy

A decline in muscular working capacity and contractile strength gradually develops in skeletal muscles with increasing age. The most general change is the decrease of muscle mass, owing to muscle atrophy and loss of fibres. However, differences in physiological as well as biochemical changes were reported depending on the type of muscle considered (6,14). Mammalian fast and slow muscles differ in respect to their structural, contractile and metabolic characteristics. In young rats muscles predominantly fast are rich in sarcoplasmic reticulum and show high levels of myosin ATPase and of glycolitic enzymes,while slow muscles are characterized by a large complement of mitochondria, a prevalent oxydative metabolism and a low myosin ATPase activity. In old rats such differences be - tween the two types of muscles appear reduced (3,6). By contrast, this phenomenon is not observed in the diafragm, a continuously working muscle composed by a mixed population of fibres in which neither the metabolic nor the contractile properties seem to be significantly affected by aging processes (3,7).

Although a lot of information on the age-related modifications which occur in mammalian muscles and even in insect muscles has so far been acquired, little is yet known about avian muscles. The iris muscle of the chick, however, has recently been the object of numerous studies,because the ciliary ganglion and its target the iris muscle are a particularly suitable model for investigations on development and aging of cholinergic mechanisms (9-13).

The iris muscle, known to be of ectodermal origin, is in the chick as well as in all Birds a striated muscle (1) innervated by cholinergic terminals of "en grappe" type (Fig.1).During post-natal growth it undergoes structural modifications similar to the maturative changes reported for skeletal muscles (2).In the young adult animal its fine structure appears similar to that of a muscle resistant to fatigue (Mussini et al., unpublished observations): for instance, all the muscle fibres are rich in mitochondria which form either intermyofibrillar rows or subsarcolemmal aggregates, thus suggesting a prevalence of the oxydative metabolism.However,the muscle mass seems reduced,whereas the iris organ appears two-times

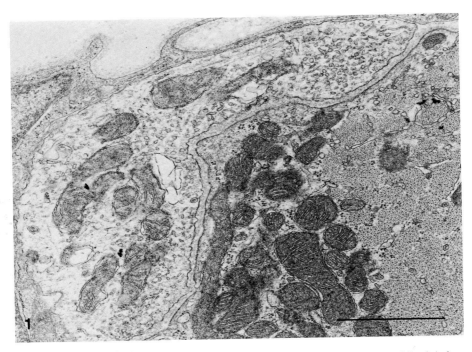

FIG. 1. Cross section of an iris muscle fibre of a 2-month-old chicken showing the "en grappe" type of innervation.
When not otherwise specified the scale bar indicates 1μm.

larger than at birth. As early as 15 days after hatching degenerative signs are observed in muscle fibres: fat droplets accumulate in the inter myofibrillar spaces, mostly associated with mitochondria aggregates (Fig.2). This accumulation progressively increases, developing characters of fatty degeneration, which results in a loss of fibres and connective tissue replacement. Degenerative phenomena are observed involving the mitochondria: glycogen particles accumulation in the matrix,sequestration of entire mitochondria into digestive vacuoles (Fig.3).

In association with lipid storage in many of the iris myofibres of a 4-year-old hen peculiar alterations were found in form of anomalous struc tures. These show to be lamellar cisterns with a regular thickness, a highly variable length and shape and a prevalent orientation according to the long axis of the muscle cell (Fig.4). In some fibres these structures occupy the main part of the cell. The Golgi apparatus is hypertrophic and the activity of the lysosomal system appears increased. Cytoplasmic deg- radation and autophagic processes are more extensive where the lamellae are more numerous (Fig.5). Nevertheless, limited areas of still well pre- served contractile material are seen among the degenerating lamellae .

The lamellar structures yet represent a unique observation, because they were found in the iris muscle of the only very old animal so far

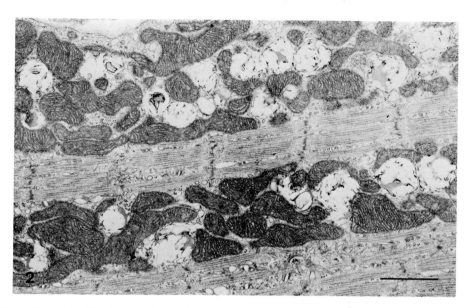

FIG.2. Longitudinal section of an iris muscle fibre of a 15-day-old chick
Note the accumulation of fat droplets (partially extracted by the dehydra
tion procedures), interspersed with mitochondria.

studied. Their membraneous nature is demonstrated also by the presence of
residual bodies engulfed by pseudo-myelin figures (Fig.5), end-products
of proteolytic digestion of large amounts of membranes. Either the origin
or the significance of such anomalous membranes remains obscure. The slow
ly progressive fatty degeneration of the iris fibres was found and follow
ed in chickens of different strains. It can, therefore, be considered as
a feature of very precocious involution of this muscle and/or a sign of
its adaptive reaction to altered metabolic conditions.

The presence of lipid droplets associated with mitochondria aggregates
was found in pigeon breast muscle, a fast acting muscle resistant to fatigue. In this muscle the mitochondria undergo marked ultrastructural
changes and great reduction in number very early after denervation before
any sign of atrophy takes place (15). On the other hand, storage of glyco
gen particles into the mitochondrial matrix, which was found to be one of
the main changes in insect heart muscle during senile involution (16),
was also observed in skeletal muscle fibres of old rats undergoing cytoplasmic degradation (8). We still lack information on the modifications
of the contractile properties of the chick iris muscle during aging. The
reduction in the working capacity of aging mammalian muscles has been related to alterations of the aerobic part of the energy metabolism (4). We
can, therefore, expect that at least the fatigability of the iris muscle
of the chick appears modified with increasing age.

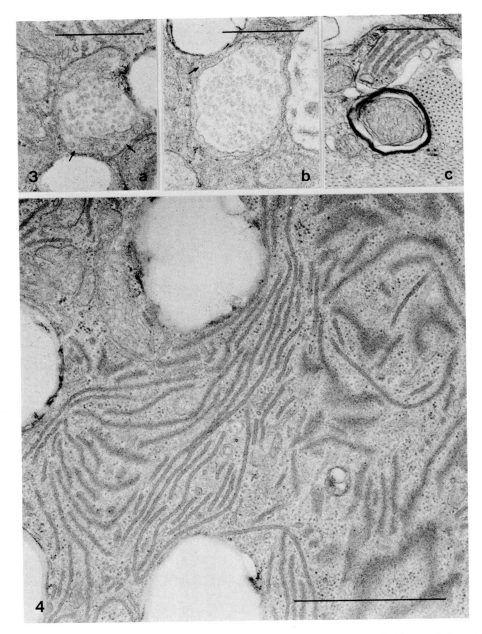

FIG. 3. Degenerative aspects of mitochondria. The accumulation of large
amounts of glycogen particles (a,b) displaces the mitochondrial cristae,
which appear tubular in shape (arrows). In c, a lysosomal vacuole contain
ing a mitochondrion. Scale bar: 0.5μm.
FIG. 4. Longitudinal section of an iris muscle fibre of a 4-year-old hen.
Proliferation of anomalous lamellar structures associated with a lipid
droplets accumulation.

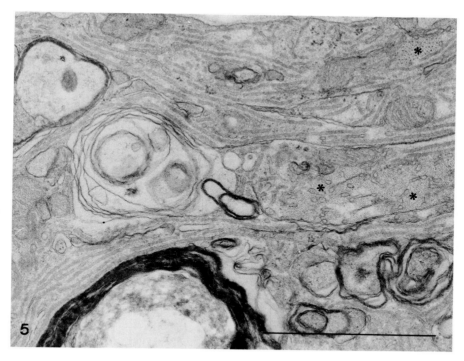

FIG. 5. Four-year-old hen. Cross section of an iris muscle fibre showing the formation of large residual bodies due to proteolytic digestion of anomalous membranes. Small myofibrills (asteriscs) are still observed in the area.

Changes in structure and function of the synapse were reported in rats suggesting a disturbance of the neurotrophic relations between nerve and muscle during old age (5-7). In the chick iris the muscle fibres, even when seriously involved by regressive phenomena, seem to maintain their innervation.However, the nerve endings observed in the oldest animal are seen to contain synaptic vesicles which often appear "agglutinated" or polymorphic in shape and size (Fig.6), similar to those found by Gutmann et al. (7) in motor end-plates of old rats.

Much is known on the changes of the acetylcholine metabolism which occur during development and aging of the iris muscle of the chick. Giacobini and coworkers have demonstrated that the levels and the uptake mechanism of the neurotransmitter and its precursor continuously increase, from the first week of incubation up to adulthood (1-2 years of age),during a period of "continuous synaptic growth" (9,10,12), which is followed by a period of "synaptic regression". This is characterized by a marked and progressive decrease in ACh and Ch levels (9). Concomitantly, ChAc and AChE activities are significantly impaired, thus supporting the view "of the peripheral terminals of autonomic neurons as a site of selective vulnerability to aging processes" (11).

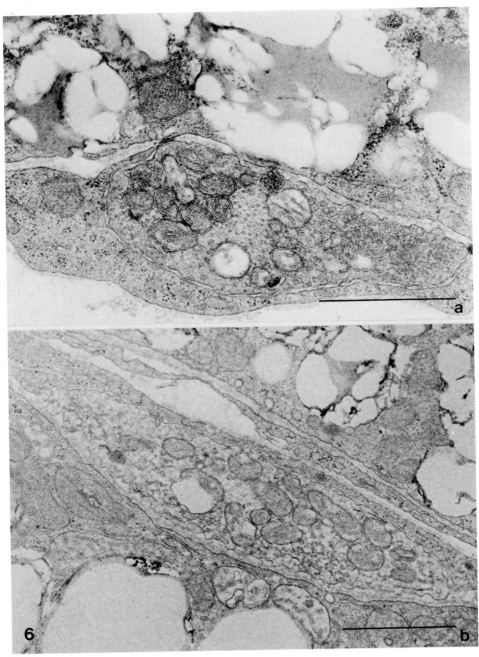

FIG. 6. Four-year-old hen. The nerve endings contain synaptic vesicles
which appear either agglutinated (a) or polymorphic in shape and size (b).
Compare with Fig. 1.

A good correlation seems to appear between this timing and the occurrence in the iris muscle of most pronounced regressive changes in more advanced ages, when also morphologically evident modifications of the neuromuscular junctions are found. However, more experimental work and more ultrastructural studies are needed in order to find out the largest number of morphological events which can be related to modifications of the ACh metabolism during aging.

ACKNOWLEDGMENTS

This work was supported by funds from the Consiglio Nazionale delle Ricerche to the Centro di Studio per la Biologia e Fisiopatologia Muscolare and, in part, by a grant from the Muscular Dystrophy Association of America to Prof. M. Aloisi.

REFERENCES

1. Aloisi, M., and Mussini, I. (1980): In: Multidisciplinary Approach to Brain Development, edited by C. DiBenedetta, pp. 463-464, Elsevier/ North Holland Biomedical Press.
2. Aloisi, M., Mussini, I., and Simeoni, M.L. (1976): 5th Meet. Europ. Muscle Club, Abstr. 32
3. Bass, A., Gutmann, E., nad Hanzlikova, V. (1975): Gerontologia, 21: 31-45
4. Ermini, M. (1976): Gerontology, 22: 301-316
5. Gutmann, E., and Hanzlikova, V. (1965): Gerontologia, 11: 12-24
6. Gutmann, E., and Hanzlikova, V. (1976): Gerontology, 22: 280-300
7. Gutmann, E., Hanzlikova, V., and Vyskocil, F. (1971): J. Physiol. Lond. 216: 331-343
8. Hanzlikova, V., and Gutmann, E. (1975): Adv. Expl. Med. Biol., 53: 421-429
9. Marchi, M., and Giacobini, E. (1980): Dev. Neurosci., 3: 39-48
10. Marchi, M., Giacobini, E., and Hruschak,K. (1979): Dev.Neurosci., 2: 201-212
11. Marchi, M., Hoffman, D.W., Giacobini, E., and Fredrickson, T. (1980): Dev. Neurosci., 3: 235-247
12. Marchi, M., Hoffman, D.W., Mussini, I., and Giacobini, E. (1980): Dev. Neurosci., 3: 185-198
13. Marchi, M., Yurkewicz, L., Giacobini, E., and Fredrickson, T. (1981): Dev. Neurosci., 4: 258-266
14. McCarter, R. (1978): In: Aging in Muscle, edited by G. Kaldor, and W.J. DiBattista, pp. 1-21, Raven Press, New York
15. Muscatello, U.,and Patriarca,P.L.(1968):Am.J.Pathol.,52: 1169-1189
16. Sohal, R.S. (1978): In: Aging in Muscle, edited by G. Kaldor and W.J. DiBattista, pp. 211-226. Raven Press, New York

The Aging Brain: Cellular and Molecular Mechanisms of Aging in the Nervous System, edited by E. Giacobini et al., Raven Press, New York © 1982.

Phospholipid Biosynthesis in the Aging Brain

G. Porcellati, A. Gaiti, and M. Brunetti

Biochemistry Department, The Medical School, Perugia University, 06100 Perugia, Italy

Aging in the brain is a complex process which is characterized by morphological and neurochemical alterations in man and other animal species. The morphology and composition of the central nervous system during aging is rather well known (5, 10).   On the other hand, brain tissue consists of different cell types with distinct biochemical and functional features and the interactions among cells may be quite complex during aging.   Losses have been observed in cell number, particularly in the neuronal population of the cerebbelar cortex both in rats and humans, and suggestion has also been made that the loss of neurons may be compensated for by an increase of other cells such as glial cells.

The process of aging involves biochemical changes in neural substrates, membranes, molecules, and ions which have behavioral correlates during aging.   The most important task in the study of these changes is to find out their functional significance in terms of mechanisms responsible for aging (3, 12).   Recently, the concept of lysosomal involvement in cell damage during aging has gained much attention (3, 12).   On the other hand, the loss during aging of neurons may alter the interactions among cells and complicates the neurochemical findings.   This is probably the main limiting factor about the knowledge of the chemical and biochemical changes in the aging brain.

There has been up to now little work done on age-related changes of structure and turnover of lipid in experimental animals.   On the other hand, the role of lipids is very important according to the hypothesis which relates the catalytic activity of membrane-bound enzymes to membrane structure and composition.

Brain cells are continuously synthesizing new molecules of ethanolamine phosphoglycerides (EPG) and choline phosphoglycerides (CPG), the two more abundant phospholipid classes, from low molecular weight precursors by a "net synthesis" process.   Some of these precursors are freely soluble in the cell, some are membrane-bound.   The rate of synthesis of these two lipids may depend from several factors, as enzyme activity, availability of substrates and intermediates, energy requirements, composition of substrates, membrane structure.

This chapter examines the synthesis of the main rat brain phospholipids, CPG and EPG, including plasmalogens, at different ages.   It is shown that one of the possible causes of the decrease of the rate of CPG and EPG synthesis during aging is a variation in the structure of lipid substrates, rather than changes in enzyme activity or substrate concentration.

SYNTHESIS OF CPG AND EPG IN BRAIN MICROSOMES

The rate of the de novo synthesis of CPG and EPG has been examined by measuring the activities of choline and ethanolamine phosphotransferases (EC 2.7.8.1 and 2.7.8.2) in brain microsomes from wistar rats of different ages in the presence of labelled CDP-choline or CDP-ethanolamine (4).   No exogenous diacyl glycerol was added to the incubation medium in vitro.   By this means the measured activities were dependent only on the concentration of the membrane-bound endogenous microsomal diacyl glyceroils.   The activity of both phosphotransferases decreases noticeably during the first part of the rat life span, as shown in Fig.1.   No additional other changes occurred in brain microsomes of rats older than 20 months of age, and rather large scattering of data took place after this time.   It is interesting to mention that the 18 months represent about the middle, or more, of the normal rat lifespan, and that this age is indicated to represent the stage at which the initial aging phoenomena have already begun (11).   Fig. 1 indicates that the decrease of the rate of synthesis of both CPG and EPG is around 40 %.

It is known that CPG and EPG represent the whole class of choline and ethanolamine phospholipids.   Subsequent experiments have been carried out therefore by examining the rate of incorporation of CDP-choline and CDP-ethanolamine into subclasses of CPG and EPG of microsomal membranes of 18 months old-rats in comparison to controls.   Incubation has been carried out essentially as described by Brunetti et al. (4) and fractionation of CPG and EPG into the correspondent diacyl- and alkenylacyl-derivatives (plasmalogens) was performed as reported elsewhere (6).

Table 1 shows that the variation between the control and aged rats was very significant and that the rate of synthesis of choline and ethanolamine plasmalogens was even more severely depressed by aging (50-55%). These results, together with those reported in Fig.1, indicate a noticeable effect of aging on the rate of phospholipid synthesis in the rat brain endoplasmic reticulum, where most of lipid production occurs.   It must be observed, at this point, that the phosphotransferases which transfer phosphorylcholine or phosphorylethanolamine from their correspondent cytidine nucleotides to the endogenous diacyl glycerol, represent

the last step in the <u>de novo</u> synthesis of CPG and EPG in brain, only one
of the various steps in the overall pathway.   It is worth mentioning, in
this connection, that the enzymic reaction catalyzed by the cytidylyl-
transferases (EC 2.7.7.14 and 2.7.7.15) is most probably the really rate-
limiting step in the whole process (9).

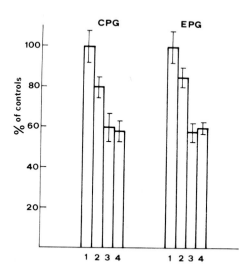

FIG. 1. Conversion to corresponding CPG
and EPG of CDP–choline and CDP–ethanolamine in rat brain microsomes during
aging.   Experiments have been carried
out as described elsewhere (9).   Data
are represented as change per cent of
controls (2 months rats) and are means
of 9 experiments for CPG synthesis and
5 for EPG synthesis.   Bars represent
data with their standard deviation values.
1, 2, 3 and 4 mean 2, 12, 18 and 20 months
of age.   See text, for further details.

DIACYL GLYCEROL COMPOSITION OF BRAIN MICROSOMES

It was shown with the previous section that a significant variation
between adult and aged rat brains takes place as regard to the <u>in vitro</u>
diacyl glycerol utilization for lipid synthesis.   With parallel experiments it was also observed that the kinetics of diglyceride utilization
by the brain microsomes of the aged rats was essentially similar to that
already reported elsewhere for adult rats (1, 9).   Moreover, CDP–choline
and CDP–ethanolamine concentrations used in the incubation experiments
were certainly saturating (9), and therefore do not affect <u>per se</u> the
results reported in Fig.1 and in Table 1.   Finally, the main concentra-

TABLE 1. The rate of synthesis of CPG and EPG subclasses in brain microsomes of adult and 18 months old-rats

Lipid subclass	Adult rats	Aged rats	Decrease (%)
Diacyl-GPC	1.13 (9)	0.70 (5)[a]	– 38
Alkenylacyl-GPC	0.33 (9)	0.17 (5)[b]	– 49
Diacyl-GPE	1.01 (5)	0.59 (5)[a]	– 41
Alkenylacyl-GPE	0.13 (5)	0.06 (5)[b]	– 54

Data are reported as nmoles lipid synthesized/mg protein/40 min. Number of experiments betwwen brackets. Adult rats : 2 months old-rats. Aged rats : 18 months old-rats. See the text for additional details.
[a]$P < 0.01$; [b]$P < 0.001$.

tion value of diacyl glycerol content in the brain microsomes of aged rats of 18, 20 or 24 months was similar to that reported elsewhere (2) for adult rats, *i.e.* about 9–10 nmoles/mg protein.

It is not valid, therefore, to indicate as responsible for the changes reported in the previous section a variation of diacyl glycerol concentration in brain microsomes, nor does it seem possible to indicate as responsible a catalytic change of some enzymes related to phospholipid synthesis in brain.

A series of experiments has been subsequently carried out by determining the fatty acyl composition of the brain microsomal diacyl glycerol pool in adult and 18 months old-rats, in order to relate possible variations of this composition to the different rates of the phosphotransferase reaction (Fig.1 and Table 1).   Table 2 indicates that the percent of content of monoenoic and dienoic species increases noticeably during aging in rat brain microsomal diglycerides, whereas that of arachidonic acid decreases.

The variations reported in Table 2 may influence the phosphotransferase reaction described in Fig. 1 and Table 1, since previous work had reported that different reaction rates occur in brain with the use of single different diacyl glycerols as substrate (7).   As a consequence, the variation of the molar distribution of the microsomal diacyl glycerol molecular species, reported in Table 2, may change the rate of synthesis of CPG and EPG in brain observed in the first section of this work.

In order to prove this hypothesis and to confirm the results reported in this and in the previous section, the saturating concentration of externally added diacyl glycerols was checked on the light of previous observations (8, 9).   It was thus found that no significant differences exist between values of saturating diacyl glycerols if these substrates were added to microsomal membranes of either adult or aged rat brains. Subsequent experiments have been therefore carried out with exogenously added diacyl glycerols, and results will be reported in the next section.

TABLE 2. The composition of brain microsomal diacyl glycerol in the adult and aged rats

Fatty acid	Adult rats	Aged rats	Variation (%)
16:0	24.7	23.3	–
16:1	5.7	9.5	+ 67
18:0	27.0	25.0	–
18:1	17.3	20.9	+ 21
18:2	1.7	3.2	+ 88
18:3	traces	traces	–
20:4	22.7	17.9	– 21
22:6	traces	traces	–

Microsomal diacyl glycerol composition was estimated by GLC of the corresponding methyl esters using a Fractovap Mod GCV gas liquid chromatograph (Carlo Erba, Milan, Italy). The stationary phase was 5 % ethylene glycol adipate on sylanized Chromosorb-W (100–200 mesh) in 200 x 0.2 cm glass columns. Nitrogen flow was 20 ml/min, and column and detector temperatures were 180°C and 230°C, respectively. Quantitation was done as reported elsewhere (2).

THE EFFECT OF DIACYL GLYCEROL ADDITION ON MICROSOMAL PHOSPHOLIPID SYNTHESIS DURING AGING

On the light of previous observations, experiments were then performed by incubating the microsomal membranes from 18 months old-rat brain in the presence of saturating concentrations of diacyl glycerols. This type of experiment was done in order to minimize the contribution of the small amount of endogenous microsomal diacyl glycerols in the overall rate of reaction in both aged and control rats.

By comparing the data with those reported in Table 1, the variation found in the rate of CPG and EPG synthesis from CDP-choline and CDP-ethanolamine between control and aged rat brain microsomes was not at all significant (Table 3). In other words, much smaller variation is seen between adult and ageing brains, when their microsomes are supplemented with exogenous diglycerides.

All the evidence produced in this and in the previous sections suggests that the composition of the endogenous diglyceride pool in brain microsomes, rather than an enzymic defect, may affect the rate of the phosphotransferase reaction during ageing. The variation found in Table 2 further convalidates this hypothesis, because a change was observed in the fatty acyl composition of diacyl glycerols between rat brain of different ages.

TABLE 3.   The rate of synthesis of CPG and EPG in brain microsomes of adult and aged rats after adding exogenous diacyl glycerol

Lipid class	Diacyl glycerol added (mM)	Adult rats	Aged rats	(%)[a]
EPG	6.5	134	118	−12
	7.8	139	117	−15
	10.5	145	126	−13
CPG	5.0	143	120	−16
	10.5	143	114	−20

See Table 1 for explanation and details.   Data from three to four experiments.   Variation in the aged rats were not statistically significant, if compared to adult rat values.   Diacyl glycerols were added and prepared as reported elsewhere (4).

[a] Decrease per cent.

SYNTHESIS OF CPG AND EPG IN NEURONS AND GLIA DURING AGING

Interactions among cells of different origin and function in brain are very critical and complex.   Although the results of the previous section were rather clear, it could be argued that the differences found in whole brain microsomes between adult and aged rats might be due to a decrease of the neuronal population, where the rate of phospholipid synthesis is higher (1), and/or to an increase of glia, where this rate is lower (1).

With subsequent experiments, the total phospholipid concentration, the DNA content and other parameters were thus determined in neuronal and glial cells of 2 months old- (controls) and 18 months old-rat brains. Table 4 clearly indicates that no evident variation was visible on these parameters from either adult or aged animals, and only a slight decrease of the DNA content was found in neurons when expressed on a protein basis.

TABLE 4.   Lipid and DNA composition of neuronal and glial cells from adult and aged rat brains

Component	Neurons		Glial cells	
	Adult rats	Aged rats	Adult rats	Aged rats
DNA	67.1 ± 0.9	60.4 ± 1.2	7.6 ± 1.3	7.5 ± 1.7
Phospholipid P	9.3 ± 2.2	9.5 ± 2.8	16.2 ± 3.5	16.3 ± 2.4
Diacyl glycerols	10.4 ± 3.2	8.4 ± 1.2	23.4 ± 5.0	24.0 ± 4.4

DNA and phospholipid P are expressed as μg/mg protein ± S.D.   Diacyl glycerols are expressed as nmol/mg protein ± S.D.   Data represent means from six experiments.

The activities of choline and ethanolamine phosphotransferases were successively examined by incubating neuronal and glial cell homogenates with labelled CDP-choline or CDP-ethanolamine without adding exogenous diglycerides, following described procedures (1). Fig. 2 indicates that a significant decrease of choline phosphotransferase takes place in rat neurons up to 18 months of age with no further change after this age.

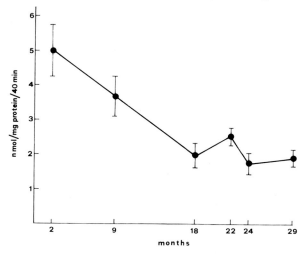

FIG. 2. The incorporation of CDP-choline into CPG of neuronal cell homogenates. See the text for experimental details. No diacyl glycerols were added in the incubation medium. Each data is the mean from at least five experiments.

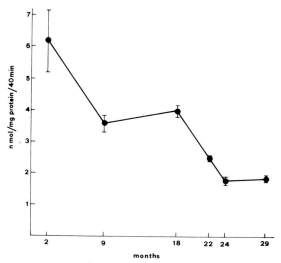

FIG. 3. The incorporation of CDP-ethanolamine into EPG of neuronal cell homogenates. No diacyl glyrol added. See the text and Fig.2 for other details.

Fig. 3 shows that also EPG synthesis in the absence of added diacyl glycerol is affected by aging in rat neurons, and that the rate of conversion of CDP-ethanolamine into EPG sharply decreases even after 18 months of age.   Interestingly, no changes either in the rate of CPG synthesis or in that of EPG were found as regard to glial activity, as shown in Table 5.

From the results so far obtained, conclusion is drawn that neurons possess a much lower rate of phosphotransferase activity during aging, and hence a much lower rate of phospholipid synthesis, whereas glial cell does not show any differences throughout the examined life span.   The main lipid composition of neurons, which did not change with aging (see also Table 4) could not influence the activity of the enzymes tested, and the slight decrease of the DNA content in neurons could not account for the differences in the rate of synthesis in terms of cell reduction alone. Probably, the reason for the change in neuronal enzyme activity during aging resides on changes of composition of endogenous substrates.   This hypothesis is also related to the results reported in the previous sections of this chapter.

TABLE 5.   The rate of synthesis of CPG and EPG in glial homogenates from rat brain during aging

Age (months)	CPG synthesis	EPG synthesis
2	1.78 ± 0.23 (9)	2.18 ± 0.45 (10)
9	1.31 ± 0.24 (7)	1.59 ± 0.19 (10)
18	1.81 ± 0.50 (11)	2.06 ± 0.69 (12)
22	1.37 ± 0.16 (5)	1.70 ± 0.11 (5)
24	1.56 ± 0.11 (5)	1.61 ± 0.16 (5)
29	1.70 ± 0.47 (5)	1.64 ± 0.06 (5)

Incubations were carried out as reported elsewhere (9).   Data expressed as nmol/mg protein/40 min ± S.E.M.   Number of experiments between brackets.

Accordingly, a series of experiments was performed by preparing diglycerides from aged and adult rat brain cortex CPG and adding them in proper saturating concentrations (1) to homogenates of glia and neurons from adult rats and then crossing the experiments.   On performing these cross-experiments no more differences were found in the rate of CPG synthesis between adult and aged (18 months old) neurons (Table 6).   This result is in line with those obtained with microsomes from adult and aged rat brain (compare the data of Table 6 with those of Tables 1 and 3).

With parallel experiments it was shown that the diacyl glycerols prepared from adult or aged rat brain cortex were rather rich in polyunsaturated fatty acids.   The results of the cross-experiments, reported in Table 6, are to be interpreted therefore keeping in mind this composition.

It is known, in fact, that the molecular species of diglycerides are utilized at different rates by brain microsomes (2, 7) and that a certain degree of enzyme specificity for different diglycerides exists in brain (2, 7). The addition, therefore, of diglycerides prepared from whole brain cortex, which are rather rich in polyunsaturated fatty acids, is capable of almost completely restoring the choline phosphotransferase activity (Table 6), which was noticeably decreased in aging neurons as reported in Fig.2.

TABLE 6. The effect of the addition of brain diglyceride on the rate of synthesis of choline phosphoglycerides in neuronal cells of adult and aged rats

Diglyceride (mM)	Brain lecithin source	Choline Phosphoglycerides Synthesis	
		2 months	18 months
0.6	adult	45.9	45.2
0.6	aged	46.6	40.1
1.2	adult	47.4	43.0
1.2	aged	49.0	45.0
2.4	adult	52.4	47.4
2.4	aged	51.3	46.2

The results are expressed as nmoles/mg protein/40 min, and represent mean values from three experiments. See the text for further details.

From these results we conclude that aging of the nervous system is characterized by a decrease, mainly in the neuronal cells, of the ability to synthesize in vitro the main phosphoglycerides. One of the possible causes of the differences in the de novo synthesis between adult and aged rats could be the lesser availability of endogenous polyunsaturated diglycerides in aged rat brain neurons. This assumption is in line with the results of the previous sections, which demonstrated significant differences in the fatty acid composition of endogenous diglycerides between microsomes from 2 months- and 18 months-old rat brains.

CONCLUSION

The synthesis of choline phosphoglycerides and ethanolamine phosphoglycerides is affected by aging in brain microsomes of the Wistar rats. The decrease of these metabolic activities is essentially limited to the neurons. The addition of diacyl glycerols to the incubation medium restores noticeably these activities, both in microsomes and neurons. The effect of adding exogenous diglycerides, together with the data on its microsomal composition, suggests that one of the causes of the decrease of the rates of CPG and EPG synthesis is a variation of essential lipid substrates.

ACKNOWLEDGEMENT

This work was supported by a grant from the Consiglio Nazionale delle Ricerche, Rome (contract No. 80.00543.04/115). The technical assistance of Mr. Edmondo Giovagnoli is gratefully acknowledged.

REFERENCES

1. Binaglia, L., Goracci, G., Porcellati, G., Roberti, R., and Woelk, H. (1973) : J. Neurochem., 21 : 1067–1082.
2. Binaglia, L., Roberti, R., and Porcellati, G. (1978) : In : Enzymes of Lipid Metabolism, edited by S. Gatt, L. Freysz, and P. Mandel, pp. 353–366, Plenum Press, New York.
3. Brody, H., Harman, D., and Ordy, J.M., editors (1975) : Clinical, Morphological and Neurochemical Aspects in the Aging Central Nervous System. Raven Press, New York.
4. Brunetti, M., Gaiti, A., and Porcellati, G. (1979) : Lipids, 14 : 925–931.
5. Dhopeshwarkar, G.A., and Mead, J.F. (1975) : In : Aging, edited by H. Brody, D. Harman, J.M. Ordy, Vol.1, pp. 108–132. Raven Press, New York.
6. Gaiti, A., De Medio, G.E., Brunetti, M., Amaducci, L., and Porcellati, G. (1974) : J. Neurochem., 23 : 1153–1159.
7. Porcellati, G. (1973) : In : Advances in Enzyme Regulations, Vol.X, edited by G. Weber, pp. 83–100, Pergamon Press, London.
8. Porcellati, G., Biasion, M.G., and Arienti, G. (1970) : Lipids, 5 : 725–733.
9. Porcellati, G., Biasion, M.G., and Pirotta, M. (1970) : Lipids, 5 : 734–742.
10. Scheibel, M.E., and Scheibel, A.B. (1975) : In : Aging, edited by H. Brody, D. Harman, and J.M. Ordy, Vol.1, pp.11–38. Raven Press, New York.
11. Shelanski, M.L. (1976) : In : Neurobiology of Aging, edited by R.D. Terry, and S. Gershon, pp. 339–349. Raven Press, New York.
12. Terry, R.D., and Gershon, S., editors (1976) : Neurobiology of Aging, Raven Press, New York.

The Aging Brain: Cellular and Molecular Mechanisms of Aging in the Nervous System, edited by E. Giacobini et al., Raven Press, New York © 1982.

Phospholipid Methylation, ³H-Diazepam, and ³H-GABA Binding in the Cerebellum of Aged Rats

G. Calderini and G. Toffano

Department of Biochemistry, Fidia Research Laboratories, 35031 Abano Terme, Italy

γ-aminobutyric acid (GABA) is the major inhibitory neurotransmitter in the mammalian central nervous system. Since GABA containing neurons are abundant in virtually all brain regions where they interact with most of the other neurotransmitter systems, an impairment of the GABAergic activity may play a role in the alterations of cerebral functions during the aging process.

Loss of normal synaptic inhibitory tone is probably involved in many pathological conditions such as epilepsy, Parkinson's disease, Huntington's chorea and neuropsychiatric disorders whose incidence increases with age (16). The synaptic GABAergic function is affected by benzodiazepines (BDZ) primarily through an interaction with specific recognition sites, proposed as BDZ receptors (14, 17), which are part of the complex GABA/BDZ receptor unit (4). As to the molecular mechanism of the BDZ action, it has been recently reported that BDZ receptor occupancy enhances phospholipid methylation (18), and conversely that the addition of S-adenosylmethionine to crude synaptic plasma membranes increases both ³H-Diazepam and ³H-GABA binding (3). Since phospholipid methylation is suggested to be an important metabolic process influencing the internalization of many biological signals (1Q), we thought interesting to study whether changes of phospholipid methylation, ³H-GABA and ³H-Diazepam binding do occur in senescent rats. Furthermore clinical reports have indicated that elderly patients are more susceptible to anxiolytic drugs (7), although inconsistent data have been reported on both ³H-Diazepam (13, 15) and ³H-GABA binding (2, 8, 12) in aged rats.

MATERIALS AND METHODS

Sprague-Dawley rats of different ages obtained from the "Italian Study Group on Brain Aging", were maintained in standard environmental conditions with free access to food and water and a light-dark cycle of 12 hours. The animals were sacrified by decapitation and the brains were quickly removed and dissected. Tissue samples were stored at -60°C till assays were performed.

Membrane preparation and receptor binding assays

Crude synaptic plasma membranes were prepared according to Enna and Snyder (6) as modifed by Toffano et al (19).

H-Diazepam binding was performed according to Möhler and Okada (14) on 1 ml of frozen-thawed membranes incubated at 4°C for 20 minutes with various amounts of radioactive ligand (H-Diazepam, S.A. 64.06 Ci/mmol). The reaction was terminated by rapid filtration through Whatman GF/B glass filters. The filters were washed twice with 5 ml ice-cold 50mM Tris-citrate buffer pH 7.1 and the radioactivity was measured by liquid scintillation spectrometry. The specific H-Diazepam binding was calculated by correcting the amount of radioactivity found in the presence of H-Diazepam with that found during incubation with H-Diazepam plus 10^{-5} M cold Diazepam.

High affinity H-GABA binding was performed on 200-300 μg protein of frozen-thawed and Triton X-100 treated crude synaptic membranes incubated at 4°C for 5 minutes with amounts of radioactive ligand (H-GABA, S.A. 40 Ci/mmol) from 5 to 30 nM (19). The reaction was terminated by centrifugation, the supernatant was removed and the pellet was quickly rinsed with cold distilled water and solubilized in NCS. The radioactivity was measured by liquid scintillation spectrometry. The specific binding of H-GABA was calculated by subtracting from the amount of radioactivity found in the presence of H-GABA, that occurring in the presence of H-GABA plus 10^{-5} M cold GABA. The kinetic constants were calculated according to the Scatchard's analysis.

Membrane phospholipid methylation

Crude synaptic membrane fractions of pooled cerebella were assayed for phosphomethyltransferase 1 (PMT1) activity according to Crews et al (5). Briefly, incorporation of H-methyl groups were assayed on crude synaptic plasma membranes incubated at 37°C for 30 minutes with 0.7 μM S-adenosyl-[H-methyl] methionine (H-SAM). The reaction was stopped with 10% trichloroacetic acid and the samples were centrifuged at 10,000 rpm for 10 minutes. Phospholipids were extracted with chloroform/methanol (2:1) and washed twice with 0.1M KCl in 50% methanol. One millimeter of the chloroform phase was evaporated to dryness and the radioactivity counted by liquid scintillation spectroscopy. Products were identified using thin-layer chromatography (5).

Protein

Proteins were determined according to Lowry et al (11).

RESULTS

^{3}H-Diazepam and ^{3}H-GABA binding in the cerebellum of rats at different ages

An age-dependent increase of ^{3}H-Diazepam binding occurs in crude synaptic plasma membrane from rat cerebella (Table 1). The kinetic analysis indicates that the modification in the binding properties of benzodiazepine recognition sites is due to an increase of their apparent number (Bmax) rather than to changes in their apparent affinity (Kd).

Table 1. Binding of ^{3}H-Diazepam to crude synaptic plasma membranes from rat cerebellum

Age (months)	Kd (nM)	Bmax (pmol/mg prot)	% increase
1	7.24	1.100	
3	7.31	1.280	+ 16
13	7.35	1.360	+ 24
17	7.82	1.500	+ 36
21	7.88	1.550	+ 41

Kinetic constants of ^{3}H-Diazepam binding to crude synaptic plasma membranes prepared from rat cerebellum at various ages. H-Diazepam binding was assayed with 0.3 - 0.5 mg prot and H-Diazepam at concentrations ranging from 0.75 to 9nM. Each value determined by Scatchard's analysis is the mean of 3 determinations, each determination was carried out in triplicate using 5 pooled cerebella. Standard error is less than 10%.

In 21 month old rats, Bmax increases of about 40% with respect to the 1 month old group. The phenomenon is present at a minor extent also in the 13 and 17 month old groups (24% and 36% increase respectively). The apparent Kd slightly increases with age without reaching significant difference.

In contrast the high affinity ^{3}H-GABA binding is essentially unmodified in the cerebella of young and old animals in agreement with previous reports (2, 8, 12). As shown in Table 2, neither Bmax nor Kd change with age.

Table 2. Binding of ^{3}H-GABA to crude S.P.M. from rat cerebellum

Age (months)	Kd (nM)	Bmax (pmol/mg prot)
3	15	3.20
21	13	3.40

^{3}H-GABA binding assay was done using 0.2 - 0.3 mg prot of a frozen thawed and Triton X-100 treated membrane preparation and ^{3}H-GABA at concentrations ranging from 5 to 30nM.

Phospholipid methylation and aging

The methylation of membrane phospholipids was studied by measuring the incorporation of $\left[^3\text{H-methyl}\right]$ group from S-adenosyl-$\left[^3\text{H-methyl}\right]$ methionine into lipids extracted by methanol-chloroform as described by Hirata et al. (9). The aging process stimulates the activity of PMT1, the rate limiting enzyme of the methylation pathway. The activation of the enzymatic conversion of phosphatidyl-ethanolamine (PE) into phosphatidylcholine (PC) by aging is confirmed by the identification of the methylated derivatives by thin-layer chromatography indicating that the mono- and dimethylated forms of PE and PC increase with age.

Table 3. ^{3}H-methyl-group incorporated into phospholipidic fraction of crude S.P.M. from rat cerebellum at various ages

Age (months)	Total phospholipids	PC	PNNE	PNE
3	6960	2189	2261	2510
13	12313	4020	4322	3971
17	12839	3561	4642	4636
21	12158	3207	4820	4131

Values are expressed as dpm/mg prot. Phospholipid methylation was studied by incubating 0.7 μM ^{3}H-SAM. Phosphatidylcholine (PC), monophosphatidyletha-nolamine (PNE), and dimethylphosphatidylethanolamine (PNNE) were separated by TLC as reported in "Materials and Methods".

The incorporation of the methyl groups in the total phospholipidic fraction (PNE + PNNE + PC) increases more than 70% at 13 months of age and then remains constant. In the case of phosphatidylcholine, the phase of increase is followed by a decline indicating that activation of the catabolism of this phospholipid may occur with aging.

DISCUSSION

An age-dependent increase of 3H-Diazepam binding, due to an increase in the apparent number of binding sites, occurs in rat cerebellum. The increased density of benzodiazepine binding sites with age may be significant since it may represent the biochemical basis for the increased sensibility to anxyolitic drugs of elderly patients [7], even if the differences in pharmacokinetics have also to be taken into account. However this hypothesis, although attractive, needs further confirmation. Our results contrast with those of Pedigo et al. [15] who found no change of ^{3}H-Flunitrazepam binding in the brain of senescent Fischer rats. Using the Sprague-Dawley strain an age-dependent increase of benzodiazepine receptor binding sites has been found in the hippocampus [13] and in the retina (Biggio, G.: manuscript in preparation). The difference in strain as well as in the experimental procedures may explain these discrepancies. That benzodiazepine binding sites may increase with aging is also supported by the increased density of ^{3}H-Flunitrazepam binding sites in the cerebellum and cerebral cortex of patients affected by Huntington's chorea [21].

[3]H-GABA binding has been found constant in the cerebellum of aging rats confirming previous reports by Maggi et al. [12] and by Govoni et al. [8]. Yet, in view of the functional coupling existing between GABA and BDZ receptors, we favour the concept that the modification of BDZ binding during aging reflects an impairment of the whole GABA/BDZ receptor complex. Support to this suggestion is provided by the observation that in aged rats when one of the two sites is occupied by the specific ligand, GABA and benzodiazepine receptor response is quantitatively different [1, 3]. In this context the activation of the methylation pathway by aging may be worth of attention. We have recently demonstrated that in rat cerebellum, benzodiazepine binding sites increase when membrane phospholipid methylation is stimulated [20].

In conclusion we have seen that aging increases ^{3}H-Diazepam binding and stimulates methyltransferase 1 activity. These two biochemical parameters may together participate in the homeostatic preservation of cerebellar GABAergic function. However impairment of GABAergic functions may result also from modifications not directly involving the GABAergic binding sites.

REFERENCES

1. Bonetti, A.C., Calderini, G., Aldinio, C., Balzano, M., Di Perri, B., and Toffano G. (1981): in press to Raven Press.
2. Calderini, G., Aldinio, C., Crews, F., Gaiti, A., Scapagnini, U., Algeri, S., Ponzio, F., and Toffano ,G. (1981): In: Apomorphine and Other Dopaminomimetics: Clinical Pharmacology, edited by G.U. Corsini, and G.L. Gessa, pp. 235-242. Raven Press, New York.
3. Calderini, G., Bonetti, A.C., Aldinio, C., Savoini, G., Biggio, G., and Toffano, G. (1981): submitted.
4. Costa, E., and Guidotti, A. (1979): Ann. Rev. Pharmacol. Toxicol., 19:531-545.
5. Crews, F., Hirata, F., and Axelrod, J. (1980): J. Neurochem., 34:1491-1498.
6. Enna, S.J., and Snyder, S.H. (1977): Molec. Pharmacol., 13:442-453.
7. Epstein, L.J. (1978): In: Psychopharmacology: A Generation of Progress, edited by M.A. Lipton, A. DiMascio, and K.F. Killam, pp. 1517-1523. Raven Press, New York.
8. Govoni, S., Memo, M., Saiani, L., Spano, P.F., and Trabucchi, M. (1980): Mech.

Age. Dev., 12:39-46.

9. Hirata, F., Viveros, O.H., Diliberto, E.J. Jr., and Axelrod, J. (1978): Proc. Natl. Acad. Sci. USA, 75:1718-1721.

10. Hirata, F., and Axelrod, J. (1980): Science, 209:1082-1090.

11. Lowry, O.H., Rosebrough, N.J., Lewis Farr, A., and Randall, R.J. (1951): J. Biol. Chem., 193:265-275.

12. Maggi, A., Schmidt, M.J., Ghetti, B., and Enna, S.J. (1979): Life Sci., 24:367-374.

13. Memo, M., Spano, P.F., Trabucchi, M. (1981): J. Pharm. Pharmacol., 33:64.

14. Möhler H., and Okada T. (1977): Science, 198:849-851.

15. Pedigo, N.W., McDougal, J.N., Burks, T.F., and Yamamura, H.I. (1981): Fed. Proc., 40:311, abstract n° 439.

16. Roberts, E., Chase, T.N., and Tower, D.B., editors (1976): GABA in Nervous System Function, Raven Press, New York.

17. Squires, R.F., and Braestrup, C. (1977): Nature, 266:732-734.

18. Strittmatter, W.J., Hirata, F., Axelrod, J., Mallorga, P., Tallman, J.F., and Henneberry, R.C. (1979): Nature, 282:857-859.

19. Toffano, G., Guidotti, A., and Costa, E. (1978): Proc. Natl. Acad. Sci. USA, 75:4024-4028.

20. Toffano, G., Battistella, A., Teolato, S., Bonetti, A.C., Di Perri, B., and Calderini G. (1981): submitted.

21. Yamamura,H.I.,Reisine,T.D.,andBeaumont,K.(1980): BrainRes.Bull.,5:773-775.

The Aging Brain: Cellular and Molecular Mechanisms of Aging in the Nervous System, edited by E. Giacobini et al., Raven Press, New York © 1982.

Aging, Receptor Binding, and Membrane Microviscosity

D. Samuel, D. S. Heron, M. Hershkowitz, and *M. Shinitzky

*Departments of Isotope Research and *Membrane Research, The Weizmann Institute of Science, 76100 Rehovot, Israel*

The ability of the central nervous system (CNS) to maintain homeostasis is crucial for its proper function. In response to fluctuating physiological or environmental conditions, changes can occur at the neuronal level by dendritic proliferation or sprouting (15), or at the synaptic level by altered rates of transmitter turnover or changes in receptor number and characteristics (23). An impaired ability to adapt has been suggested as one of the main causes for the aging of the CNS (2).

One mechanism of homeostasis is the process of "homeoviscous adaptation" (22), which is responsible for keeping the lipid fluidity of many cell membranes constant. This process has been shown to operate, for example, when the environmental temperature of poikilotherms or bacteria is changed (22) or in mammalian systems after chronic exposure to agents which fluidize membranes, such as alcohol (3) or morphine (13). We suggest that homeoviscous adaptation is also impaired with increasing age, causing a decrease in the membrane lipid fluidity of many tissues. In brain this occurs, for instance, mainly due to an increase in the mole ratio of cholesterol to phospholipids (C/PL) or of sphingomyelin to lecithin (S/L) (18), which are the main determinants of membrane fluidity (20). Nagy has already suggested that increased membrane rigidity may play a key role in the process of aging, by causing an imbalance in the regulatory processes of many cells (16).

In fact, membrane fluidity has been shown to modulate the action of many membrane-bound proteins (14). We have previously reported (8,9) that ligand binding to serotonin and to opiate receptors from mouse brain can change when the synaptic membrane microviscosity (the reciprocal of fluidity) is altered. These neurotransmitter systems, which are crucial for many physiological phenomena, may be involved in many of the problems of increasing age, such as changes in the pattern of sleep, alterations in mood, decreased libido, elevated pain threshold, etc. (4). We have, therefore, investigated the changes in ligand binding to these two receptor systems in aged animals, and correlated them with changes in lipid fluidity of synaptic membranes.

Crude homogenates were prepared from the forebrains (i.e. whole brain without the cerebellum) of young adult (6-8 weeks) and old (24-27 months) C57Bℓ mice and incubated with different lipid suspensions in polyvinyl-pyrrolidone (PVP), as described previously (8,9,21). Cholesteryl-hemi-succinate (CHS) was used for increasing membrane viscosity and egg-lecithin (Sigma) for decreasing it. The affinity and number of opiate

(17) and serotonin (1) receptor sites in these membranes were determined by conventional techniques, using (^{3}H)-D-ala-enkephalinamide or (^{3}H)-serotonin. Membrane microviscosity, $\bar{\eta}$, was measured by fluorescence depolarization, using 1,3,5-diphenyl-hexatriene (DPH) as a probe (8,9). The C/PL ratio was also determined in some samples.

The results are presented in Table 1. It is apparent that the microviscosity of membranes from most brain regions is higher in preparations from old mice as compared to those from young ones. The differences are largest in cortex caudate and hippocampus, where there is also an increase in the measured C/PL ratio.

TABLE 1. Membrane lipid microviscosity ($\bar{\eta}$) and cholesterol to phospholipid mole ratio (C/PL) of several brain regions from young (2-3 months) and old (24-27 months) C57Bℓ mice.

Brain region	Preparation	$\bar{\eta}$, 25°C (poise)[b]		C/PL	
		Young	Old[a]	Young	Old[a]
Whole brain	Crude homogenate	5.3±0.2	6.0±0.3	–	–
Hypothalamus	Dissociated cells	5.4±0.4	6.0±0.3	–	–
Cerebellum	" "	5.5±0.2	6.0±0.3	–	–
Brain stem	" "	6.8±0.2	7.2±0.3	–	–
Hippocampus	" "	5.0±0.3	6.0±0.3	0.44±0.04	0.61±0.18
Caudate	" "	5.1±0.2	6.3±0.3	0.43±0.02	0.59±0.07
Thalamus	" "	5.4±0.4	6.1±0.3	–	–
Cerebral cortex	" "	4.8±0.2	5.3±0.2	0.42±0.04	0.59±0.01

[a] $p < 0.01$ in all cases of old vs. young.
[b] The data represent the mean ± S.D. of 3 separate experiments with 4-7 animals in each group. Determinations were carried out in duplicate for each animal separately.

The effect of changing the microviscosity of membranes on (^{3}H)-serotonin binding of homogenates from young and old mice is shown in Figure 1. Control (untreated or vehicle-treated) samples from old mice are clearly more viscous and possess a higher capacity for serotonin-binding than membranes from young mice. An important point is that, as we have shown earlier, increasing the microviscosity of membranes from young mice by treatment with CHS increased the number of serotonin-binding sites up to a maximum of nearly six-fold as compared to the binding to control (untreated) membranes. In old (24-27 months) mice the increase in serotonin binding is much less, i.e. only 2.2-fold. The maximum number of serotonin-binding sites, that could be uncovered by the rigidifying treatment with CHS, is 83% higher in membranes prepared from the brains of young mice, as compared to those from old ones. These results are in agreement with the report by Shih and Young (19), of increased serotonin receptor binding, but reduced affinity, in synaptic membranes isolated from the brains of old men, as compared to those from young adults.

Similar experiments with (^{3}H)-D-ala-enkephalinamide binding are presented in Figure 2. Here, the increased microviscosity of membranes from old mice is accompanied by an increase in enkephalin-binding, as compared to young mice, though to a much lesser extent than serotonin.

The common feature of all binding profiles is the increase in ligand-binding with increasing $\bar{\eta}$, to a maximum beyond which binding sharply

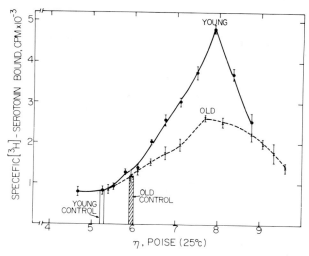

FIG. 1. Specific binding of (^{3}H)-serotonin to crude homogenates from forebrains of young (●——●) and old (X---X) C57Bℓ mice, as a function of membrane microviscosity ($\bar{\eta}$). Aliquots from a crude homogenate prepared from 5-10 forebrains were incubated with varying amounts of lipid suspensions (CHS - 0.4 mg/ml, egg-lecithin - 0.8 mg/ml, in 170 mM Tris-acetate buffer, pH 7.4, containing 3.5% polyvinyl-pyrrolidone (PVP), see Ref.14), for 2 hours at room temperature. Between 1-30 volumes of the lipid suspensions were incubated with one volume of membrane suspension (100 mg/ml). Control samples were incubated with the lipid vehicle alone. All samples were thoroughly washed after the lipid treatments and assayed simultaneously for membrane fluidity by fluorescence depolarization, using 1,3,5-diphenyl-hexatriene (DPH) as a probe, and for serotonin-binding (9). All binding assays were done in triplicates, together with triplicates containing also 2.5 µM (final concentration) unlabeled serotonin to correct for non-specific binding. All fluidity measurements were done in duplicates, which varied between them by less than 2%. Each point represents the mean ± S.D., from at least two experiments.

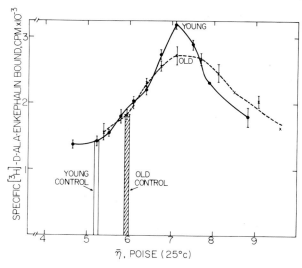

FIG. 2. Specific binding of (^{3}H)-D-ala-enkephalinamide to crude homogenates from forebrains of young (●——●) and old (X---X) C57Bℓ mice, as a function of membrane microviscosity ($\bar{\eta}$). Experiments were done as in Fig.1. The binding assay was performed according to (9,17). Each point represents the mean ± S.D., from at least two experiments.

declines. This can be due to the increasing exposure of the receptors out of the plane of the membrane, with increasing microviscosity until a critical point is reached, beyond which the receptors are shed into the surrounding medium (8). For the receptors we have examined, this critical point is at the same absolute value of membrane microviscosity in both young and old mice. This suggests that membrane-bound proteins occupy an equilibrium position, determined to a large extent by the fluidity of the lipid region adjacent to it (8,9).

An increase in the microviscosity of synaptic membranes could result in one or more of the following possibilities: (a) increased ligand binding; (b) decreased affinity for agonists; (c) decreased lateral encounters with adenylate-cyclase; (d) changes in ion (potassium, etc.) permeability; (e) long-term changes in electrical activity; (f) increased vulnerability to degradation by proteases; or (g) a greater potential for being "shed". The two latter possibilities will, in the long run, cause a reduction in the number of receptors. Obviously, any combination of these possibilities will result in a loss of function. The increase in membrane microviscosity with age may be due to the gradual accumulation of cholesterol with time, or to a compensatory process for loss of function. This might, in fact, be the cause of the reported decrease in the levels of several neurotransmitters (5) and of their synthesizing enzymes (24) with age.

It is not yet clear whether the reduction in the potential binding capacity in membranes of old mice as compared to young ones is the result of a reduced rate of receptor protein synthesis, or from an increased rate of degradation. What is clear, however, is that the synaptic membranes of aged mice contain a lower capacity for versatility, i.e. for receptor modulation. This is in accord with the results of Greenberg and Weiss (6,7), who report of an impairment in the ability of aged rats to increase β-adrenergic receptors of brain, in response to decreased adrenergic input.

Our results may be of importance in understanding the process of aging of the central nervous system. Furthermore, they suggest a method for pharmacological intervention. Rehabilitation of the aging nervous system, in an animal model by reducing excess membrane lipid viscosity with an active lipid fraction, is now being studied in our laboratory.

REFERENCES

1. Bennett, J.P., Jr., and Snyder, S.H. (1976): Mol.Pharmacol., 12:373.

2. Birnbaum, L.S., and Baird, M.B. (1978): Exp.Gerontol., 13:299.

3. Chin, J.H., and Goldstein, D.B. (1977): Science, 196:684.

4. Feinberg, I. (1976): In: Neurobiology of Aging, edited by R.D. Terry, and S. Gershon, Raven Press, New York.

5. Finch, C.E. (1973): Brain Res., 52:261.

6. Greenberg, L.H., and Weiss, B. (1978): Science, 201:61.

7. Greenberg, L.H., and Weiss, B. (1979): J.Pharmacol.Exp.Ther., 211:309.

8. Heron, D.S., Shinitzky, M., Hershkowitz, M., and Samuel, D. (1980): Proc.Natl.Acad.Sci.USA,

9. Heron, D., Israeli, M., Hershkowitz, M., Samuel, D., and Shinitzky, M. (1981): Eur.J.Pharmacol., 72:361-364.

10. Heron, D.S., Hershkowitz, M., Shinitzky, M., and Samuel, D. (1980): In: Neurotransmitters and Their Receptors, edited by U.Z. Littauer et al., p.125, John Wiley & Sons, Ltd.

11. Heron, D.S., Shinitzky, M., Hershkowitz, M., Israeli, M., and Samuel, D. (1981): Molec.Pharmacol. (in press).

12. Hershkowitz, M., Heron, D., Samuel, D., and Shinitzky, M. (1981): Progress in Brain Research, Vol.10 (in press).

13. Hosein, E.A., Lapalme, M., and Vadas, E.B. (1977): Biochem.Biophys. Res.Commun., 78:194.

14. Luly, P., and Shinitzky, M. (1979): Biochemistry, 18:445.

15. Merrill, E.G., and Wall, P.D. (1978): In: Neuronal Plasticity, edited by C.W. Cotman, p.97, Raven Press, New York.

16. Nagy, I.Zs. (1979): Mech.Aging & Development, 9:237.

17. Pasternak, G.W., Wilson, H.A., and Snyder, S.H. (1975): Mol.Pharmacol., 11:478.

18. Rouser, G., and Yamamoto, Y. (1968): Lipids, 3:284.

19. Shih, J.C., and Young, H. (1978): Life Sci., 23:1441.

20. Shinitzky, M., and Barenholz, Y. (1978): Biochim.Biophys.Acta, 515:367.

21. Shinitzky, M., Skornick, Y., and Haran-Ghera, N. (1979): Proc.Natl. Acad. Sci.USA, 76:5313.

22. Sinensky, M. (1974): Proc.Natl.Acad.Sci.USA, 71:522.

23. Sporn, J.R., Harden, T.K., Wolfe, B.B., and Molineff, P.B. (1976): Science, 194:624.

24. Vernadakis, A. (1973): In: Neurobiological Aspects of Maturation and Aging: Progress in Brain Research, edited by D.H. Ford, Vol.40, pp.341-354, Elsevier, Amsterdam.

The Aging Brain: Cellular and Molecular Mechanisms of Aging in the Nervous System, edited by E. Giacobini et al., Raven Press, New York © 1982.

Ten-Nanometer Filament Proteins in Neural Development and Aging

Amico Bignami and Doris Dahl

West Roxbury Veterans Administration Medical Center, Boston, Massachusetts 02132 and Department of Neuropathology, Harvard Medical School, Boston, Massachusetts 02115

Ten-nanometer filaments are present in a variety of vertebrate cells. They are usually called intermediate-sized filaments (IFs) because their diameter is in between that of microtubules and actin microfilaments, the other two major components of the cytoskeleton. In the nervous system, IFs are abundant in all myelinated axons, certain non-myelinated axons and axonal terminals (e.g. basket axons and their terminals forming the baskets surrounding Purkinje cells in the cerebellar cortex), certain large neuronal perikarya (e.g. motor neurons in spinal cord and sensory neurons in posterior root ganglia), in fibrous astroglia throughout the brain and spinal cord, and in Schwann cell processes surrounding non-myelinated axons in peripheral nerve. It is only in recent years that major advances have been made concerning the biochemistry of IFs. Although IFs in different cell types are morphologically similar, the proteins which form the filaments are relatively cell-specific with one notable exception, i.e. the major IF protein in fibroblasts.

Cell-specific IF proteins are: i, α-keratin in stratified squamous epithelium (39, 41); ii, desmin (25) or skeletin (37) in muscle; iii, GFA protein in astrocytes (1, 17, 32); and iv, a triplet of polypeptides at approximately 200K, 150K and 70K daltons in neurons (23, 33). As to neurofilaments and glial filaments, it is interesting to note that their cell-specificity had been established well before anything was known concerning their polypeptide composition. Two major neurohistological stains developed at the turn of the century, that is Weigert's stain for astroglia and Cajal's silver nitrate impregnation for neurons are based on the selective decoration of glial and neurofilaments, respectively. The idea underlying the development of these methods was that glial fibrils and neurofibrils are made of specific substances (see for example Weigert, 1895) (47). Neurofibrils and glial fibrils correspond to neurofilaments and glial filaments at the electron microscopic level.

Vimentin (19) or decamin (40) is the non-specific IF protein originally reported as the major IF protein of fibroblasts (19). Vimentin was subsequently localized in a variety of cells maintained in tissue culture including epithelium (27), astroglia (8, 28) and neuroblastoma (46). Later in this presentation, we will report on some remarkable transitions from non-specific to specific IF proteins during neural development in vivo.

IF PROTEINS IN DEVELOPMENT

Neuroglia

Recent findings in this laboratory (13, 14) indicate that glial cells undergo a remarkable IF transition during development, a finding that may be relevant to the study of genome-cytoskeletal interactions (7) and that may provide some clues towards the understanding of morphogenesis at the molecular level. In accordance with other investigators, we found that astrocytes in rat brain not only contain their cell-specific IF protein, i.e. GFA, but also vimentin (12, 35, 49). However, fewer astrocytic progresses stained with anti-vimentin, as compared to anti-GFA. Glial fibers maintaining in adult brain the radial arrangement characteristic of immature glia (34), i.e. Bergmann glia of cerebellum and tanycytes of hypothalamus were exceptions in this respect, that is they stained equally well with anti-GFA and anti-vimentin antisera. Conversely, in newborn rat brain, where only few GFA positive astrocytes are present (2, 3), glioblasts in the non-myelinated white matter, in the periventricular germinal zone and spanning the entire thickness of the cerebral hemispheres (radial glia) were intensely vimentin positive. (Similar findings concerning the immunohistological localization of vimentin in immature glia have been reported in another laboratory) (35). Since quantitation by immunostaining is notoriously difficult, we tried a different approach to substantiate these findings. Extraction with triton, a non-ionic detergent, is a common procedure to prepare IF-enriched fractions from cells maintained in culture (38). The triton-insoluble fraction is called a cytoskeletal preparation. Using this procedure we were able to show that vimentin is a major cytoskeletal component in newborn rat brain and that the same is true for GFA protein in adult brain (13). As to the time of the transition, in rat brain it occurs during the second and third week of postnatal development, that is at the time of rapid myelination (14). This was not an unexpected finding since we previously reported that in white matter tracts glioblasts differentiate into GFA positive interfascicular astrocytes at the time of myelination (2). Considering that the majority of fibrous astrocytes reside in white matter, it was thus not surprising that in whole brain cytoskeletal preparations the vimentin-GFA transition became apparent during this period.

A vimentin-neurofilament transition in embryonal development?
We previously demonstrated that neurofilament proteins are expressed relatively late in embryonal development, that is on day 3 in the chicken (4) and on day 12 in the rat (31). In accordance with previous findings obtained with the silver neurofibrillary staining (43), we found that motor neurons are among the first to differentiate according to this criterion (sensory neurons in the posterior root ganglia differentiate one day later in both chicken and rat). With vimentin antisera, the findings were completely different from what we expected (15). We thought that the embryos would start to express vimentin rather early in development. In fact, rat embryos remained completely negative up to day 11. The trophoblast was a notable exception since it was already intensely stained with vimentin antisera in the younger embryos we examined, that is on day 9, counting the day of mating as day 0. Vimentin

positive cells were first observed on day 11 but even at this stage no immunofluorescence was found in the neural tube. On day 12, concomitant with the sudden appearance of neurofilament staining in the anterolateral regions of the neural tube up to the diencephalic fissure and in the anterior roots emerging from these regions, vimentin positive fibers made their appearance throughout the CNS including the cerebral vesicles. An unexpected finding was that in regions of the CNS containing neurofilament-positive material, the staining patterns obtained with the 2 antisera (anti-neurofilament and anti-vimentin) were similar. This apparent localization of both vimentin and neurofilament proteins in neurons was observed only for a limited period. As of day 15, neurofilament and vimentin antisera selectively decorated neurons and glia, respectively. These findings were confirmed by experiments conducted in vitro (Bignami, Raju and Dahl, in preparation). Neurons dissociated from 13 and 14 day embryos expressed both neurofilament and vimentin in monolayer culture as indicated by double labeling experiments. On day 15 and later, vimentin was no more demonstrated in neurofilament positive cells.

IF PROTEINS IN AGING

Neuroglia

A marked increase in fibrous astrocytes is a constant feature in the senile brain (45). In the cerebral cortex, the increase in glial fibers is first seen in the molecular layer (marginal gliosis of Chaslin) but as senile atrophy becomes more severe, it extends to involve the remaining cortical layers where glial fibers are scarce under normal conditions. A recent report on the changing properties of the C-6 glioma cell line as a function of passage in culture (29) may provide a clue as to the possible significance of the fibrous transformation of neuroglia in aging (see also in this volume: A. Vernadakis, Glial cells in the central nervous system in aging). It was found that with successive passages the oligodendrocytic properties of C-6 cells progressively decreased and the astrocytic properties concomitantly increased, a phenomenon described with the term of "transdifferentiation". It would be interesting to know if a similar phenomenon occurs in the senile brain. Satellite glia surrounding neurons in the cerebral cortex do not contain filaments and they are traditionally interpreted as oligodendrocytes although they do not form myelin. It is tempting to speculate that "transdifferentiation" of these cells into astrocytes may play a role in the pathogenesis of senile dementia.

Neurons

The neurofibrillary tangle is a distinctive histological change of the neuronal perikaryon occurring in several neurological conditions of the advanced age and, to a lesser extent, in "normal" aging of the brain (5). In Alzheimer's disease, the most frequent form of senile dementia, the tangles are formed by bundles of filaments approximately 20 nm in diameter and characterized by constrictions about 10 nm in diameter at 80 nm intervals (24, 44). These have been interpreted as paired filaments coiled as double helixes making a full turn every 160 nm (24); alternatively, as constricted microtubules, for which the term twisted tubules was proposed (44).

The chemical composition of the Alzheimer's neurofibrillary tangle still remains to be elucidated (18, 22) (see also in this volume K. Iqbal, Neuronal fibrillary changes in aging). In collaboration with Pierluigi Gambetti (Case Western Reserve University) and Dennis J. Selkoe (Harvard Medical School and McLean Hospital) we have tried to characterize the tangles by immunohistochemical methods (16, 20). Antisera to GFA protein, vimentin and desmin failed to decorate the tangles, and the same was true for a keratin antiserum prepared in our laboratory. Neurofilament antisera raised to degraded antigen isolated from urea extracts of chicken brain by hydroxyapatite chromatography heavily stained the tangles. The antisera reacted with the 70K and 150K neurofilament polypeptides by immunoaffinity chromatography (10) and with all 3 components of the neurofilament triplet (70K, 150K and 200K) as indicated by immunostaining of brain filament preparations resolved on SDS-PAGE (16, 20). (By immunoaffinity chromatography the 200K polypeptide was absorbed to the column but eluted under less than drastic conditions. It was thus not possible to rule out non-specific absorption). Conversely, antisera to gel purified 150K neurofilament protein failed to decorate the tangles or did so very weakly, as previously reported for neurofibrillary tangles experimentally induced by aluminum or mitotic spindle inhibitors (9, 11). It should be noted, however, that failure to demonstrate the 150K neurofilament protein in the tangles does not necessarily indicate an abnormality in polypeptide composition compared to normal neurofilaments. It has been our experience that neuronal perikarya displaying a typical neurofibrillary pattern with the anti-chicken brain neurofilament antisera failed to react with anti-150K or did so very weakly while adjacent nerve fibers appeared well stained. We thus suggested that 150K is mainly a component of the axonal neurofilament (11). Recent findings indicating that isolated motor neuron perikarya mainly synthetize the 70K neurofilament component appear consistent with this hypothesis.

Gambetti et al. have recently studied the reactivity with anti-chicken brain neurofilament antisera of neurofibrillary tangles occurring in other neurological conditions, that is, post-encephalitic parkinsonism, and progressive supranuclear palsy (21). Two cases of Pick disease were also investigated (in this form of presenile dementia the intraneuronal argyrophilic material, called a Pick body, is globular in shape rather than forming a tangle). In post-encephalitic parkinsonism, the tangles are formed by filaments morphologically identical to those observed in Alzheimer's disease (48) while in Pick disease the filaments are similar to IFs in normal neurons (6). As to progressive supranuclear palsy, the tangles are made of 150 Å filaments which have been interpreted as abnormal IFs or as microtubules (30, 42). It was found that all lesions stained with the anti-chicken brain neurofilament antisera by the PAP procedure.

In conclusion, these data suggest that the degradation of neurofilament proteins may be deranged in a number of pathological conditions of the advanced age, resulting in the accumulation of filaments within neurons. As to the correlation between clinical symptoms and the distribution of the neurofibrillary changes, it may be noted that the hippocampus is most severely affected in Alzheimer's dementia and the brain stem in progressive supranuclear palsy. Recent findings by Selkoe and his collaborators (36) may provide a clue as to the nature of the biochemical change responsible for the formation of the tangles. It was found that in Alzheimer's disease the tangles remain insoluble after exposure to sodium dodecylsulfate, β-mercaptoethanol, urea and guanidine, thus suggesting that the filaments in the tangle are crosslinked by non-disulfide covalent bonds into a rigid intracellular polymer. It was also noted by Selkoe et al. that covalently crosslinked protein polymers have been described in the lens during senile cataract formation and in terminally differentiated skin keratinocytes.

REFERENCES

1. Bignami, A., Eng, L.F., Dahl, D., and Uyeda, C.T. (1972): Brain Res., 43:429-435.

2. Bignami, A., and Dahl, D. (1973): Brain Res., 49:393-402.

3. Bignami, A., and Dahl, D. (1974): J. Comp. Neurol., 153:27-38.

4. Bignami, A., Dahl, D., and Seiler, M.W. (1980): Develop. Neurosci., 3:151-161.

5. Blackwood, W., and Corsellis, J.A.N. (1976): Greenfield's Neuropathology. Arnold, London.

6. Brion, S., and Mikol, J. (1971): Revue Neurologique, 125:273-286.

7. Cervera, M., Dreyfuss, G., and Penman, S. (1981): Cell, 23:113-120.

8. Chiu, F-C., Norton, W.T., and Fields, K.L. (1981): J. Neurochem., 37:147-155.

9. Dahl, D., Bignami, A., Bich, N.T., and Chi, N.H. (1980): Acta Neuropathol., 51:165-168.

10. Dahl, D. (1981): Biochim. Biophys. Acta, 668:299-306.

11. Dahl, D., Bignami, A., Bich, N.T., and Chi, N.H. (1981): J. Comp. Neurol., 195:659-666.

12. Dahl, D., Crosby, C.J., and Bignami, A. (1981): Exp. Neurol. 71: 421-430.

13. Dahl, D., Rueger, D.C., Bignami, A., Weber, K., and Osborn, M. (1981): Eur. J. Cell Biol., 24:191-196.

14. Dahl, D. The vimentin-GFA protein transition in rat neuroglia cytoskeleton occurs at the time of myelination. Submitted.

15. Dahl, D., and Bignami, A. Cytoskeletal transitions in neural development. Submitted.

16. Dahl, D., Selkoe, D.J., Pero, R.T., and Bignami, A. Immunostaining of neurofibrillary tangles in Alzheimer's senile dementia with a neurofilament antiserum. Submitted.

17. Eng, L.F., Vanderhaeghen, J.J., Bignami, A., and Gerstl, B. (1971): Brain Res., 28:351-354.

18. Eng, L.F., Forno, L.S., Bigbee, J.W., and Forno, K.I. (1980): In: Aging of the Brain and Dementia, edited by L. Amaducci, A.N. Davison, and P. Antuono, pp. 49-54. Raven Press, New York.

19. Franke, W.W., Schmid, E., Osborn, M., and Weber, K. (1978): Proc. Natl. Acad. Sci. USA, 75:5034-5038.

20. Gambetti, P., Velasco, M.E., Dahl, D., Bignami, A., Roessmann, U., and Sindely, S.D. (1980): In: Aging of the Brain and Dementia, edited by L. Amaducci, A.N. Davison, and P. Antuono, pp. 55-63. Raven Press, New York.

21. Gambetti, P., Ghetti, B., Hirano, A., and Dahl, D. Neurofibrillary changes in human brain. Submitted.

22. Grundke-Iqbal, J., Johnson, A., Wisniewski, H.M., Terry, R.D., and Iqbal, K. (1979): Lancet, 1:578-579.

23. Hoffman, P.N., and Lasek, R.J. (1975): J. Cell Biol., 66:351-366.

24. Kidd, M. (1963): Nature, 197:192-193.

25. Lazarides, E., and Hubbard, B.D. (1976): Proc. Natl. Acad. Sci. USA, 73:4344-4348.

26. Nakayama, T. (1981): J. Neurochem., 36:1398-1405.

27. Osborn, M., Franke, W.W., and Weber, K. (1980): Exp. Cell Res., 125:37-46.

28. Paetau, A., Virtanen, I., Stenman, S., Kurki, P., Linder, E., Vaheri, A., Westermark, B., Dahl, D., and Haltia, M. (1979): Acta Neuropathol. (Berl.), 47:71-74.

29. Parker, K.K., Norenberg, M.D., and Vernadakis, A. (1980): Science, 208:179-182.

30. Powell, H.C., London, C.W., and Lampert, P. (1974): J. Neuropathol. Exp. Neurol., 33:98-106.

31. Raju, T., Bignami, A., and Dahl, D. (1981): Dev. Biol., 85:344-351.

32. Rueger, D.C., Huston, J.S., Dahl, D., and Bignami, A. (1979): J. Mol. Biol., 135:53-68.

33. Schlaepfer, W.W., and Freeman, L.A. (1978): J. Cell Biol., 78: 653-662.

34. Schmechel, D.E., and Rakic, P. (1979): Anat. Embryol., 156:115-152.

35. Schnitzer, J., Franke, W.W., and Schachner, M. (1981): J. Cell Biol. 90:435-446.

36. Selkoe, D.J., Ihara, Y., and Salazar, F.J. Alzheimer's disease: partial purification of paired helical filaments and demonstration of insolubility in SDS, urea and guanidine. Submitted.

37. Small, J.V., and Sobieszek, A. (1977): J. Cell Sci. 23:243-268.

38. Starger, J.M., Brown, W.E., Goldman, A.E., and Goldman, R.D. (1978): J. Cell Biol., 78:93-109.

39. Steinert, P.M. (1978): J. Mol. Biol., 123:49-70.

40. Steinert, P.M., Idler, W.W., Cabral, F., Gottesman, M.M., and Goldman, R.D. (1981): Proc. Natl. Acad. Sci. USA., 78:3692-3696.

41. Sun, T-T., and Green, H. (1978): J. Biol. Chem., 253:2053-2060.

42. Tellez-Nagel, I., and Wisniewski, H.M. (1973): Arch. Neurol., 29:324-327.

43. Tello, J.F. (1923): Trav. Lab. Rech. Biol. (Madrid), 21:1-93.

44. Terry, R.D. (1963): J. Neuropathol. Exp. Neurol., 22:629-642.

45. Timiras, P.S., and Bignami, A. (1976): In: Special Review of Experimental Aging Research. Progress in Biology, edited by M.F. Elias, B.E. Eleftheriou, and P.K. Elias, pp. 352-378. Ear, Inc., Bar Harbour.

46. Virtanen, I., Lehto, V.-P., Lehtonen, E., Vartio, T., Stenman, S., Kurki, P., Wager, O., Small, J.V., Dahl, D., and Bradley, R.A. J. Cell. Sci, in press.

47. Weigert, C. (1895): Moritz Diesterweg, Frankfurt a.M.

48. Wiśniewski, H.M., Terry, R.D., and Hirano, A. (1970): J. Neuropath. Exp. Neurol., 29:163-176.

49. Yen, S.-H., and Fields, K.L. (1981): J. Cell Biol., 88:115-126.

The Aging Brain: Cellular and Molecular Mechanisms of Aging in the Nervous System, edited by E. Giacobini et al., Raven Press, New York © 1982.

Biochemical and Behavioral Parallels in Aging and Hypoxia

Gary E. Gibson and Christine Peterson

Department of Neurology, Cornell University Medical College, Burke Rehabilitation Center, White Plains, New York 10605

Aging leads to cognitive changes that resemble those which occur in metabolic encephalopathies, a group of disorders in which mental function declines secondarily to systemic changes (72). Hypoxia (i.e. low oxygen), hypoglycemia, heavy metal intoxication, some inborn errors of metabolism and certain nutritional deficiencies may all be regarded as metabolic encephalopathies. Since these diseases have many similar clinical symptoms, despite diverse etiologies, they may share a common molecular basis. Thus, an understanding of one metabolic encephalopathy may lead to an understanding of the others as well. With this in mind, we have studied the molecular changes that occur during hypoxia and used these results as a guide to examine aging. We found many parallels and distinctions between aging and hypoxia. In addition, we examined the effects of hypoxia on the aged brain to see if it is more vulnerable to metabolic insults than the younger mature brain.

McFarland (54) suggested that "the sensory and mental impairment which occurs in both normal and clinical subjects under experimental conditions

TABLE 1. <u>Similarity in the behavioral changes due to hypoxia and aging</u>

Behavorial variable	Effect	Age	Level of hypoxia Height (ft.)	$\% O_2$	References
Dark adaptation	delayed	40	11,500	13%	3
		50	15,400	12%	58
		60	17,500	10%	57
Flicker frequency	threshold decreased				55 77
Visual ability with glare	decreased	80			55
Hearing: low frequency high frequency	none decreased	50	17,500	10%	53
Paired associations	decreased	55	10,000	15%	53

107

of oxygen deprivation simulate very precisely the behavioral changes observed in the aging process". A delay in dark adaptation, a decreased ability to detect a flickering light and an inability to visualize an object in the presence of glare showed that light responses were the most sensitive to aging and hypoxia. Optical measurements suggest that these decreases are due to neural changes and not to pupil or lens alterations (TABLE 1). Delayed dark adaptation ($r=-0.89$) and diminshed critical flicker frequency ($r=-0.65$ to -0.80) correlated with aging. Other subjective measures which decrease with aging and hypoxia include attention, judgement, the ability to calculate, immediate memory and emotional stability (56).

The decline in mental function with mild hypoxia has been well documented for decades but its pathophysiological basis is still unknown. Many hypotheses have been postulated to explain this decline in cognitive function with low oxygen (TABLE 2). The most widely investigated explanation is that hypoxia produces an energy failure. However, in even severe hypoxic hypoxia ATP levels are maintained. A precise comparison of the various hypotheses is complicated because varying degrees and models of hypoxia have been used. Impaired neurotransmitter function is an attractive mechanism to explain the effects of hypoxia because we understand how disruptions in their metabolism can alter neural regulation (i.e. compared to disruption caused by elevated lactate). In addition, we also have some knowledge of how to pharmacologically manipulate neurotransmitter interactions.

TABLE 2. Hypotheses to explain the effects of hypoxia

Biochemical variable	Supporting or negating evidence	Reference
Energy failure	No change in ATP	39, 40, 80
Energy utilization	Decreased $\sim$P use	19
Lactate	Increased concentrations	66
Free radicals	Thio-disulfide status altered	14, 22
Redox state	Reduced in cytosol and mitochondria	26, 27, 79, 84
Cyclic nucleotides	Increased cyclic GMP Unchanged cyclic AMP	25, 28
K^+ efflux	Increased	64
Ca^{2+} metabolism	Decreased in stimulated smooth muscle	20
Fatty acids	Increased	25

A disruption in ACh metabolism may explain some of the cognitive deficits in hypoxia and other metabolic encephalopathies (TABLE 3). Quastel and his colleagues (51,52,53) demonstrated in the 1930's that glucose and oxygen were required for ACh synthesis in vitro. This appears to be more than just a general requirement for oxygen and glucose to maintain tissue viability. The closeness of the relation between ACh and oxidative metabolism became apparent when it was found that inhibition of carbohydrate oxidation caused a proportional decline in ACh formation even though less than 1% of the oxidized substrate was converted to ACh (31,45,46). These results suggested that alterations in glucose or oxygen availability may limit ACh metabolism <u>in vivo</u>. In 1943, Welsh observed that hypoxia and hypoglycemia decreased the concentration of ACh in rat brain. His studies suggested that alterations in ACh metabolism were important in the pathophysiology of hypoxia and hypoglycemia. However, the concentrations of ACh or other neurotransmitters may not accurately reflect functional changes in a particular neurotransmitter pathway. Turnover measurements monitor dynamic changes in neurotransmitter metabolism more accurately (7). Chemical hypoxia, hypoglycemia (29) and levels of hypoxic-hypoxia (29,37) that decrease mental function in man reduced ACh synthesis (FIG 1.), but did not alter its concentration in whole brain.

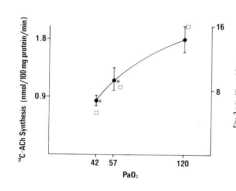

FIG 1. <u>In vivo</u> synthesis of whole brain ACh during mild hypoxic hypoxia.

Incorporation of $[^2H_4]$choline and $[U-^{14}C]$glucose into ACh was determined in whole rat brain after 15 min of 30% O_2 (PaO_2 = 120 mm Hg), 15% O_2 (PaO_2 = 57 mm Hg) or 10% O_2 (PaO_2 = 42 mm Hg; 29).

TABLE 3. <u>Evidence of a role for ACh in hypoxia.</u>

ACh Metabolism	System	References
Requires oxygen and glucose	Brain slices Ganglia	27, 51, 52, 73 43
Closely linked to oxidative metabolism	Brain slices	6, 31, 45, 46
Concentrations in hypoxia no change	Rat <u>in vivo</u>	8, 26, 27, 49
decreased	Rat <u>in vivo</u>	91
Synthesis during hypoxia decreased (NaNO$_2$-)	Rats/mice <u>in vivo</u>	26, 27 37
decreased (low O_2)	Rats/mice <u>in vivo</u>	29, 37
Anticholinergics drugs induce hypoxic-like symptoms	Man	18

Although hypoxia interrupts oxidative metabolism as shown by an accumulation in brain lactate concentrations, it increased glucose utilization as measured with $[U-^{14}C]$glucose (15% oxygen; 29) or 2-deoxyglucose (10% oxygen; 63).

The synthesis of non-cholinergic neurotransmitters are also altered by hypoxia. The rate limiting steps in norepinephrine and serotonin synthesis depend upon molecular oxygen and thus decline with hypoxia (TABLE 4). The percent reduction in their formation was not as large as ACh synthesis at the same level of hypoxia, but this does not necessarily reflect their physiological significance. However, when animals are stressed, the syntheses of the catecholamines, no longer depends upon oxygen; thus, the physiological importance of the hypoxic-induced decrease is unclear (5,12). The behavioral relevance of the increase in adenosine concentration with hypoxia has not been established (92).

TABLE 4. Metabolism of non-cholinergic neurotransmitters in hypoxia.

Neurotransmitter	% O_2	Percent Change in metabolism	Reference
Catecholamine	10%	-20 (synthesis)	11
Serotonin	10%	-26 (synthesis)	11
Alanine, aspartate glutamate, GABA	5%	-55 (synthesis)	93
Adenosine	10%	+13 (levels)	92

TABLE 5. Neurotransmitter synthesis from $[U-^{14}C]$glucose in mild anemic hypoxia and hypoxic hypoxia.

	Anemic Hypoxia % Methemoglobin		Hypoxic Hypoxia % O_2	
	12	31	15	10
ACh	65 ± 9[a]	42 ± 5[a]	69 ± 3[a]	54 ± 6[a]
Alanine	82 ± 10	66 ± 13[a]	62 ± 11	48 ± 9[a]
Aspartate	88 ± 12	51 ± 10[a]	70 ± 4[a]	49 ± 10[a]
GABA	77 ± 14	38 ± 4[a]	82 ± 8	58 ± 15[a]
Glutamine	70 ± 8[a]	41 ± 7[a]	119 ± 8	57 ± 2[a]
Glutamate	76 ± 11[a]	49 ± 7[a]	89 ± 7	66 ± 11[a]
Serine	63 ± 10[a]	63 ± 16[a]	44 ± 3[a]	42 ± 9[a]

Anemic hypoxia was produced by $NaNO_2$ injection. Hypoxic hypoxia was induced by decreasing oxygen in the gas mixture for 15 min. ACh and amino acid values are mean percent $\pm$ S.E.M. of non-hypoxic control d.p.m./nmol. [a]Denotes value differs (P<0.05) from non-hypoxic control.

Hypoxia also reduced the synthesis of the other glucose derived neuro transmitters (i.e. the amino acids: alanine, aspartate, glutamine, glutamate, γ-aminobutyrate and serine). Previous studies demonstrated a decrease in their synthesis in severe hypoxia (i.e. 5% oxygen; TABLE 4; 93). In mild anemic hypoxia (i.e. $NaNO_2$ injections) or hypoxic-hypoxia (15% and 10% oxygen) their synthesis declined in parallel with the ACh formation (TABLE 5). Studies on the synthesis of all the glucose derived neurotransmitters with varying degrees of chemical hypoxia demonstrated that the curvilinear correlation between the decline in the synthesis of ACh and the amino acids was greater than 0.97. Thus, the cholinergic system is not the only neurotransmitter system that is altered by hypoxia.

In spite of this lack of selectivity, the decline in ACh synthesis appears to be physiologically important. Studies with isolated superior cervical ganglia show that cholinergic transmission is blocked by anoxia long before there are decreases in axonal conduction (17) or concentrations of ATP (40). The similarity between the memory impairment with anticholinergic drugs (e.g. scopolamine; 18) and hypoxia (56) suggests that the hypoxic induced deficits in cognitive function may be due to impaired ACh metabolism. Furthermore, pretreatment with the acetylcholinesterase inhibitor, physostigmine, prolonged the time until siezures and death in hypoxic (76) and anemic hypoxic (26) animals. These latter studies employed severe degrees of hypoxia and crude behavioral tests. Thus, the behavioral importance of the cholinergic system during mild hypoxia was re-examined with a tight rope test, a sensitive behavioral indicator that can detect early changes in the metabolic encephalopathies (1). The tight rope test measures a mouse's ability to traverse an elevated taut string. Performance decreased linearly with increasing levels of hypoxia and brain lactate concentration (FIG. 2) and has proven to be a simple reproducible behavioral test that is sensitive to metabolic insults.

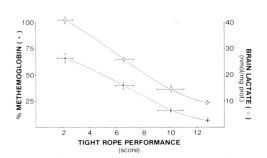

FIG 2. **Tight rope test performance during anemic hypoxia.**

Mice were injected with various concentrations of $NaNO_2$ which converts hemoglobin to methemoglobin, and 30 min later they were either tight rope tested or microwaved for brain lactate determinations.

The decline in tight rope performance during hypoxia can be manipulated with cholinergic drugs (FIG 3.). Performance improved by pretreatment with the acetylcholinesterase inhibitor physostigmine, which acts centrally and peripherally, but not by neostigmine, which acts primarily in the periphery. Both a muscarinic and nicotinic component appears to be important in this hypoxic-induced deficit. The beneficial effects of physostigmine was blocked by pretreatment with the muscarinic blocker atropine or the nicotinic antagonist mecamylamine. Injection of either nicotine or the muscarinic agonist, arecoline, significantly improved tight rope test scores by hypoxic mice. These interactions (32) are more complicated than described here, but they lead to two major conclusions: 1. The deficit in cholinergic function during hypoxia is behaviorally important 2. The decline in performance is not exclusively a cholinergic dysfunction since cholinergic therapies could not totally overcome the deficits.

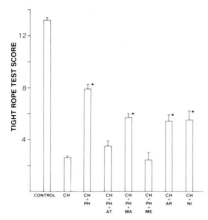

FIG 3. **Cholinergic treatment of the hypoxic-induced decline in tight rope test performance.**

Chemically hypoxic (CH) mice (150 mg/kg of $NaNO_2$) were pretreated with physostigmine (PH), PH + atropine (AT), PH + mecamylamine (ME), nicotine (NI), or arecoline (AR) (32)

The precise biochemical linkage between ACh synthesis and oxidative metabolism is unknown.   Hypotheses include metabolic compartmentation (30), a coupling with the transmitochondrial redox potential (17,26) and a reduction in the release of ACh (33), but they are not necessarily exclusive.   The latter postulate is based upon the observation that during hypoxia in vivo the synthesis of ACh declined without a corresponding reduction in its concentration.   This hypothesis was directly tested in vitro by varying oxygen tensions during a Ca^{2+}-dependent K^+-stimulated release incubation with brain slices or synaptosomes (33,34; FIG 4).

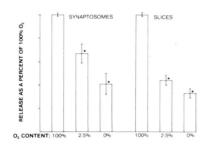

FIG 4. **Hypoxia and the Ca^{2+}-dependent-K^+-stimulated release ACh.**

Release of ACh was measured after prelabelling the ACh in brain slices or synaptosomes with $[U-^{14}C]$glucose in low K^+ (5 mM) buffer. They were then incubated with high K^+ (31 mM) to measure the release of ACh under various oxygen tensions.

Only the K^+-stimulated-Ca^{2+}-dependent release of ACh was decreased by low oxygen.   The low K^+ release and high K^+ release without Ca^{2+} were unaffected by low oxygen.   This decline in release during hypoxia could be partially reversed by agents that stimulate Ca^{2+} influx into nerve terminals (e.g. the aminopyridines; FIG 5).   This same concentration of 4-aminopyridine improved tight rope test performance in hypoxic mice from 2.3 to 7.3 (32), which suggests that the decline in the Ca^{2+}-dependent release of ACh during hypoxia is behaviorally important.
    Since hypoxia and aging produce similar behavioral and cognitive deficits, we studied these same variables in aged mice.   Several studies

suggest that aging alters oxidative metabolism (TABLE 6). The interpretation of <u>in vivo</u> studies are complicated by age-related diseases, but

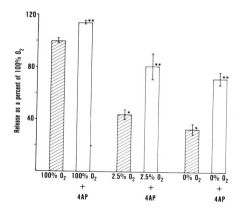

FIG 5. Promotion of Ca^{2+}-entry by
4-aminopyridine and the
hypoxic-induced decline in
the release of ACh.

4-Aminopyridine (10 $\mu\underline{M}$) was added
to the hypoxic release incubation
after the brain slices were preincubated with [U-^{14}C]glucose to
label the releasable ^{14}C-ACh
(33,34).

TABLE 6. <u>Changes in brain oxidative metabolism with age</u>

Measures of Oxidative Metabolism	Species	Effect of Aging	References
In vivo			
glucose utilization	man	decreased	7
~P utilization	mouse	striatum (-52%)	21
	mouse	cerebellum (-28%)	50
2-deoxyglucose	rat	decreased (<30%)	48, 82
Slices			
O_2 consumption	dogs	decreased	41
	rat	cortex (-13%)	70
		hippocampus(-20%)	
	mice	decreased (-21%)	68
CO_2 production			
glucose	man	unchanged	81
	mice	decreased (-28%)	68
	rat	decreased (-40%)	69
3-hydroxybutyrate	rat	decreased (-40%)	69
Homogenates			
O_2 consumption	rat	decreased (-38%)	74
Mitochondria			
CO_2 production			
pyruvate	rat	nonsynaptic(-34%)	15
		synaptic (-18%)	
3-hydroxybutyrate	rat	nonsynaptic no change	15
		synaptic (-48%)	

carefully controlled studies in man demonstrated that aging decreased the
cerebral metabolic rate for glucose but not oxygen (9). Recent studies
with rats found that senescence reduced 2-deoxyglucose utilization, but

many of these age related changes occurred by middle age and were restricted to a few brain nuclei (e.g. striatum, pons, inferior colliculus and inferior olivary nucleus; 48,82). High energy phosphate utilization in the striatum (21) and in the cerebellum (50) declined with aging. Oxidative metabolism also diminished with aging *in vitro*, where the cardiovascular factors that complicate *in vivo* studies can be minimized. Brain slices from aged animals consumed less oxygen (41) and produced less CO_2 from glucose or ketones bodies than those from young animals (16). Oxidative metabolism also decreased with senescence in cell free systems such as homogenates (74) or mitochondria (69). We examined whole brain glucose utilization *in vivo* in two strains (C57BL and BALB/c) of aged mice (3, 10 and 30 month) of age (TABLE 7). Although glucose utilization did not decrease with aging in either strain, carbohydrate metabolism was altered since brain lactate concentrations increased. These results with aging paralleled the effects of mild hypoxia on lactate production and whole brain glucose utilization as measured with [U-^{14}C]glucose (24) or 2-deoxyglucose (63).

TABLE 7. Brain glucose utilization and lactate concentration

	Age (Months)		
	3	10	30
Glucose Utilization (nmole/mg protein/min)			
BALB/c	7.35 ± 0.52	8.26 ± 0.57	8.27 ± 1.04
C57BL	7.25 ± 0.90	6.86 ± 0.69	8.19 ± 0.05
Lactate (nmole/mg protein)			
BALB/c	9.38 ± 1.00	11.50 ± 1.82	13.93 ± 1.78*
C57BL	10.44 ± 0.95	11.94 ± 1.19	30.15 ± 5.47*

Glucose utilization was from [U-^{14}C]glucose (24). Values are means ± S.E.M. *Denotes value differs from 3 month old control (P<0.05).

Since impaired oxidative metabolism decreases ACh synthesis and aging diminishes the brain's oxidative capacity, a decrease in ACh synthesis with aging seemed plausible. Age related changes in the concentrations of ACh, choline acetyltransferase, acetylcholinesterase and cholinergic receptors have been reported (TABLE 8). These alterations are generally small (i.e. seldom more than 20%). Furthermore, changes in concentrations or enzyme activities do not necessarily reflect the dynamics of the cholinergic system. Small decreases in the high affinity choline uptake in the mammalian central nervous system (78), ACh synthesis by the superior cervical ganglia and heart atria (89), and ACh release at the neuromuscular junction (82) occurred with aging.

An omission in these studies was the *in vivo* synthesis of ACh in the aging central nervous system. ACh formation from isotopic precursors provides a sensitive indication of cholinergic activity (7). We measured whole brain ACh formation *in vivo* with [U-^{14}C]glucose to label the acetyl moiety and [^{2}H$_4$]choline to label the choline moiety of ACh (36). The injection of [U-^{14}C]glucose also allowed a simultaneous estimate of whole brain glucose utilization (TABLE 7). The incoporation of both isotopes into ACh decreased in 10 and 30 month old mice compared to 3 month old mice (TABLE 9).

TABLE 8. The mammalian cholinergic system during aging.

Cholinergic Marker	Effect of aging	References
Choline acetyltransferase activity	Decrease in caudate and cortex	60, 61
	Increase in ganglia	75
Acetylcholinesterase activity (humans, mice, rats)	Decreased	10, 23, 42, 41, 61, 65, 67, 89, 90
Muscarinic receptor binding	Decreased in hippocampus	47
Acetylcholine levels	No change	62, 88
High affinity choline uptake	Decreased	78
Acetylcholine release	Decreased	83
Acetylcholine synthesis ganglia	Decreased	81
human cortex	No change	23

TABLE 9. ACh rate of synthesis during senescence.

	Age (Months)		
	3	10	30
[U-^{14}C]Glucose (nmol/100 mg protein/min)			
C57BL	6.9 ± 0.4	3.5 ± 0.3	2.2 ± 0.3
BALB/c	5.3 ± 0.3	3.0 ± 0.3	1.8 ± 0.3
[^{2}H$_{4}$]Choline (nmol/100 mg protein/min)			
BALB/c	6.6 ± 0.9	3.3 ± 0.5	1.6 ± 0.4

Values are mean ± S.E.M. All age groups differ ($P < 0.05$).

Since the formation of ACh and the amino acids decreased in parallel during hypoxia, we their synthesis with senescence. Age-related changes in the amino acid neurotransmitters have not been examined as extensively as the cholinergic system. Glutamate decarboxylase activity (61) and amino acid levels declined with aging (85). Synthesis has been reported to be either unchanged (13) or decreased (87) depending upon which precursor was employed. We examined the incorporation of [U-^{14}C]glucose into the amino acid neurotransmitters in senescent mice. Significant

decreases were observed in the formation of glutamine and GABA (TABLE
10), although a general decline was observed in the others.

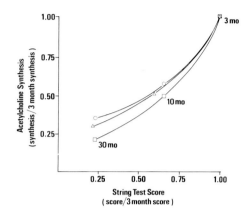

FIG 6. The relation of ACh
synthesis and tight rope
performance in aged mice.

Each age group varies signifcantly
from the others. Symbols represent
synthesis of ACh from [U-^{14}C]glu-
cose (Δ,C57BL; $\square$,BALB/c) and [^{2}H$_{4}$]-
choline (O,BALB/c).   Figure is
from Gibson et al. (36) with per-
mission of _Science_.

TABLE 10. Amino acid synthesis in senescent C57BL mice.

	Age (Months)		
	3 Month	10 Month	30 Month
Alanine	100 + 19	95˙ + 17	80 + 17
Aspartate	100 + 15	61 + 8*	77 + 15
GABA	100 + 13	102 + 10	54 + 10*
Glutamine	100 + 14	67 + 11	55 + 8*
Glutamate	100 + 13	90 + 12	69 + 13
Serine	100 + 17	61 + 11	88 + 16

Synthesis was determined from [U-^{14}C]glucose. Values
are mean percent ± S.E.M. of 3 month old mice. * Denotes
value differs ($p<0.05$) from 3 month old mice.

The biochemical mechanisms that underlie these in vivo changes remain
unclear. We used brain slices to examine oxidative metabolism and neurotransmitter release in these age related deficits.   During in vitro incubation with low K^{+}, senescence reduced oxidative metabolism (FIG 7.),
whether it was measured by ^{14}CO$_2$ production from [U-^{14}C]glucose (i.e.
overall glucose oxidation), [3,4-^{14}C]glucose or [1-^{14}C]pyruvate (i.e.
measures of flux though pyruvate dehydrogenase with low or high pyruvate
concentrations, respectively).   Similar decreases in carbohydrate
oxidation occurred when brain slices or synaptosomes from young animals
were incubated under low oxygen (FIG 4.; 45,46). However, brain slices
from aged animals (30 months old) responded more to K^{+}-stimulation, so

that the differences between oxidation by slices from young and old brains in high K^+ buffer was less than 10% (35). Thus, the magnitude of the decrease in oxidative metabolism with senescence in high or low K^+ buffer was not adequate to account for the decline in ACh synthesis in vivo.

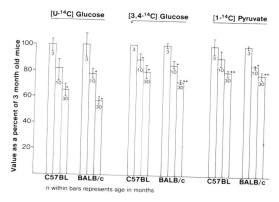

FIG 7.   **Oxidative metabolism with low K^+ buffer during aging.**

Brain slices were incubated with 5 mM-K^+ and CO_2 was collected from the indicated isotopes. *Denotes value differs from 3 month old mice ($p<0.05$). **Denotes value differs from 3 and 10 month old mice ($p<0.05$).

Although the synthesis of ACh in vivo declined with senescence, its concentrations did not change. Thus, by analogy with our hypoxia experiments, we examined the release of ACh by brain slices from aged mice (FIG 8.). The high-K^+-Ca^{2+}-dependent release declined by 10 months and decreased even further at 30 months. The non-Ca^{2+}-dependent release and the release with low K^+ were not altered by senescence.

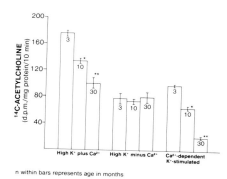

FIG 8.   **Decreases in the Ca^{2+}- dependent release of ACh with senescence.**

Brain slices were preincubated in low K^+ buffer with [U-^{14}C]glucose to label the ACh that was released by incubation with high K^+ (35)

The percent decrease in Ca^{2+}-dependent release with aging paralleled the decline in synthesis of ACh in vivo, however its physiological importance has not been demonstrated directly. Both the tight rope test performance and passive avoidance behavior as measured by Bartus (2; FIG 9.) decline in parallel with the decreases the in vitro release and in vivo synthesis of ACh.

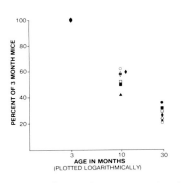

FIG 9.   Relation of ACh
          synthesis and
          release to behavioral
          changes with aging

○ *IN VITRO* ACh RELEASE Balb/c
● *IN VIVO* ACh SYNTHESIS Balb/c
□ *IN VITRO* ACh RELEASE C57Bl
■ *IN VIVO* ACh SYNTHESIS C57Bl
▲ TIGHT ROPE PERFORMANCE Balb/c
◊ TIGHT ROPE PERFORMANCE C57Bl
♦ PASSIVE AVOIDANCE LATENCY C57Bl

Few studies have examined the relative susceptibility of the aged brain to metabolic insults. Thus, the sensitivity of the aged brain to hypoxia was determined. Although the aged brain has a diminished response to spreading depression (84) it does not have an increased sensitivity to ischemic insults as reflected by increases in brain lactate (86). The response of senescent animals to other metabolic encephalopathies (i.e. hypoglycemia, hyperammonemia or nutritional deficits) has not been investigated. Chemical hypoxia decreased the synthesis of ACh in aged animals by about the same percent as the young mice. Since ACh synthesis was already reduced in the aged mice, the rate of sythesis in the hypoxic aged mouse was only 10% of that in a three month old non-hypoxic mouse (FIG. 10).

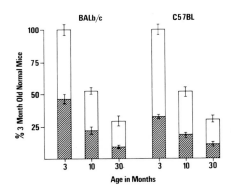

FIG 10.   ACh synthesis in normal
          and mildly hypoxic aged
          mice.

Mice of the indicated ages were made hypoxic by injection of $NaNO_2$ (75 mg/kg). ACh synthesis was determined from $[U-^{14}C]$glucose.

The synthesis of the amino acids during hypoxia was inhibited similarly in all three age groups, however, the residual synthesis was greater than that observed for ACh (TABLE 11). Metabolic compartmentation of these amino acids complicates the interpretation of this inhibition since it is difficult to know if we are examining the neurotransmitter pool of these amino acids.

TABLE 11. Amino Acid Synthesis During Anemic Hypoxia in
Senescent C57BL Mice

	Age(Months)		
	3 Month	10 Month	30 Month
Alanine	42 + 9	22 + 2	18 + 1
Aspartate	54 + 7	32 + 3	28 + 2
GABA	42 + 5	49 + 12	54 + 10
Glutamine	47 + 3	25 + 8	55 + 8
Glutamate	39 + 6	22 + 4	20 + 2
Serine	22 + 4	17 + 6	22 + 6

Values (percents of 3 month old nonhypoxic mice ± S.E.M.) differ
significantly (P<0.05) from 3 month old nonhypoxic mice.

In conclusion, hypoxia and aging caused similar declines in ACh metabolism in vivo and in vitro. These decreases can be highly correlated to
deficits in tight rope test performance and reductions in the Ca^{2+}-depen-
dent-K^+ stimulated release of ACh.   In both aging and hypoxia, alterations in carbohydrate metabolism may participate in the production of
these changes in ACh as well as the decreases in amino acid metabolism.
The synthesis of ACh in the aged animals appears to be particularly vulnerable to hypoxic insults.   There appears to be many parallels between
these biochemical changes in aging and those in hypoxia.   Thus, hypoxia
may serve as a useful model of the metabolic encephalopathies and aging.
Since decreases in pyruvate dehydrogenase (71), oxidative enzymes (4) and
in the cerebral metabolic rate for oxygen (9) occur in Alzheimer's type
dementia, these results may also have implications in the pathogenesis of
the dementias.

Supported in part by grants NS03346 and NS16997 the Winifred Masterson
Burke Relief Foundation, the Brown and Williamson Company and the Will
Rogers Institute.

References

1. Barclay,L.L., Gibson,G.E., and Blass,J.P. (1981): Pharm. Biochem.
Behav., 14:153-157.
2. Bartus,R.T., Dean,R.L., Goas,J.A. and Lippa,A.S. (1980): Science,
209:301.
3. Birren,J.E., Bick,M.W., and Fox,C. (1948): J. Geront., 3:267-271.
4. Bowen,D.M., Goodhardt,M.J., Strong,A.J., Smith,C.B., White,P.,
Branston,N.M., Symon,L. and Davison,A.N. (1976): Brain Res.,
117:503-507.
5. Brown,R.M., Snider,S.R., and Carlsson,A. (1974): J. Neur. Trans. 35:
293-305.

6.   Browning,E.T., and Schulman,M.P. (1968): J. Neurochem.,
     15:1391-1405.
7.   Cheney,D.L. and Costa,E. (1977): Ann. Rev. Pharmac. Toxicol.,
     17:369-386.
8.   Cortell,R., Feldman,J. and Gellhorn,E. (1941): Amer. J. Physiol.,
     132:588-593.
9.   Dastur,D.K., Lane,M.H., Perlin,S. and Sokoloff,L. (1963): In:
     Human Aging: a Biological Study, edited by J.E.Birrin, R.N.Butler,
     S.W.Greenhouse, L.Sokoloff, M.R.Yarrow, p. 59. U.S. Government
     Printing Office, Washington, D.C.
10. Davies,P. and Maloney,A.J.F. (1976): Lancet II, 1403.
11. Davis,J.N. and Carlsson,A. (1973): J. Neurochem., 20:913-
12. Davis,J.N., Giron,L.T., Stanton,E. and Maury,W. (1979): Adv.
     Neurol., 26:219-223.
13. DeKoning-Verest,I.F. (1980): Mech. of Aging and Develop., 13:83-92.
14. Demopoulos,H., Flamm,E., Seligman,M., Power,R., Pietronigro,D. and
     Ransohoff,J. (1977): In: Oxygen and Physiologic Function, edited by
     F.F.Jobsis, pp. 491-508. Professional Information Library, Dallas,
     Texas.
15. Deshmukh,D.R., Owen,D.E. and Patel,M.S. (1980): J. Neurochem.,
     34:1219-1224.
16. Deshmukh,D.R. and Patel,M.S. (1980): Mech Aging Dev., 13:75-81.
17. Dolivo,M. (1974): Fed. Proc. Am. Soc. Exp. Biol., 33:1043-1048.
18. Drachman,D.A. (1978): In: A Generation of Progress, edited by
     M.A.Lipton, A.DiMascio and K.F.Killam, pp. 651-662. Raven Press,
     New York.
19. Duffy,T.E., Nelson,S.R. and Lowry,O.H. (1972): J. Neurochem.,
     19:959-977.
20. Ebigbe,A.B., Jennett,S. and Pikard,J.D. (1979): Proc. Physiol. Soc.,
     18P.
21. Ferrendelli,J.A., Sedgwick,W.G. and Suntziff,V. (1971): J.
     Neuropath. and Exp. Neurol., 30:638-649.
22. Fridovich,I. (1979): Adv. in Neurology, 26:255-266.
23. Frolkis,V.V. and Berzrukov,V.V. (1973): Gerontologia, 19:45.
24. Gaitonde,M.R. (1965): Biochem. J., 95:803-810.
25. Gardiner,M., Nilsson,B., Rehncrona,S. and Siesjo,B. (1981): J.
     Neurochem., 36: 1500-1505.
26. Gibson,G.E. and Blass,J.P. (1976): J. Neurochem., 27:37-42.
27. Gibson,G.E. and Blass,J.P. (1976): J. Biol. Chem., 251:4127-4130.
28. Gibson,G.E. and Blass,J.P. (1978): J. Neurochem., 30:71-76.
29. Gibson,G.E. and Duffy,T.E. (1981): J. Neurochem., 36:28-33.
30. Gibson,G.E., Blass,J.P. and Jenden,D.J. (1978): J. Neurochem.,
     30:71-76.
31. Gibson,G.E., Jope,R. and Blass,J.P. (1975): Biochem J., 148:17-23.
32. Gibson,G.E., Pelmas,C. and Peterson,C. (1981 a): submitted.
33. Gibson,G.E. and Peterson,C. (1981a): Fed. Proc., 40:207.
34. Gibson,G.E. and Peterson,C. (1982): Biochem. Pharm. 31:111-114.
35. Gibson,G.E. and Peterson,C. (1981c): J. Neurochem. 37: 978-984.
36. Gibson,G.E., Peterson,C. and Jenden,D.J. (1981 b): Science,
     213:674-676.
37. Gibson,G.E., Peterson,C. and Sansone,J. (1981 c): J. Neurochem.,
     37:192-201.
38. Gibson,G.E., Shimada,M., and Blass,J.P. (1978): J. Neurochem.,
     31:757-760.
39. Gurdjian,E.S., Stone,W.E. and Webster,J.E. (1944): Arch. Neurol.
     Psychiatr., 54:474-477.

40. Harkonen,M.H.A., Passonneau,J.V. and Lowry,O.H. (1969): J. Neurochem., 16:1439-1450.
41. Himwich & Himwich (1959): In: Aging and the Individual, edited by J.E.Birren, pp. 187-215. Univ. of Chicago Press, Chicago, Illinois.
42. Hollander,J. and Barrows,C.H.,Jr. (1968): J. Geront, 23:174.
43. Kahlson,G. and MacIntosh,F.C. (1939): J. Physiol., 96:277-292.
44. Kaur,G. and Kanungo,M.S. (1970): Ind. J. Biochem., 7
45. Ksiezak,H.J. and Gibson,G.E. (1981a): J. Neurochem., 37:88-94.
46. Kseizak,H.J. and Gibson,G.E. (1981b): J. Neurochem. 37:307-315.
47. Lippa,A.S., Critchett,D.J., Ehlert,F., Yamamura,H.I., Enna,S.J. and Bartus,R.T. (1981): Neurobiology of Aging, 2:3-8.
48. London,E.D., Nespor,S.M., Ohata,M. and Rapoport,S.I. (1981): J. Neurochem., 37:217-221.
49. MacIntosh,F.C. (1939): J. Physiol., 96:16P.
50. Maker,H.S., Lehren,G.M., Silides,P.J. and Weiss,C. (1973): Prog. in Brain Res., 40:293-307.
51. Mann,P.J.G., Tennenbaum,M. and Quastel,J.H. (1938): Biochem. J., 33:822-835.
52. Mann,P.J.G., Tennenbaum,M. and Quastel,J.H. (1939): Biochem. J., 243-261.
53. McFarland,R.A. (1937): Arch. Psychol., 145:135.
54. McFarland,R.A. (1952): In: The Biology of Mental Health and Disease, pp. 335-355. Paul B. Hoeber, Inc., New York.
55. McFarland,R.A. (1962): Ergonomics, 5:123-131.
56. McFarland,R.A. (1963): Ergonomics, 6: 340-366.
57. McFarland,R.A., Domey,R.G., Warren,A.B. and Ward,D.C. (1960): J. Geront., 15:149-154.
58. McFarland,R.A. and Fisher,M.B. (1955): J. Geront., 10:424-428.
59. McFarland,R.A.. Warren,A.B. and Raris,C. (1958): J. Exp. Psychol., 56:529-538.
60. McGeer,P.L. and McGeer,E.G. (1976): In: Nutrition and the Brain Vol. 5, edited by A.Barbeau, J.H.Growden and R.J.Wurtman, pp. 177-199. Raven Press, New York.
61. McGeer,E.G., Gibiger,H.C., McGeer,P.L. and Wickson,V. (1971): Exp. Gerontol., 6:391-396.
62. Meek,J.L., Bertelsson,L., Cheney,D.L., Zsilla,G. and Costa,E. (1977): J. Gerontol., 32:129-131.
63. Miyaoka,H., Shinohara,M., Kennedy, C. and Sokoloff,L. (1979): Trans. Am. Neurol. Assoc. (In Press).
64. Morris,M.E. (1974): Can J. Physiol. Pharmacol., 52:872-882.
65. Moudgil,V.K. and Kanungo,M.S. (1973): Biochem Biophys. Acta., 329:211.
66. Myers,R.E. (1979): Adv. in Neurology, 26:195-213.
67. Ordy,J.M. and Schjeide,O.A. (1973): In: Progress in Brain Research, edited by D.H.Ford. pp. 25-52. Elsevier, New York.
68. Parmacek,M.S., Fox,J.H. Harrison,W.H., Garron,D.C. and Swenie,D. (1979): Gerontology, 25:185-191.
69. Patel,M.S. (1977): J. Geront., 32:643-646.
70. Peng,M.T., Peng,Y.I. and Chen,F.N. (1977): J. Gerontology, 32:517-522.
71. Perry,E.K., Perry,R.H., Blessed,G. and Tomlinson,B.E. (1977): Lancet i, 189.
72. Plum,F. (1975): In: The Nervous System, edited by D.Tower, pp. 193-201. Raven Press.
73. Quastel,J.H., Tennenbaum,M. and Wheatley,A.H.M. (1936): Biochem. J., 30:1668-1681.

74. Reiner,J.M. (1947): J. Geront., 2:315-320.
75. Reis,D.J., Rosa,R.A. and Joh,T.H. (1977): Brain Res., 136:465-474.
76. Scremin,A.M.E. and Scremin,O.U. (1979): Stroke, 10:142-143.
77. Seitz,C.P. (1940): Arch. Psychol., 36 (257):1-38.
78. Sherman,K., Dallob,A., Dean,R.L., Bartus,R.T. and Freeman E. (1980):
     Fed. Am. Soc. Exptl. Biol., 39:508.
79. Siesjö,B. and Berntman,L. (1979): Adv. in Neurology, 26:319-323.
80. Siesjö,B.K. and Nilsson,L. (1971): Scand. J. Clin. Lab. Invest.,
     27:83-96.
81. Sims,N.R., Bowen,D.M. and Davison,A.N. (1981): Biochem J.,
     6:867-876.
82. Smith,C.B., Goochee,C., Rapoport,S.I. and Sokoloff,L. (1980):
     Brain, 103:351-365.
83. Smith,D.O. (1979): Exp. Neurol., 66:650-666.
84. Sylvia,A.L. and Rosenthal,M. (1979): Brain Res., 165:235-248.
85. Timaras,P.S., Hudson,D.B. and Oklund,S. (1973): Prog. in Brain Res.,
     40:267-275.
86. Tamaki,K., Fujishima,M., Ogata,J., Nakatomi,Y., Ishitsuka,T.,
     Sadoshima, S. and Omae, T. (1979) Brain Research 170:368-371.
87. Tyce,G.M. and Wong,K.L. (1980): Exp. Geront., 15:527-532.
88. Vasko,M.R., Domino,L.E. and Domino,E.F. (1974): Eur. J. Pharmcol.
     27:145-147.
89. Verkhratsky,N.S. (1970): Exp. Geront., 5:49-56.
90. Valcana,T. and Timiras,P.S. (1969): In: Proc. 8th Int. Congr. of
     Gerontology, Vol. II, p. 24. International Assoc. of Gerontology,
     Washington.
91. Welsh,J.H. (1943): J. Neurophysiology., 329-336.
92. Winn,H.R., Welsh,J.E., Rubio,R. and Berne,R.M. (1980): Circulation
     Res., 47:568-577.
93. Yoshino,Y. and Elliot,K.A.C. (1970): Can. J. Biochem., 48:228.

The Aging Brain: Cellular and Molecular
Mechanisms of Aging in the Nervous System,
edited by E. Giacobini et al., Raven Press, New
York © 1982.

Physiological and Structural Changes at the Neuromuscular Junction During Aging

Dean O. Smith

Department of Physiology, University of Wisconsin, Madison, Wisconsin 53706

Senescence, the process of becoming old, is manifest in many ways. In the nervous system aging is particularly evident, for there are distinct behavior changes. Sensory acuity, attention span, short-term memory, and motor coordination decline predictably with age. For example, the rates and the magnitudes of various reflex responses, including simple movements of a finger or a foot, generally decrease during senescence. These changes in behavior reflect changes in the structure and the function of the nervous system at the cellular and the subcellular level. The underlying mechanisms have been studied in both the peripheral and the central nervous system.

Particular attention has focused on age-related decreases in neurotransmitter levels in the presynaptic nerve terminals. Neurochemical evidence indicates decreased transmitter levels in many, but not all, regions of the central nervous system (16,18,41,43). In the peripheral nervous system, smaller amounts of acetylcholine (ACh) have been assayed in the autonomic ganglia and iris of the chick (36) and inferred at the neuromuscular junction (20).

Age-related decreases in the rate of synthesis could explain the lower levels of transmitter. The most widely studied has been choline acetyltransferase (CAT) which catalyzes production of ACh. In the spinal cord (61), the sympathetic ganglia (49), the caudate (40), and the hippocampus (67) the activity declined during senescence. However, in the cerebellum (40,65,67) and the neuromuscular junction of the phrenic nerve (63) there were no age-related changes in CAT activity. Similar diversity has been reported for other enzymes involved in transmitter synthesis (40,49,65). Thus, reduced enzyme activities cannot explain all cases of altered transmitter levels.

Limited availability of the substrate choline appears to underlie the lower amounts of ACh in both the central and the peripheral nervous systems. These include rat cerebellum (44) and chick sympathetic ganglia and iris (35). In the chick, reduced availability of choline for ACh synthesis has been attributed to an age-related decline in V_{max} of the high-affinity uptake system for choline (36); however, values of K_m are unchanged with advancing age. This suggests that there may be a drop in the number of active transport proteins in the membrane.

Physiologically, aged animals exhibit a decreased capability to sustain synaptic transmission. At the neuromuscular junction, there is a much greater tendency for action potential propagation failure to occur in the presynaptic nerve terminals (54). Also, there is a marked increase in the extent of synaptic depression during repetitive action potential discharge in senescent animals relative to young controls (cf. 30). The rate of spontaneous transmitter release increases until advanced senescence, when it drops considerably (24,54). Furthermore, in cerebellar Purkinje cells, the rate of spontaneous action potentials is slower (50) and the inhibition by noradrenergic afferents is less intense (37).

Attention has also focused on deterioration and loss of synaptic structures. In the brain, a reduced number of dendritic processes has been observed (17,23,42,52; cf. 7), and this is mirrored by a more general reduction in the number of synapses (22,26,28,66). At the neuromuscular junction of the soleus muscle, fewer nerve terminals characterize senescence (46,64). Furthermore, following denervation by lesions or pharmacological agents, compensatory sprouting of undamaged terminals, which occurs in young animals, is considerably diminished in aged animals (46; cf. 11).

A composite description of the changes in synaptic structure and function during senescence appears to emerge from these various data. Namely, there is a trend for transmitter levels to decline, synaptic transmission to become less effective, and synapses to degenerate. However, the details have been obtained from many different preparations, and for any particular synaptic system this vraisemblance may be misleading. Furthermore, in the absence of cohesive data from a single synapse, the temporal sequence of events and the functional interactions between age-related changes cannot be readily deduced. Thus, in my laboratory we have begun a comprehensive series of experiments (54,56,57) to elucidate the mechanisms of the aging process at a single, identified synapse, the neuromuscular junction.

All experiments were performed on tissue obtained from the widely studied phrenic nerve-diaphragm muscle of rats. Use of this vital system precludes the possibility that significant disuse atrophy may affect the results. Barrier-reared, male Fischer 344 rats were obtained from the Aged Animal Colonies at the Charles River Breeding Laboratory (Wilmington, Massachusetts). The ages of the old and the control rats were 28 mos and 10 mos, respectively. All animals were used within several days after receiving them from the breeders.

SYNAPTIC DEPRESSION

The postsynaptic responses to repetitive stimulation of the phrenic nerve were recorded to determine the extent of synaptic depression in both the aged and the control rats. Experiments were performed in tissue from 5 rats of each age group. After blocking muscle contraction with about 10^{-7} g/ml of curare added to the bath saline, 1000 end-plate potentials (e.p.p.s) were evoked by stimulation of the phrenic nerve at a rate of 3 impulses/s.

The extent of the synaptic depression, which is characteristic for this preparation (33), was more pronounced in the aged rats. In both age groups, the amplitudes of the e.p.p.s became progressively smaller until a relatively stable value was attained after about 5 impulses. However, the rate of decline in e.p.p. size was faster and the steady state amplitude was lower in the aged rats (56). These results are consistent with observations obtained using paired stimulus pulses reported in a previous study (54).

ACh CONTENT OF NERVE TERMINALS

Freshly Dissected Tissue

An initial set of experiments was performed to determine the ACh content in freshly dissected tissue from both control and aged rats. Concerted efforts were made to minimize any possible changes in ACh levels during the dissection or the early states of the experiment. Following anesthesia, the tissue samples were quickly removed from the animal, and the small strips were obtained for the assay and for counting the number of fibers and, consequently, the number of end plates (57) to be assayed. This was accomplished in less than 10 min, and the heart was beating strongly throughout this period. The excised tissue was placed immediately in cold HCl for subsequent analysis using the radiochemical techniques developed by McCaman and Stetzler (38). This stabilized the ACh by preventing hydrolysis due to endogenous AChE. Nonetheless, the values of ACh measured during this set of experiments may underestimate slightly the content of intact preparations due to hydrolysis during the dissection.

The total amount of ACh per end plate was found to be less in the aged animals. In this freshly dissected tissue, average values (±s.e.) of 54.4 ± 7.5 and 26.6 ± 8.9 fmol/end plate were assayed in the control and aged rats, respectively. Thus, the ACh in the end plates of the aged rats was about 49% the amount in the control animals. This reduction is significant statistically ($P < 0.05$).

Stimulated Tissue

The amount of ACh released in response to action potentials in the presynaptic axon was determined in 8 animals from each age group. After the quick dissection, the tissue was placed in an experimental chamber and bathed in circulating, oxygenated physiologic saline. Two small strips of tissue were prepared. The phrenic nerve innervating one strip was cleaned of connective tissue and drawn into a suction electrode for stimulation at 3 impulses/s for 1000 impulses. The other was maintained in the bath under similar conditions but not stimulated. Cutting the tissue strips, cleaning the nerve, and stimulation usually required about 15 min, after which the samples were placed in cold HCl for the assay. The amount of ACh released was calculated by subtracting the ACh content of the stimulated piece of tissue from that of the nonstimulated piece.

As in the freshly dissected tissue, the amount of ACh in the nonstimulated preparations was less in the older animals by an amount which is statistically significant ($P < 0.05$). The values, summarized in Table 1, were higher following 15 min in the physiologic saline than immediately following dissection. This could be attributed to synthesis during this period. However, for both the control and the aged animals the differences between the two averages were tested using the t statistic and were not found to be statistically significant ($p < 0.2$ for both age groups).

Following stimulation, the ACh within the tissue dropped to a lower level in older rats (Table 1). The difference between the two age groups is statistically significant ($P < 0.05$). These levels of ACh following stimulation presumably reflect values of ACh within the intramuscular and terminal axon regions of both age groups at which release is balanced by synthesis.

TABLE 1. Amounts of ACh at the phrenic nerve-diaphragm muscle neuromuscular junction following 15 min in physiologic saline[a]

Age (mos)	ACh (fmol/end plate)			
	Non-stimulated	Stimulated	Released	Fraction released
10	82.0 ± 5.8	53.3 ± 4.1	28.7 ± 7.1	0.35
28	35.9 ± 3.6	25.0 ± 2.2	10.9 ± 4.2	0.30

[a]Stimulation of the phrenic nerve consisted of 1000 impulses
at a rate of 3 impulses/s. Each value of the ACh results is the
average (±s.e.) of 8 measurements from different animals. These
data were compared using a two-sided, paired-sample t test; in
each case, the differences were statistically significant (P<0.05).
The fractions released were obtained by dividing the amount released into the amount in nonstimulated tissue; these ratios were
not compared statistically.

The amount of ACh released was estimated by subtracting the ACh content of the stimulated piece of tissue from that of the nonstimulated
piece. It was found that less ACh was released during 1000 impulses from
the nerves of the aged animals (Table 1). The tissue obtained from
senescent rats released about 28% as much ACh as those taken from younger
controls. This decrease is significant statistically (P <0.05).
The fraction of the total ACh that was released in response to the
1000 impulses was obtained by dividing the amount released into the
amount in the nonstimulated tissue (Table 1). These calculations indicated that the fraction released was about 5% less in the older animals.
Thus, in the aged rats a slightly smaller fraction of a smaller amount of
ACh is released than in the control animals in response to 1000 action
potentials.

Effects of Hemicholinium

Hemicholinium (HC-3) has been shown to block the high affinity uptake
of choline into the terminals (47). The effects of suppressing the high
affinity uptake of exogenous choline were studied by determining the ACh
content and the amount of ACh released when HC-3 (2 x 10^{-5}M) had been
added to the physiologic saline (56). After about 20 min in this saline,
the tissue which was either nonstimulated or stimulated at 3 impulse/s
for 1000 impulses was assayed for ACh.
There were no significant differences between the amount of ACh
assayed in nonstimulated or stimulated tissue from the two age groups.
Consequently, the calculated levels of ACh released and the fraction released from nerves of the senescent rats did not differ significantly
from control values. This is in contrast to the data obtained when HC-3
had not been added (Table 1). Thus, addition of HC-3 has in some way
reduced the quantitative differences in the results which had been obtained from young and aged animals in normal saline.
The effects of HC-3 were examined more specifically by subtracting
the ACh levels observed after the addition of HC-3 from the levels

observed in normal physiologic saline. The results indicated that in
the control animals HC-3 led to reduced amounts of ACh in stimulated tissue and to a smaller fraction of ACh released (47). However, similar
changes were not observed in the aged rats. Thus, the sensitivity of
stimulated tissue to HC-3 apparently declines during senescence.

Activity of Choline Acetyltransferase

Reduced amounts of ACh in the older animals could be due to lower activity of the enzyme (CAT) which catalyzes synthesis of ACh from the substrates choline and acetyl-CoA. To test this possibility, small strips
of tissue were obtained from each preparation, and the activity of CAT
was assayed (48). Possible CAT in nonneuronal components of these samples was also tested by assaying muscle tissue strips which had no nerve
terminals. There was no significant nonneuronal CAT activity in any of
the samples tested.

The CAT activities measured in tissue obtained from the aged and the
control animals did not differ significantly. This result was found, re-
gardless of whether the activities are normalized for the number of end
plates or the amount of protein in the sample. Thus, paucity of the enzyme CAT does not appear to underlie the reduced levels of ACh observed
in the aged animals.

Activity of Acetylcholinesterase

Unequal rates of hydrolysis of ACh in the synaptic cleft regions of
tissue from the two age groups could possibly underlie the observed differences in synaptic depression. To test this possibility, the activity
of acetylcholinesterase (AChE) was assayed. Both junctional and extra-
junctional AChE were tested.

The activity of AChE was not significantly different in either the
innervated or the noninnervated tissue obtained from the two age groups.
The average (±s.e.) ratio of AChE in innervated/noninnervated tissue obtained from these data are 3.15 (±0.93) and 4.49 (±1.06) for the control
and the aged animals, respectively. The difference between these ratios
is not significant statistically. Thus, the changes in AChE activity do
not seem to be an important factor in the aging process in this preparation. This is consistent with similar results obtained from rat sciatic
nerve (39).

Conclusion

It is concluded that in the phrenic nerve terminals of aged rats there
is a smaller amount of ACh released per action potential. This is
accompanied by results suggesting that there is not only less ACh per
terminal but also a slightly smaller fraction of it is released. Furthermore, evidence is presented which indicates that this may result in part
from lower levels of substrate required for ACh synthesis in the senescent animals.

Do the changes in ACh levels associated with senescence contribute to
the enhanced synaptic depression observed in the aged animals? The
answer to this question is probably yes, for the amount of ACh released
presumably depends on the quantity contained within the terminal (32),
and significant age-related differences are observed. However, synaptic
depression has also been attributed to progressive depletion of the
fraction of this quantity which is available for release (14,45,60). In
aged rats, the fraction released is not much less than in the young

animals. These data are averaged over 1000 impulses, though, and this
may mask large differences shortly after the onset of stimulation. Thus,
definite conclusions are premature, and other possible causes must also
be considered.

RESTRICTED DIFFUSION OF EXTRACELLULAR K^+

The more pronounced synaptic depression in aged animals is associated
with not only smaller quantities of ACh released per action potential
but also onset of presynaptic conduction blocks at lower frequencies of
nerve stimulation (54). In the older animals, the membrane potentials
are also lower, and the rate of spontaneous transmitter release is faster
(54).

One or more of these differences between aged and young rats could be
explained by age-related differences in the extent of extracellular K^+
accumulation during repetitive nerve stimulation. Levels of K^+ in the
immediate vicinity of nerve cells increase during action potential discharge (19). This increase should result in greater spontaneous (31) and
evoked (10,27) transmitter release. In addition, it should cause membrane depolarization which has been proposed to underlie blockage of
action potentials due to Na^+ channel inactivation (55,59).

Direct measurements of K^+ activity, a_K, in the immediate vicinity of
the axon membrane are unfeasible in this preparation. However, measurements of changes in K^+ levels at a site quite near (<50 μm) the membrane
should provide an indirect indication of changes in a_K at the membrane
(58). Thus, the activity of extracellular K^+ near the axon terminal at
the neuromuscular junction was measured during repetitive nerve stimulation using K^+-sensitive microelectrodes in aged and young rats.

Distance and Time Relationships

The activity was recorded at different distances from neuromuscular
junctions in 4 animals of each age group. Within 1s after the onset of
repetitive stimulation of the phrenic nerve, a_K recorded by the electrode
began to rise. It attained a peak value whose magnitude depended on the
distance between the axon terminal region and the electrode tip and the
frequency of stimulation. This maximum value was then maintained for as
long as 5 min, usually with no significant decline (cf. 34), until stimulation was discontinued. The value of a_K then decayed to levels observed before stimulation.

Peak values of a_K varied with the distance between the electrode tip
and the axon terminal region. At longer distances, lower peak values
of a_K were recorded. For any distance, the peak values measured in the
aged preparations were generally greater than those obtained from the
control animals.

The rate of change in a_K was slower as the distance from the terminal
increased. Thus, the time interval between the onset of stimulation and
the initial response at the K^+-sensitive electrode was longer at greater
distances. Also, the time for a_K to rise to one-half of the maximum
value was longer at greater distances. From these results, it is apparent that at equal distances the changes in a_K at the electrode tip occur
more slowly in the aged rats.

Decay of a_K following termination of stimulation was also slower in
the older animals. The half-times for decay following stimulation at
75 impulses/s were measured at sites located 25 (±3) μm from the axon
terminal in 4 animals from each age group. The averages (±s.e.) were
1.08 (±0.18) and 1.50 (±0.20)s in the control and the aged rats,

respectively. This difference is marginally significant at the 0.10 level.

Frequency Dependence

For both age groups, an increase in the frequency of stimulation resulted in a larger maximum value of a_K. The frequencies required to obtain a measurable change in a_K were generally higher in the older animals. Frequencies of at least 50 impulses/s were required to obtain a measurable change in a_K in the old rats. However, rates as low as 20 impulses/s produced detectable changes in a_K in the control rats.

Effects of Collagen and Protease

Collagen and other constituents of the extracellular environment may change with age, posing a barrier to ionic diffusion (53). A series of experiments were performed in each animal to examine this possibility. With the K^+-sensitive electrode located 25 ± 3 μm from an axon terminal, the stimulation frequency was progressively increased. The frequency at which a change in a_K was first detected at the electrode was then recorded. Subsequently, changes in a_K were measured during stimulation at 75 impulses/s. Stimulation was then discontinued, and the preparation was soaked for 1 hr in 0.1% collagenase; in one rat from each age group, this was followed by an additional 30 min in 0.025% protease (Sigma, Type VII). The tissue was rinsed with fresh saline, stimulation was begun again, and the minimum frequency at which a change in a_K could be seen as well as the maximum response at 75 impulses/s were recorded and compared with values obtained before proteolysis. During these procedures, care was taken to preclude any movement of the electrode tip.

The maximum values of a_K attained during stimulation decreased following collagenase treatment. The addition of the protease did not yield results significantly different from those obtained following collagenase alone, so the data were pooled. In each age group, lower peak values of a_K were recorded following treatment with collagenase; however, the decrease was considerably larger in the aged rats (41%) than in the controls (8%). Furthermore, the minimum rate of stimulation required to produce a measurable change in a_K dropped following collagenase. The extent of this decrease was also more pronounced in the aged (19%) than in the control (6%) animals.

The kinetics of the a_K response were faster after treatment with collagenase. The time to reach one-half the maximum a_K was reduced by 83% and 78% in the aged and the control rats, respectively. Also, following termination of stimulation, the times for the a_K response to decay by one-half declined by 13% and 19% in the old and the young animals, respectively.

Effects of Acetylcholine on the Electrode Response

The ion-exchanger resin is also sensitive to ACh, the transmitter agent at the end plate. Indeed, the selectivity for ACh relative to K^+ is about 100:1 (3), and in phrenic nerve terminals the molar quantity of ACh released per impulse is about 10 times that of K^+ efflux (29,47). Such high levels of ACh could lead to spurious results. This possibility is not too likely, however, for considerably less ACh is released in these Mg^{2+}-blocked preparations. Furthermore, ACh is hydrolyzed readily, although the extent of hydrolysis is not known (cf. 56). In contrast, collagenase produces an irreversible drop in the activity of AChE (4), which may augment any ACh effect.

Because of the uncertainty introduced by the presence of ACh, two additional experiments were performed as controls in each preparation. (i) While keeping the K^+-sensitive microelectrode in the same location as in the preceding collagenase experiments, the amount of ACh released during stimulation was reduced even further by addition of Mg^{2+} to the bath until the evoked e.p.p.s became just indistinguishable from the noise of the recording equipment (20 to 30 µV). The Mg^{2+} concentration was elevated to about 16 to 18 mM in these cases. Maximum values of a_K were again measured during stimulation at 75 impulses/s. The results obtained did not differ significantly from those measured previously at the same site. (ii) Subsequently, the hydrolysis of ACh was inhibited by adding the anticholinesterase physostigmine (60 µM) to the saline. If ACh had been affecting the electrode response, this effect should be potentiated under these conditions. However, the results did not differ significantly from those obtained in the preceding experiments. It was concluded that ACh had not interfered seriously with the reported measurements of a_K.

Muscle Fiber Density

The amount of K^+ diffusing from the axon terminal region to the K^+-sensitive electrode has been found to be less in the aged than in the control rats. A possible explanation is that in the aged rats there might be excessive diffusion of K^+ along a gradient through spaces between loosely packed underlying muscle fibers, away from the electrode.

To test this possibility, the density of muscle fibers was measured in preparations from both age groups. Strips of fresh muscle tissue were dissected from each diaphragm studied. They were then pinned at "resting length" in a transparent dish and viewed in cross section under the light microscope. The size of the tissue was measured, and the number of muscle fiber profiles present were counted. Subsequently, the number of muscle fibers/cm^2 of tissue was calculated for each preparation.

The muscle fiber density was slightly higher in the aged rats. The average values (±s.e.) obtained from 62 samples from old rats and 73 samples from control rats were 0.715 (±0.021) and 0.651 (±0.022) fibers/cm^2, respectively. Thus, it seems quite unlikely that there could be significant differences in the spacing of muscle fibers underlying the K^+-sensitive electrode which could explain the results.

Conclusions

It is concluded that diffusion of K^+ away from the nerve ending is slower in aged than in young rats. This suggests that the accumulation of extracellular K^+ at the nerve terminal membrane during repetitive stimulation is greater in aged than control rats. However, this result cannot readily explain conduction block, for the kinetics of the K^+ buildup, and the corresponding membrane depolarization, are considerably faster than the onset of conduction block. In the aged animals, conduction failure was observed to occur only after 2 min of repetitive stimulation at 50 impulses/s; the times were much longer (>10 min) for the control rats (54). Although they are statistically significant, the small differences (<0.5s) between the half-times for K^+ accumulation in the old and the young rats are not large enough to explain readily the age-related differences in the time to conduction block.

Furthermore, accumulation of more K^+ extracellularly, with correspondingly greater membrane depolarization, does not readily explain the enhanced synaptic depression observed in the older animals. In this preparation, a rise in extracellular K^+ causes the quantal content of the e.p.p. to increase. However, less ACh is released per action potential in the aged rats. Without the increased K^+ buildup, synaptic depression might actually be more pronounced in the older rats. Whether some other aspect of the release process is affected by the K^+ accumulation is not known.

NUMBER OF PRESYNAPTIC TERMINALS

The reduced amounts of ACh at the end plates could be associated with fewer nerve terminals per end plate. To assess this possibility, end-plate architecture was examined in young and old rats. The end-plate region and the nerve terminals were visualized using a cholinesterase stain and silver-gold impregnation, respectively. Specific details of the methods used to prepare the tissue for light and electron microscopy are presented in Smith and Rosenheimer (57).

Nerve Terminal Architecture

To determine the extent of axon terminal growth within the end plate and the effects of aging upon the innervation pattern, tissue was obtained from 5 animals in each age group. Twelve end plates were examined from each animal. The criteria for selecting a particular end plate to study were that it appeared to be (i) incorporated completely within the section and (ii) located in a plane parallel to that of the section. It was necessary to view the tissue at high magnification (1000x) and to adjust the focal plane frequently to delineate accurately the sites of origin and termination of the axon terminal branches. The terminal branches, which are nonmyelinated, were characterized by their small diameters (<3 μm) and, occasionally, by a small bouton. Length and area measurements obtained from these preparations may be underestimates of values in vivo due to tissue shrinkage during the histological procedures.

Number and Length of Nerve Terminals

The number of terminal branches in each end plate was counted in animals of both age groups. In addition, the length of each terminal branch was measured from the point of origin at the bifurcation to its ending. These lengths were then summated to obtain the total length of nerve terminal within the end-plate region.

The average number (±s.e.) of terminals per end plate was 13 ± 1 and 18 ± 1 in the young and the aged rats, respectively. This was also manifest as a significantly (P <0.005) greater total length of terminal branches per end plate in the older animals. However, the average length of the terminal did not differ by an amount which is significant statistically (p <0.4), indicating that the difference in total length of terminal branches is due to the existence of more individual arborizations.

Number of Axon Branches Entering the End-Plate Region

To determine if the large number of terminals in the older animals was due to a greater number of collaterals projecting into the end-plate region or to more extensive branching within the end plate, the number of myelinated and nonmyelinated axon branches innervating each end plate was

counted. Most of these collaterals were myelinated, although nonmyelinated branches were observed to project into 19% and 11% of the end plates
in the aged and the control rats, respectively. There were no cases in
which more than one nonmyelinated branch innervated an end plate.

The number of motor axon collaterals, from which the terminal branches
emanate, projecting into the end plates was not significantly different
for the two age groups. Thus, the increased number of terminal endings
in the old rats is due to more frequent branching within the end-plate
region and not to a greater number of collaterals projecting to the end
plate.

In some preparations, axon collaterals formed a second end plate on a
single muscle fiber. This was observed to occur in 1.7% of the 402 muscle fibers examined in the control rats and 1.6% of the 375 muscle fibers
in the aged animals. The difference between these two values is not significant statistically (P <0.3). More than two end plates were never observed on a single muscle fiber.

End Plate Area

To determine if the increased number of nerve terminals in aged rats
was associated with larger end plates, the areas of the end-plate regions
which stained for cholinesterase were measured with an electronic planimeter. The sizes of the end-plate regions of the young and the old age
groups were found to be 737 ± 59 μm^2 and 835 ± 49 μm^2, respectively; these
values are not significantly different. The values measured may be underestimates because they were obtained from two-dimensional representations of the cylindrical muscle fiber. However, if the diameters of the
muscle fibers in the two age groups are not substantially different this
underestimation should not affect conclusions drawn from comparisons between control and aged rats.

The diameters of the muscle fibers were measured, and those of the
aged rats were smaller by an amount which was statistically significant
(P <0.05). The values are 42.7 ± 0.94 μm and 40.1 ± 0.89 μm in the young
and the old rats, respectively. However, the magnitude of the difference,
6%, is quite small. Thus, it is not expected to have biased significantly the measurements of end-plate area.

Degeneration of Axon Terminals

Within the end-plate region, indications of axon terminal degeneration
were observed. Degenerating terminals are characteristically swollen.
They end in inflated, irregularly shaped boutons, in contrast to the thin
processes commonly associated with "normal" terminals (57; cf. 1). To
determine whether degeneration was more extensive in either age group, the
number of end plates showing any indication of this phenomenon was counted.

Terminal degeneration was seen more frequently in the younger animals.
In 43% and 23% of the end plates in control and aged rats, respectively,
some evidence of terminal regression was observed. Similar results were
obtained in cat soleus muscle (64), although the values were somewhat
lower (12% and 5%, respectively). Thus, the process of degeneration is
apparently less extensive in the senescent rats.

Sprouting

To determine the extent of new nerve growth, or sprouting, the number
of nonmyelinated axon branches which appeared to terminate in growth cones
either within or close to the end plate was counted. Growth cones could

be identified readily as conical or bulbous endings on thin axon processes (57). Sprouts originated from either a node of Ranvier near the site at which the axon entered the end-plate region or a terminal branch within the end plate. These are termed nodal and terminal sprouts, respectively (cf. 1,64).

Sprouting was observed more frequently in the younger animals. The results are summarized in Table 2. The fraction of end plates in which either nodal or terminal sprouting was evident was significantly (P<0.001) higher in the control rats. Terminal sprouting was not observed in the end-plate region of aged animals, and nodal sprouting was seen less often in the older rats.

TABLE 2. Degeneration and sprouting at the neuromuscular junction[a]

Age (mos)	Fraction of End Plates Examined		
	Degeneration	Sprouting	Sprouting and Degeneration
10	0.426	0.408	0.113
28	0.228	0.102	0

[a]In 5 control and 5 aged animals, 111 and 62 end plates were examined, respectively. The fractions of these end plates in which degeneration or sprouting was observed are presented. In addition, the fraction of the total end plates in which both sprouting and indications of terminal degeneration were seen are presented. The fractions obtained from the control and the aged animal data were compared by testing the difference in proportions, and in each case the difference was significant at the 0.05 level.

Size and Number of Synaptic Vesicles

There is less transmitter substance per terminal yet more terminals per end plate in the aged than in the control rats. This implies that there is probably less ACh per terminal in the aged animals. At least 50% of the ACh is bound within synaptic vesicles in the terminals (69). Thus, the possibility arises that there may be smaller or fewer synaptic vesicles per nerve terminal in senescent animals.

This possibility was tested by determining the size and the number of synaptic vesicles observed in electron micrographs of synaptic sites viewed in cross section. Micrographs were taken from 10 terminals in 5 animals from each age group. The criteria for including a micrograph in the analysis were that the profile of the axon terminal appeared circular in cross section and that the active zone, characterized by the pre- and postsynaptic densities, lay in the plane of the section.

Size of Vesicles. The diameters of 500 synaptic vesicle profiles were measured. If the profile was not circular, the average value of diameters along the major and the minor axes was used for the analysis. These data were plotted in a histogram, and using stereologic techniques (70), the average values (±s.e.) were calculated. The average diameter of the vesicles was then obtained by multiplying the average profile diameters by the factor $4/\pi$ (70). Using the formula for the volume of a sphere, the average vesicle diameter was also calculated from these data.

The synaptic vesicles were slightly smaller in the aged than in the young animals. Vesicle diameters were 48.8 ± 0.3 nm and 50.4 ± 0.2 nm, respectively. The difference, about 3%, is highly significant statistically (P <0.005), although this probably does not reflect any major functional difference.

Number of Vesicles. The number of synaptic vesicle profiles was counted in micrographs of cross sections through 20 and 30 nerve terminals of aged and control rats, respectively. Using an electronic planimeter, the area, A, of each terminal profile was also measured, and the number of vesicles per μm^2 of terminal profile, N_A, was calculated. The number of synaptic vesicles per μm^3 (N_v) was then determined for each terminal correcting for the Holmes effect, which arises when the vesicle diameter is less than the section thickness (70).

There were more synaptic vesicles in the terminals of the older rats. Specifically, 712 ± 57 and 990 ± 96 vesicles/μm^2 were measured in the young and the aged animals, respectively. The difference, 38%, is significant statistically (P <0.02). Thus, in the aged animals there are not only more terminal endings but also more synaptic vesicles per terminal.

A possible technical explanation of this result was explored and rejected. Namely, if the area of the terminals in the aged rats had been consistently smaller, higher values of N_v might have been expected. This was not the case; the terminals of the aged rats were usually larger, although the difference is not significant statistically. In the control and the aged rats, the average ($\pm$s.e.) diameter of the terminals in the region measured was 1.8 ± 0.6 μm and 2.1 ± 0.8 μm, respectively. This difference is not significant statistically (P <0.4).

Conclusions

The results of this study demonstrate an increased complexity of nerve terminal arborization and ultrastructure in the end plates of senescent rats, relative to young, control animals. In particular, it has been shown that the number of nerve terminals within the end-plate region of the phrenic nerve-diaphragm muscle is greater in senescent than in younger control rats. These terminals are derived from growth within the end-plate region, suggesting that they are the result of terminal sprouting. Furthermore, greater numbers of synaptic vesicles have been observed within the nerve terminals of the older animals. Although there are more phrenic nerve terminals in the older animals, containing more synaptic vesicles, all of these terminals may not be functional. More extensive terminal arborization might be expected to occur as an indirect consequence of the decline in transmitter release during senescence. Indeed, extensive terminal formation due to sprouting is a commonly observed response following reduction of ACh release by botulinum toxin (12,62). However, sprouting was seldom observed in the aged rats, indicating that some other phenomena may be involved.

The activity of the muscle may also influence terminal growth during aging (cf. 6,13). Because of its vital function, the diaphragm muscle remains active throughout the life of the animal. Thus, changes in the frequency of sprouting observed in this preparation cannot readily be attributed to possible inactivity of the muscle.

A more compelling explanation of these results is that there is an unbalanced decrease in the rates of continual growth and regression of axon terminals in the senescent rats (cf. 5,51). Under normal conditions in younger animals, the synaptic terminals of a motor axon undergo a continual process of sprouting and degeneration, renewing the architecture of the end plate (1,64,68). In his extensive study of the dynamics of end-plate structure in the cat, Tuffery (64) concluded that the growth and regression of terminals are not necessarily coupled but are independent phenomena. In the aged rats both processes occur considerably less frequently than in younger controls. If the rate of decline of the occurrences of sprouting were slower than that of degeneration, the number of nerve terminal·endings within the end-plate region would be higher in the older animals. The results of this study are consistent with this particular relationship.

In different nerves, the converse relationship may exist. For example, in the soleus nerve of aged rats (46; cf. 21), fewer nerve terminals were observed per end-plate region. This may indicate that in that preparation, the rate at which sprouting occurs declines faster than that of degeneration. Indeed, the relative rates at which either process declines may vary considerably throughout the nervous system and they may also be influenced by environmental or other factors (9). Thus, variability in the axon terminal architecture within synaptic regions of different nerves may be expected due to an imbalance in the rates at which sprouting and degeneration decline (cf. 52).

There may also be an imbalance which underlies the increased number of synaptic vesicles observed within the terminals of aged animals. The rate at which vesicle membrane is synthesized, or reclaimed from terminal axolemma (cf. 25), may exceed the rate at which it is degraded during senescence. This would lead to a rise in the number of synaptic vesicles. Until the fate of synaptic vesicle membrane is better understood, however, further speculation may be misdirected.

Whether each vesicle in the senescent animals is fully loaded with ACh is difficult to determine precisely. They may not be, for there is less total ACh per end plate in the aged rats. When ACh levels are low in frog, due to impaired synthesis, there is a corresponding decrease in the amount contained within the synaptic vesicles (8). Clearly, however, further studies are necessary to determine the functional status of the terminals and synaptic vesicles observed in the senescent animals.

ACKNOWLEDGMENTS

This work was supported by NIH grants AG01572 and NS00380 (R.C.D.A.) and by the Alfred P. Sloan Foundation. The invaluable assistance of Ms. Curry Gibson and Ms. Julie Rosenheimer is gratefully acknowledged.

REFERENCES

1. Barker, D. and Ip, M.C. (1965): Proc. R. Soc. B. 163: 538-554.
2. Barnes, C.A. and McNaughton, B.L. (1980): J. Physiol., London, 309: 473-485.
3. Baum, G. (1971): Anal. Biochem. 39: 65-72.
4. Betz, W. and Sakmann, B. (1973); J. Physiol., London, 230: 673-688.
5. Black, M.M. and Lasek, R.J. (1979): Expl. Neurol., 63: 108-119.
6. Brown, M.C., Goodwin, G.M., and Ironton, R. (1977): J. Physiol., London, 267: 42P-43P.
7. Buell, S.J. and Coleman, P.D. (1979): Science, 206: 854-856.
8. Ceccarelli, B. and Hurlbut, W.P. (1975): J. Physiol., London, 247: 163-188.
9. Connor, J.R., Diamond, M.C., and Johnson, R.E. (1980): Expl. Neurol., 68: 158-170.

10. Cooke, J.D. and Quastel, D.M.J. (1973): J. Physiol., London, 228: 435-548.
11. Cotman, C.W. and Scheff, S.W. (1979): Mech. Age. Devel., 9: 103-117.
12. Duchen, L.W. (1970): J. Neurol. Neurosurg. Psychiat., 33: 40-54.
13. Duchen, L.W. and Tonge, D.A. (1977): J. Anat., 124: 205-215.
14. Elmqvist, D. and Quastel, D.M.J. (1965): J. Physiol., London, 178: 505-529.
15. Erulkar, S.D. and Weight, F.F. (1977): J. Physiol., London, 266: 209-218.
16. Estes, K.S. and Simpkins, J.W. (1980): Brain Res., 194: 556-560.
17. Feldman, M.L. (1976): In: Neurobiology of Aging, edited by R.D. Terry and S. Gershon, pp. 211-227. Raven Press, New York.
18. Finch, C.E. (1973): Brain Res., 52: 261-276.
19. Frankenhaeuser, B. and Hodgkin, A.L. (1956): J. Physiol., London, 131: 341-376.
20. Frolkis, V.V., Martynenko, O.A., and Zamostyan, V.P. (1976): Gerontol., 22: 244-279.
21. Fujisawa, K. (1976): Exp. Geront. 11: 43-47.
22. Geinisman, Y. and Bondareff, W. (1976): Mech. Age. Devel., 5: 11-23.
23. Geinisman, Y., Bondareff, W., and Dodge, J.T. (1978): Am. J. Anat., 152: 321-330.
24. Gutmann, E. and Hanzlikova, V. (1972): Age changes in the neuro-muscular system. Scientechnica, Bristol.
25. Heuser, J.E. and Reese, T.S. (1973): J. Cell Biol. 57: 315-344.
26. Hinds, J.W. and McNelly, N. (1977): J. Comp. Neurol., 171: 345-368.
27. Hubbard, J.I. and Willis, W.D. (1968): J. Physiol., London, 194: 381-405.
28. Johnson, J.E. and Miquel, J. (1974): Ageing Dev., 3: 203-224.
29. Keynes, R.D. (1951): J. Physiol., London, 114: 119-150.
30. Landfield, P.W., McGaugh, J.L. and Lynch, G. (1978): Brain Res., 150: 85-101.
31. Liley, A.W. (1956): J. Physiol., London, 134: 427-443.
32. Liley, A.W. and North, K.A.K. (1953): J. Neurophysiol. 16: 509-527.
33. Lundberg, A. and Quilisch, H. (1953): Acta Physiol. Scand., 30: Suppl. III: 111-120.
34. Lux, H.D. and Neher, E. (1973): Exp. Brain Res., 17: 190-205.
35. Marchi, M. and Giacobini, E. (1980): Dev. Neurosci., 3: 39-48.
36. Marchi, M., Hoffman, D.W., Giacobini, E. and Fredrickson, T. (1980): Brain Res., 195: 423-431.
37. Marwaha, J., Hoffer, B., Pittman, R., and Freedman, R. (1980): Brain Res., 201: 85-97.
38. McCaman, R.E. and Stetzler, J. (1977): J. Neurochem., 28: 669-671.
39. McMartin, D.N. and O'Connor, J.A. (1979): Mech. Age. Devel., 10: 241-248.
40. McGeer, E.G., Fibiger, H.C., McGeer, P.L. and Wickson, V. (1971): Exp. Geront. 6: 391-396.
41. Meek, J.L., Bertilsson, L., Cheney, D.L., Zsilla, G., and Costa, E. (1977): J. Gerontol., 32: 129-131.
42. Mehraein, P. and Yamada, M. (1975): In: Physiology and Pathology of Dendrites, edited by G.W. Kreutzberg. Raven Press, New York.
43. Meier-Ruge, W., Reichlmeier, K., and Iwangoff, P. (1976): In Neurobiology of Aging, edited by R.D. Terry and S. Gershon, pp. 379-387. Raven Press, New York.
44. Mohan, C. and Radha, E. (1978): Exp. Geront. 13: 349-356.

45. Otsuka, M., Endo, M., and Nonomura, Y. (1962): <u>Jap. J. Physiol</u>. 12: 573-584.

46. Pestronk, A., Drachman, D.B., and Griffin, J.W. (1980): <u>Expl. Neurol</u>. 70: 65-82.

47. Potter, L.T. (1970): <u>J. Physiol., London</u>, 206: 145-166.

48. Rand, J.B. and Johnson, C.D. (1981): <u>Anal. Biochem</u>., in press.

49. Reis, D.J., Ross, R.A., and Joh, T.H. (1977): <u>Brain Res</u>., 136: 465-474.

50. Rogers, J., Silver, M.A., Shoemaker, W.J., and Bloom, F.E. (1980): <u>Neurobiology of Aging</u>, 1: 3-11.

51. Scheff, S.W., Benardo, L.S., and Cotman, C.W. (1978): <u>Science</u>, 202: 775-778.

52. Scheibel, M.E., Lindsay, R.D., Tomiyasu, U., and Scheibel, A.B. (1975): <u>Exptl. Neurol</u>., 47: 392-403.

53. Sinex, F.M. (1968): In: <u>Treatise on Collagen</u>, Vol. 2 (Biology of Collagen), edited by B.S. Gould, pp. 409-448. Academic Press, N.Y.

54. Smith, D.O. (1979): <u>Expl. Neurol</u>., 66: 650-666.

55. Smith, D.O. (1980): <u>J. Physiol., London</u>, 301: 243-259.

56. Smith, D.O. and Gibson, C.T. (1982): <u>J. Neurophysiol</u>.: in press.

57. Smith, D.O. and Rosenheimer, J.L. (1982): <u>J. Neurophysiol</u>.: in press.

58. Somjen, G.G. (1979): <u>Ann. Rev. Physiol</u>., 41: 159-177.

59. Spira, M.E., Yarom, Y. and Parnas, I. (1976): <u>J. Neurophysiol</u>., 36: 882-899.

60. Theis, R. (1965): <u>J. Neurophysiol</u>., 28: 427-442.

61. Timiras, P.S. (1972): <u>Developmental Physiology and Aging</u>. Macmillan, New York.

62. Tonge, D.A. (1974): <u>J. Physiol., London</u>, 241: 127-139.

63. Tucek, S. and Gutmann, E. (1973): <u>Expl. Neur</u>., 38: 349-360.

64. Tuffery, A.R. (1971): <u>J. Anat</u>., 110: 221-247.

65. Unsworth, B.R., Fleming, L.H. and Caron, P.C. (1980): <u>Mech. Age. Devel</u>., 13: 205-217.

66. Vaughan, D.W. (1977): <u>J. Comp. Neurol</u>., 171: 501-516.

67. Vijayan, V.K. (1977): <u>Exp. Geront</u>., 12: 7-11.

68. Wernig, A., Pecot-Dechavassine, M., and Stöver, H. (1980): <u>J. Neurocytol</u>. 9: 277-303.

69. Whittaker, V.P., Michaelson, I.A., and Kirkland, R.J.A. (1964): <u>Biochem. J</u>., 90: 293-303.

70. Williams, M.A. (1977): <u>Quantitative Methods in Biology</u>. North-Holland, Amsterdam.

The Aging Brain: Cellular and Molecular
Mechanisms of Aging in the Nervous System,
edited by E. Giacobini et al., Raven Press, New
York © 1982.

Peripheral and Central Adrenergic
Neurons: Differences During the Aging Process

M. Marchi, L. Yurkewicz, E. Giacobini, and D. W. Hoffman

*Laboratory of Neuropsychopharmacology, Department of Biobehavioral Sciences, University of
Connecticut, Storrs, Connecticut 06268*

The peripheral nervous system of the chick has been used by this
laboratory to provide a productive model for the study of age-related
changes in the nervous system. Previous publications have described
in detail significant age-related variations in the parameters of
cholinergic neurotransmission such as choline and acetylcholine (ACh)
levels in autonomic ganglia and iris (19, 20), and choline uptake in
the autonomic terminals of the iris (21, 22, 25). Other properties of
cholinergic neurotransmission in these tissues, including the activities
of the enzymes acetylcholinesterase (AChE) and choline acetyltransferase
(ChAc) (22), binding of the receptor-ligand α-bungarotoxin (26) and
turnover of ACh (24), have been determined throughout the lifespan to
more fully define the dynamics of development and aging in our model
system.

A second innervation of the chick iris is adrenergic, and in this
same tissue we have also demonstrated the occurrence of age-related
changes in the individual characteristics of norepinephrine (NE) uptake, both at early (12) and late (14) stages of life. These changes
have been compared and correlated functionally with the levels of NE
found in these adrenergic terminals and fibers from embryonic life to
senescence (13).

In order to obtain a more complete picture of neuronal aging we have
extended our studies of the adrenergic components of both the peripheral nervous systems (PNS) and the central nervous system (CNS). The
results presented here both supplement and complement our previous
studies, and permit us to compare, in greater detail, the aging process
in both cholinergic and adrenergic neurons. In addition, we are now
able to describe and compare the relationships between the events occurring in cell bodies and those occurring in their terminals in both CNS
and PNS structures; respectively, the locus coeruleus (LC), with terminals in the cerebellum, and the lumbar sympathetic ganglia with terminals in the iris.

Present address of M.M.: Istituto di Farmacologia et Farmacognosia,
Universita di Genova, Via al Capo di S. Chiara, 16146 Genova, Italy.

TYROSINE HYDROXYLASE ACTIVITY
IN THE PERIPHERAL AND CENTRAL NERVOUS SYSTEM

Tyrosine hydroxylase (TH: tyrosine-3-monooxygenase, EC1.14.16.2), the
rate limiting enzyme for the biosynthesis of norepinephrine (NE, 18), is
synthesized in the cell soma, and then is transported to nerve terminals
where most neurotransmitter synthesis takes place (9). Therefore, TH
activity was used as a neurochemical marker of noradrenergic cell bodies
and axon terminals.
    Tyrosine hydroxylase activity was measured in the region of LC, cere-
bellum, cervical spinal cord, lumbar sympathetic ganglia and iris,
throughout most of the lifespan of the chicken (8 days of incubation to
5 years; 39). The chick cerebellar cortex has a richer noradrenergic
innervation than that of mammals (31) and in addition, endogenous NE
levels in developing chick cerebellum and cervical spinal cord have
already been reported (34, 35) allowing comparisons with these data. In
the chick, all segments of the spinal cord are innervated by noradrenergic fibers, and the development of this innervation has recently been
described (34). The cell bodies that give rise to these fibers are located solely in the brainstem and are presumed to be in the medullary
reticular formation and LC (34).
    The lumbar sympathetic ganglia, which contain noradrenergic cell
bodies, and the iris, an area richly innervated by noradrenergic fibers,
were chosen for analysis since these structures have already been well
characterized biochemically in the developing and aging chicken (7, 10,
11, 12, 13, 19, 20). In addition, the development of NE content in the
chick sympathetic ganglia and in the iris have been described. Although
the iris is directly innervated by the superior cervical ganglion (17)
and not by the lumbar sympathetic ganglia, the latter was chosen for
study since the activity of TH during the embryonic period in the chick
has already been determined in this region (7), and the lumbar sympathetic chain provides more tissue for analysis.

DEVELOPMENT IN THE CNS
TH ACTIVITY: THE LOCUS COERULEUS AND TARGET SITES.

    At 8 and 10 days of incubation (d.i. Stage 34 and 36) the cerebellum
and the section of brainstem containing the LC were dissected according
to the scheme shown in Fig. 1A. At all later stages a thin section of
brainstem containing the LC was dissected out as described in Fig. 1B.
In the following pages "LC-R" refers to this strip of the corresponding
brainstem region.
    The cervical region of the vertebral column (16) was dissected, and
the cervical segment of the spinal cord was removed and collected for
analysis. The iris and sympathetic ganglia were dissected according
to previously described methods (3, 7).
    The greatest overall increase in total TH activity in the LC-R and
the cerebellum occurred during the embryonic period. The increase in
the cerebellum was more pronounced than in the LC-R, indicating an
early active transport of the enzyme to the terminals (Fig. 2A, B).
The cervical spinal cord, in contrast, increased at approximately the
same rate in both the embryonic and post-hatching periods (Fig. 2A, B).
    In the period 8-14 d.i., TH specific activity decreases in the cere-
bellum and then remains constant to 18 d.i., whereas in the cervical
spinal cord it increases throughout this period (Fig.2C). These trends

may reflect changes in enzyme activity in the preexisting terminals or differences in the growth of the innervating fibers as well as growth of the target regions.

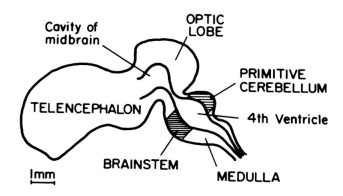

FIG. 1A. Schematic diagram of a sagittal section of a chick embryo brain at 8-10 d.i. Shaded areas illustrate the region dissected: primitive cerebellum and the section of brain stem containing presumptive LC cells.

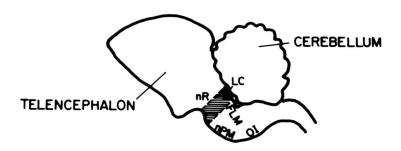

FIG. 1B. Schematic diagram of a sagittal section of a chick brain at posthatching stages, with the optic lobes removed. The shaded area illustrates the region of brain stem dissected containing the locus coeruleus (LC) referred to in the text as LC-R. Abbreviations: nR - nucleus Ruber, FLM - fasciculus longitudinalis medialis, nPM - nucleus pontis medialis, OI - nucleus olivaris inferior.

In the period just following hatching (1 day - 1 month), total TH activity continues to increase in the LC-R, whereas in the two target areas, the enzyme activity remains constant (Fig. 2A). Thus, cell bodies in the LC-R appear to accumulate the enzyme without increasing the amount transported to these two target sites. The specific activity of TH in the cerebellum during the same period shows a sharp (3-fold) decrease, probably reflecting growth of the cerebellum without a concomitant increase in the number of noradrenergic terminals, since during the same period there is a 3-fold increase in the wet weight of this region with no corresponding increase in enzyme activity (Fig. 2C).

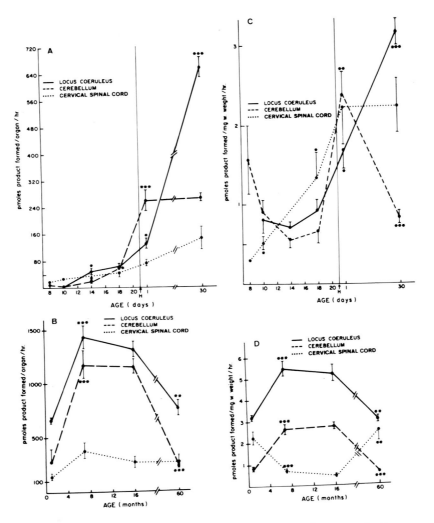

FIG. 2. Developmental pattern of tyrosine hydroxylase activity expressed as pmoles product formed/organ/hr (Fig. A,B) and as pmoles product formed/mg w.w. (Fig. C,D) in the CNS. Values are the mean $\pm$ S.E.M. A significant difference from the preceding age, based on the Student's t test, is indicated by *p < 0.05, **p < 0.01, and ***p < 0.001.

As the brain matures into adulthood (1-7 months), total TH activity in the LC-R continues to rise (Fig. 2B). This also occurs in the cerebellum where an even greater increase is observed, possibly reflecting increased transport of TH to this brain region during the adult period (Fig. 2B). During the same period, the two target areas show opposite trends in the specific activity of TH, which may indicate a difference between the two target areas in the relative growth of the noradrenergic fibers with respect to the growth of the organ (Fig. 2D).

All three brain regions (LC-R, cerebellum and cervical spinal cord) exhibit the highest total TH activity at 7 months, which remains constant thereafter, until 16 months. This may reflect the fact that during this period the target sites are completely innervated, the organs have reached their full size and the biosynthetic mechanisms are able to maintain a relatively steady-state level (Fig. 2A, B).

DEVELOPMENT IN THE PNS TH ACTIVITY:
THE SYMPATHETIC GANGLIA AND IRIS

In the PNS structures examined, the greatest increase in both total and specific TH activity occurred during the post-hatching period, with a greater rise in the cell bodies of the lumbar sympathetic ganglia than in the noradrenergic terminals of the iris (Fig. 3A, B, C, D).

The pronounced drop in TH specific activity in the sympathetic ganglia following hatching (7-14 d.i.) may be correlated with the drop in monoamine oxidase, dopadecarboxylase (DDC) and dopamineβ-hydroxylase (DBH) activities seen in the same tissue between 1-4 d.a.h. (5, 8). Such sudden and reversible change suggests that following hatching there may be an increased transport in both TH and DBH from the cell bodies to the terminals which might be responsible for the observed transient decline in both enzyme activities seen in the ganglia. The difference in the occurrence of this decline may be explained by the different rate of transport of these enzymes (1, 32, 38).

The progressive decrease in TH specific activity seen in the sympathetic ganglia from 1 month - 5 years (Fig. 3D) can be explained by a continual increase in protein content in the ganglia during this period (19).

Total TH activity reaches its highest value at 7 months in the iris, which was also observed in the CNS regions examined. However, in the period following 7 months total TH activity in the PNS structures show opposite trends (increasing in the ganglia and decreasing in the iris) whereas constant levels are maintained in the CNS structures from 7-16 months (Fig. 2B, 3B). It is interesting to note that ACh in the chick lumbar sympathetic ganglia, which is almost exclusively presynaptically located, shows a parallel increase with TH activity up to 3 months, followed by a plateau lasting up to 1 year (19).

Throughout the period studied (8 d.i. - 5 years), TH activity and NE levels per mg protein (Fig. 4) do not follow parallel trends in the iris (13). This indicates that although TH is the rate limiting enzyme for NE synthesis, other factors contribute to the regulation of NE levels.

AGING IN THE CNS AND PNS

During the aging process in the chicken (following 16 months), both total and specific TH activity decreases in the LC-R and cerebellum, with a greater decline occurring in the cerebellum (Fig. 2B, D). This suggests that noradrenergic terminals may be more affected during the aging process than the cell bodies which is consistent with observations in the aging cholinergic system in the chick (19). A decline in the number of LC cells during aging, which has been reported in humans (2) may at least partially explain the decrease in TH activity in the LC-R. Although NE levels are declining in the cerebellum between 20 months and 3 years (35), as is cerebellar TH activity, NE levels during this period are still relatively high compared to those observed at earlier stages. Vernadakis (35) has suggested that extraneuronal uptake by

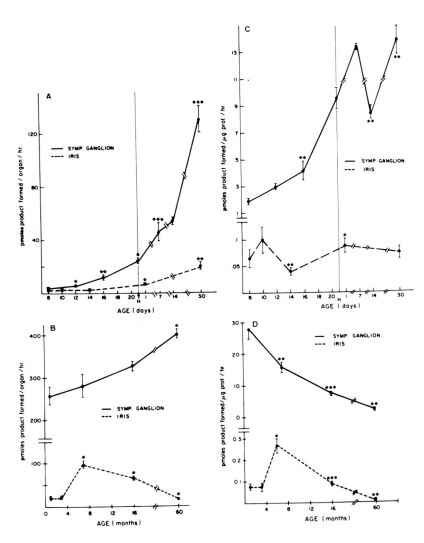

FIG. 3. Developmental pattern of tyrosine hydroxylase activity expressed as pmoles product formed/organ/hr (Fig. A, B) and as pmoles product formed/ug protein/hr (Fig. C, D) in the PNS. Values are the mean ± S.E.M. A significant difference from the preceding age, based on the Student's t test; is indicated by *p<0.05, **p<0.01 and ***p<0.001.

glial cells, which proliferate during aging, may account for these high NE levels found in the cerebellum.

In the aging cervical spinal cord total TH activity remains constant, and specific TH activity actually increases, in contrast to that observed in the cerebellum (Fig. 2B, D). Thus, these two LC target sites show different trends in TH activity during aging which may depend upon different degrees of impairment of enzyme transport from the LC cell bodies or degeneration of the noradrenergic terminals in these target sites. However, further studies are required to elucidate the mechanisms responsible for these observations.

The decrease in TH activity in the LC-R and cerebellum during aging in the chick are in agreement with other reports that demonstrate a decrease in this enzyme activity in the brains of aging humans, and aging rats (27, 28). It is interesting to note that neurochemical events associated with aging begin to occur in the same post-hatching period (1-2 years) in the noradrenergic LC-cerebellar system as well as in the cholinergic ciliary ganglion-iris system (19, 22, 23).

It appears that in noradrenergic terminals of the PNS, as in the CNS, the terminals are more affected than the cell bodies during aging since total TH activity in the iris declines whereas it continually increases in the sympathetic ganglia (Fig. 3B). This may be explained by a decrease in enzyme synthesis or in transport to the terminals as was suggested for cholineacetyltransferase in the ciliary ganglion and iris during aging (19). When comparing cell bodies and terminals, the PNS displays more marked differences in total TH activity than does the CNS. This is consistent with a report by Reis et al. (33), who found greater changes in catecholamine synthesizing enzymes in peripheral structures, such as the adrenal and superior cervical ganglion (SCG) than in various brain regions of aged rodents. In addition, these authors found elevated TH levels in the SCG of aged rats which is in agreement with the high TH levels found in the lumbar sympathetic ganglia in the aged chicken in the present study. However, Reis et al. (33) found no change in TH activity in the LC or in its terminals in the hippocampus in the aged rat.

NOREPINEPHRINE LEVELS AND UPTAKE IN PERIPHERAL NERVE TERMINALS

Significant levels of NE were found in the iris at 7 d.i. prior to the appearance of fluorescence (13-14 d.i.; 17) or Na^+-dependent uptake (10 d.i.). These levels may not be related to the noradrenergic innervation of the iris, as they do not change significantly during the period in which sympathetic innervation is established (up to 14 d.i.; Fig. 4).This NE may be derived from the yolk sac or from other parts of the embryo in which NE is synthesized at these early stages (15). It is interesting in view of the many functional roles which have been proposed for neurotransmitters in early neuro-ontogenesis (29, 37) that significant levels of neurotransmitter are present in this tissue prior to its innervation, and these levels are higher than those found in some older animals. The appearance and rapid increase to near adult levels in NE fluorescence (17) between 14-16 d.i. could be indicative of the appearance and maturation of biosynthetic and concentrative mechanisms for NE resulting in concentrations within the sensitivity of the fluorescence method.

Further changes in these NE levels appear to occur in stages, with a plateau being attained between hatching and one month after hatching,

while the iris protein content increases 3-fold. The large increase in
NE levels between one month and three months after hatching coincides
with a change in the K_m for NE uptake in the iris seen at this stage
(12). Both the change in the NE level and the change in the apparent K_m
of the uptake may reflect posthatching maturation of the retentive capa-
bilities for NE of the nerve terminals.

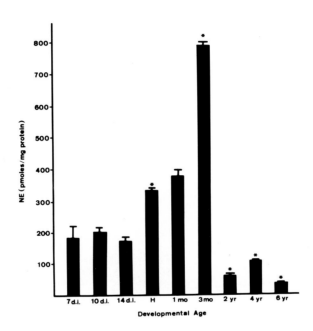

FIG. 4. NE levels in chick iris during development and aging. Each point
        represents the mean + S.E.M.of four samples in duplicate deter-
        minations. *Value significantly different from that of preceding
        age, p < 0.001.

     In the iris, the significant increases in NE levels which occur in
the period 14 d.i. to hatch are paralleled but preceded by increases in
ACh levels (20). Acetylcholine can be measured in the iris at 5 d.i.,and
the level increases between 7 and 10 d.i. to near adult values, preceding a similar rise in NE levels (Fig. 4) during the early phases of innervation in the embryo.
     In the posthatching period the age-related changes in NE levels we
describe follow a pattern very similar to that of ACh in the same iris
preparation (19, 20). Both NE and ACh increase between one month and
three months of age while the protein content of the iris does not
change. Moreover both NE and ACh decline in aging animals to levels below those found in early embryonic tissue. Our results demonstrate that
in the iris NE follows a different developmental profile than ACh during
the early embryonic period, but that these neurotransmitters in peripheral autonomic nerve terminals may share a common susceptibility to aging
     Total accumulation of ^3H-NE by the iris increases slightly from 3

months to 6 months of age (p< 0.05), and is unchanged thereafter (Fig.5). This small difference disappears when the data is normalized per dry weight of tissue, and there is no change in the amount of NE taken up over this period.

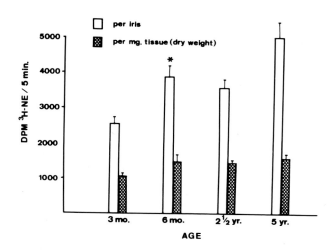

FIG. 5. Changes in NE uptake during aging. Each point represents the mean $\pm$ S.E.M. of 6-12 determinations. *Value significantly different from that of preceding age, p < 0.05.

Some of the biochemical characteristics of ^{3}H-NE uptake in the iris are described in Fig. 6 (14). Reducing the Na^+ concentration in the incubation medium from 145 mM to 25 mM inhibits uptake at all ages (p <0.001). There is, however, a significant (p <0.001) difference in the sensitivity of uptake to inhibition between 6 months and 5 years of age. There is no difference in inhibition of uptake by low Na^+ between 3 and 6 months.

Very similar age differences, though not as marked, are seen in the effects of ouabain (10^{-4}M; Fig. 6B). Uptake is inhibited by ouabain at 3 and 6 months (p <0.001) and at 5 years (p <0.001). There is again a significant (p <0.05) difference between 6 months and 5 years in sensitivity to ouabain, but not between 3 and 6 months.

In Fig. 6C the temperature sensitivity of uptake is shown as the Q_{10} value (V_{37o}/V_{27o}).This value is maintained at a value greater than 3.0 at 3 and 6 months (3.15 and 3.24 respectively) but declines to 2.13 at 5 years of age (6 months – 5 years, p <0.001). Uptake at 0°C does not change with age.

Further age-related changes are seen in the pharmacological characteristics of NE uptake in the iris. There is a steady decrease in the sensitivity of uptake to inhibition by desmethylimipramine (DMI) (Fig. 7) between 6 months and 5 years of age at each concentration (p <0.001). There is a significant difference in values for uptake between 6 months and 2½ years (p <0.01) and between 2½ and 5 years (p <0.001), except the period 2½ to 5 years at 10^{-4}M DMI.

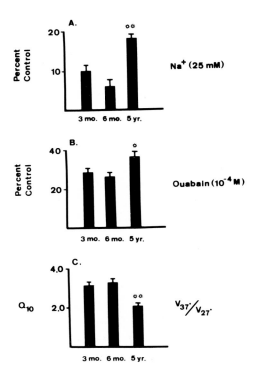

FIG. 6. Characteristics of
NE uptake in chick iris
during aging.
A. Na^+ dependence;
B. Inhibition by ouabain;
C. Temperature sensitivi-
ty. Each point represents
the mean + S.E.M. of 6-10
determinations. Value
significantly different
than that of preceding
age, *p <0.05; **p <0.001.

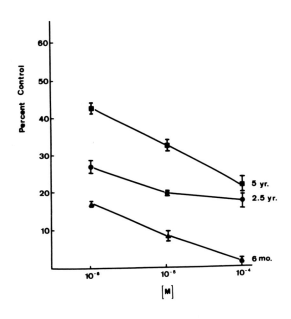

FIG. 7. Inhibition of NE
uptake in chick iris by
DMI during aging. Each
point represents the mean
+ S.E.M. of 6-8 determi-
nations. Significance is
discussed in the text.

These alterations may represent possible age-related changes in the intracellular/extracellular Na^+ gradient or its contribution to NE transport. Other changes may occur either in the general structure of the cell membrane or in intrinsic components of the membrane such as the NE transport system or the Na^+, K^+-ATPase. Changes during maturation and senescence in the relationship between these membrane constituents cannot be overlooked as possible factors.

Norepinephrine levels in the iris decline profoundly in the period between 3 months and 2 years of age (13; Fig. 4).

The levels seen at 2, 4 or 6 years are actually lower than those measured as early as 7 days of incubation, which is prior to the appearance of NE histofluorescence (17) or NE uptake (12) and is almost certainly prior to sympathetic innervation of the iris. While these findings may ·be interpreted as a discrete loss of storage capacity or synthetic activity for NE since TH activity also declines with aging (Fig. 3B, D), it is also possible to infer that a loss of peripheral adrenergic nerve terminals may occur during aging. This is reflected in the reduction in the differentiated functions which are expressed by these nerve terminals. It is less likely that the decline in uptake leads to the decline in NE levels, as levels can be maintained during pharmacological blockade of uptake (30). The state of the adrenergic innervation of the iris can not be simply verified by either histochemical fluorescence nor by autoradiographic techniques, since the observed declines with age of uptake and NE content would provide difficulties in the labeling and identification of aging adrenergic nerve terminals in the periphery. Clarification of this point may require a longitudinal morphometric study of the nerve terminals in the iris. It would be of interest to determine, if a loss of terminals does occur, and if adrenergic receptors on the iris muscle compensate functionally for this loss with a supersensitivity as is seen after denervation.

As far as our experiments can demonstrate, a concurrent loss of DMI sensitivity of NE uptake is not seen in the central nervous system (Fig. 7; 13) although age-related changes in other parameters of central adrenergic function have been reported in other preparations (33, 36). These results have interesting implications in terms of aging and mechanisms of action of drugs.

CONCLUDING REMARKS

Our studies have detailed the significant changes which occur with aging in both the cholinergic and adrenergic components which comprise the peripheral nervous system. Aging can often affect very subtly the biochemical and pharmacological characteristics of many neuronal processes. This is especially true in the central nervous system, in which the changes seem to be less marked than in the periphery, particularly in regard to the adrenergic neurons. It can be clearly seen that a common characteristic of the final period of life of the synapse is a dramatic modification in the metabolism of both ACh and NE, which is seen to occur both centrally and peripherally. The functional consequences of these changes are of great interest to gerontologists.

ACKNOWLEDGMENTS

The investigations carried out in the authors' laboratory were supported by PHS grants NS-11496, NS-11430, NS-15086, and NSF grant

GB-41475 to E.G. and by grants from the University of Connecticut Research Foundation.

REFERENCES

1. Brimijoin, S. (1972): J. Neurochem., 19:2183-2193.
2. Brody, H. (1973): In: Development and Aging of the Nervous System, edited by M. Rockstein, pp. 121-133. Academic Press, New York.
3. Chiappinelli, V., Giacobini, E., Pilar, G., and Uchimura, H. (1976): J. Physiol., 257:749-766.
4. Dahl, A., Giacobini, E., Serra, G., and Manara, L. (1980): J.Neurosci. Res., 5:73-78.
5. Dolezalova, H., Giacobini, E., Giacobini, G., Rossi, A., and Toschi, G. (1974): Brain Res., 73:309-320.
6. Enemar, A., Falck, B., and Hakanson, R. (1965): Dev. Biol., 11: 268-283.
7. Fairman, K., Giacobini, E., and Chiappinelli, V. (1976): Brain Res. 102:301-312.
8. Filogamo, G., Giacobini, E., Giacobini, G., and Nore, B. (1971): J. Neurochem., 18:1589-1591.
9. Geffen, L.B., and Rush, R. (1968): J. Neurochem.,15:925-930.
10. Giacobini, E. (1978): In: Maturation of Neurotransmission, edited by A. Vernadakis, E. Giacobini, and G. Filogamo, pp. 41-64. S. Karger, Basel.
11. Giacobini, E. (1979): In: Neural Growth and Differentiation, edited by E. Meisami, and M.A.B. Brazier, pp. 153-167. Raven Press.
12. Hoffman, D., and Giacobini, E. (1980): Brain Res.,201:57-70.
13. Hoffman, D., Salzman, S.K., Marchi, M., and Giacobini, E. (1980): J. Neurochem., 34:1785-1787.
14. Hoffman, D.W., Marchi, M., and Giacobini, E. (1980) Neurobiol.Aging, 1:48-51.
15. Ignarro, L.J., and Shideman, E. (1968): J. Pharm. Exp. Ther. 159: 38-48.
16. Jungherr, L. (1969): In: Avian Disease: The Neuroanatomy of the Domestic Fowl, pp. 107-108. The Amer. Assoc. of Avian Pathologists, Amherst, MA.
17. Kirby, M.L., Diab, I.M., and Mattio, T.G. (1978): Anat. Rec., 191: 311-320.
18. Levitt, M., Spector, S., Sjoerdsma, A., and Udenfriend, S. (1965): J. Pharmac. Exp. Ther., 148:1-18.
19. Marchi, M., and Giacobini, E. (1980): Dev. Neurosci. 3:39-48.
20. Marchi, M., Giacobini, E., and Hruschak, K. (1979): Dev. Neurosci., 2:201-212.
21. Marchi, M., Hoffman, D.W., and Giacobini, E. (1980): In: Aging of the Brain and Dementia, edited by L. Amaducci, A.N. Davison, and P. Antuono, pp. 159-166. Raven Press, New York.
22. Marchi, M., Hoffman, D.W., Giacobini, E., and Fredrickson, T. (1980): Brain Res.,195: 423-432.
23. Marchi, M., Hoffman, D.W., Giacobini, E., and Fredrickson, T. (1980): Dev. Neurosci., 3:235-247.
24. Marchi, M., Hoffman, D.W., Giacobini, E., and Volle, R. (1981): Dev. Neurosci., 6:444-453.
25. Marchi, M., Hoffman, D.W., Mussini, E., and Giacobini, E. (1980): Dev. Neurosci., 3:183-196.

26. Marchi, M., Yurkewicz, L., Giacobini, E., and Fredrickson, T. (1981): Dev. Neurosci., 4:258-266.
27. McGeer, E.G., Fibiger, H.C., McGeer, P.L., and Wickson, V. (1971): Exp. Geront., 6:391-396.
28. McGeer, P.L., and McGeer, E.G. (1976): J. Neurochem., 26:65-76.
29. McMahon, D. (1974): Science, N.Y., 185:1012-1021.
30. Molinoff, P.B., and Axelrod, J. (1971): Ann. Rev. Biochem., 40:465-500.
31. Mugnaini, E., and Dahl, A. (1975): J. Comp. Neurol., 162:417-432.
32. Oesch, F., Otten, U., and Thoenen, H. (1973): J. Neurochem., 20:1691-1706.
33. Reis, J., Ross, R.A., and Joh, T.H. (1977): Brain Res., 136:465-474.
34. Singer, H.S., Coyle, J.T., Vernon, N., Kallman, C.H., and Price, D. (1980): Brain Res., 191:417-428.
35. Vernadakis, A. (1973): In: Progress in Brain Research, Neurobiological Aspects of Maturation and Aging, edited by D.H. Ford, pp. 231-243, Elsevier Sci., Amsterdam.
36. Vernadakis, A., and Arnold, E.B. (1979): In: Advances in Cellular Neurobiology, edited by S. Fedoroff, and L. Hertz, Academic press, New York.
37. Vernadakis, A., and Gibson, D.A. (1974): In: Perinatal Pharmacology, edited by J. Dancis, and J.C. Hwang, pp. 65-76, Raven Press, New York.
38. Wooten, G.F., and Coyle, J.T. (1973): J. Neurochem., 20:1361-1371.
39. Yurkewicz, L., Marchi, M., Lauder, J.M., and Giacobini, E. (1981): J. Neurosci. Res. 6:638-647.

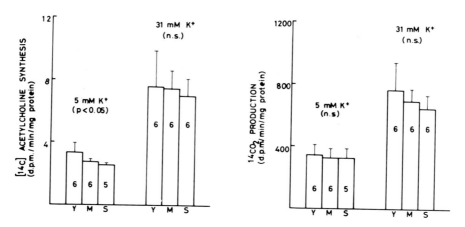

FIG.1. Effect of aging on ^{14}C-acetylcholine synthesis and $^{14}CO_2$ production in neocortex from CFY rats. Animals were divided into three age groups: young adult (Y), mean age 168 d (range 147-191 d); mature adult (M), mean age 400 d (range 365-431 d); senescent adult (S), mean age 808 d (range 739-852 d). Histograms show mean and standard deviation for the number of animals indicated. Statistical comparison of the three groups was by one way analysis of variance. Modified from Sims <u>et al</u> (27).

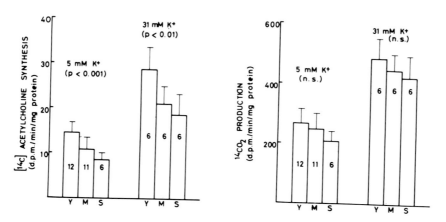

FIG.2. Effect of aging on ^{14}C-acetylcholine synthesis and $^{14}CO_2$ production in striatum of CFY rats. Other details as described in Fig.1.

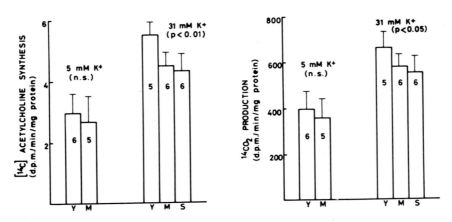

FIG.3. Effect of aging on ^{14}C-acetylcholine synthesis and $^{14}CO_2$ production in hippocampus of CFY rats. Other details as described in Fig.1.

and striatum were examined from CFY rats of three age groups and results are shown in Figs. 1-3. For all measurements made there was some tendency for a decline with age. There was no significant change in either $^{14}CO_2$ production or ^{14}C-acetylcholine synthesis in the neocortex (Fig.1) for incubations in 31 mM K^+, consistent with the findings in human brain. In 5 mM K^+, ^{14}C-acetylcholine synthesis declined significantly although the change was greater between the young adult and mature adult animals than between these and the truly senescent animals. By far the largest age-associated changes were found in the striatum where ^{14}C-acetylcholine synthesis was reduced for measurements made in both 5 mM K^+ and 31 mM K^+ in the absence of significant changes in $^{14}CO_2$ production (Fig.2). This decrease occurred over the whole of the aging period examined, although again the changes were greater between the youngest and middle groups. In the hippocampus a significant change in ^{14}C-acetylcholine synthesis was observed for incubations in 31 mM K^+ which was probably related to a decline in glucose metabolism as there was a parallel change in $^{14}CO_2$ production (Fig.3). Both changes were primarily evident between the two younger groups of animals.

Examination of these three regions in a second strain of rats (Porton-Wistar) for two age groups similar to the young adult and mature adult groups of the CFY rats confirmed the changes in the striatum and neocortex but did not show significant differences in the hippocampus (29).

In order to further assess the stability of the neocortex (when measured in 31 mM K^+) two other markers of presynaptic cholinergic function were examined. ^{14}C-acetylcholine release and the stimulation of this (presumably through presynaptic muscarinic receptors) by the muscarinic antagonist, atropine, were found not to be significantly changed between groups of Porton-Wistar rats of average ages, 189 d, 479 d and 834 d (29).

Thus the investigation of aging in rats largely confirms the relative stability of the neocortex observed in the human studies and indicates that the striatum may be more vulnerable to age-related changes. The observation that the changes found were greater between the youngest animals and mature group than between mature and senescent animals raises questions as to the relevance of these findings to functional declines in normal aging. Thus these may in fact represent late programmed developmental changes which continue at least beyond 13 m and are not related to deleterious changes in performance associated with very old age. Rats older than 3 m are commonly considered for experimental purposes to be fully mature and similar findings for other biochemical parameters may require reappraisal of this assessment. A similar pattern of age dependent change has been reported for glucose utilization in rats determined in vivo (30). One explanation suggested for these findings was that the oldest animals were selected by virtue of their survival and provided values which were not representative of the population as a whole thus possibly under-estimating the age-related change.

Alzheimer's Disease

Table 2 shows the results for samples from neocortex of patients with Alzheimer's disease compared to normal neocortex. ^{14}C-acetylcholine synthesis was reduced by approximately 50% for measurements in both 5 mM K+ and 31 mM K+. The reduction was not due to a decrease in overall glucose metabolism and was not found in a group of 6 demented patients where the biopsy samples failed to show the characteristic histological features of Alzheimer's disease. There was a correlation between the activity of the enzyme choline acetyltransferase and the production of ^{14}C-acetylcholine (28) consistent with there being a loss of functional cholinergic nerve endings in the tissue from the patients with Alzheimer's disease (such that the presynaptic cholinergic markers were lost in parallel). The remaining terminals responded in an apparently normal way to stimulation by K+.

TABLE 2. ^{14}C-acetylcholine synthesis and $^{14}CO_2$ production in biopsy samples from patients with Alzheimer's disease and controls[a,b]

	K+ (mM)	^{14}C-acetylcholine synthesis (d.p.m./min/mg protein)	$^{14}CO_2$ production (d.p.m./min/mg protein)
Controls	5	3.6 + 1.7 (19)	573 + 121 (19)
	31	7.3 + 1.4 (20)	1479 + 328 (20)
Alzheimer's disease	5	1.8 + 0.6 (9)*b	814 + 193 (9)**
	31	3.4 + 1.2 (13)**	2059 + 352 (13)**

[a] Alzheimer's disease diagnosed by presence of characteristic histological features; control samples were from apparently normal material removed to allow access to tumors.

[b] Values shown are mean + standard deviation. Results significantly different from control are indicated *p < 0.01; **p < 0.001 (Student's t-test).

Production of $^{14}CO_2$ was significantly increased in the samples from Alzheimer's disease cases. Interpretation of this requires further investigation but possible explanations include changes in the turnover rate or size of an intermediate pool (leading to a change in dilution of label without a change in actual CO_2 production), increased numbers of mitochondria or partial uncoupling of the glucose metabolism.

CONCLUSIONS

The relative stability observed for the ^{14}C-acetylcholine synthesis in the neocortex and (at least between the older groups of animals) in hippocampus leaves unexplained the close similarity between changes of cognitive and memory function associated with old age and cholinergic drug administration. The measurement of ^{14}C-acetylcholine synthesis probably reflects the potential for presynaptic cholinergic function in the tissue in that the incubations were performed in a defined media without the influences from the milieu which may occur in vivo. Furthermore electron micrographs of the prism preparation showed that the synaptic endings (which are the major site for synthesis of acetylcholine for neurotransmission) were well preserved but did not maintain connections with intact cell bodies (27), thus being largely free from influences of the neural circuitry. Hence, whilst the present studies indicate that the presynaptic synthetic capacity of these regions is largely unimpaired in aging, changes may occur in presynaptic function in vivo from the presence of inhibitory chemicals (perhaps acting through presynaptic receptors) or from a sub-optimal response because of deleterious changes in other neurotransmitter systems impinging on the cholinergic neurons. Alternatively the functional deficits may reflect changes in post-synaptic binding sites or response to acetylcholine. Binding of the muscarinic antagonist quinuclidinyl benzilate (QNB) has been found to be reduced with age in human neocortex (35) as well as rat and mouse neocortex (32) and rat hippocampus (14), the latter being accompanied by a decrease of response to iontophoretically applied acetylcholine in pyramidal cells. As the presynaptic synthetic capacity is largely maintained, identification and reversal of the defect could result in restoration of normal function.

Declines in synthesis of ^{14}C-acetylcholine in the striatum with age indicated a greater loss of presynaptic function. Several studies of choline acetyltransferase activity in aging rat brain have also shown a greater vulnerability of this region (13,17,19) although in each case changes reported were smaller (17-27%) than those found for ^{14}C-acetylcholine synthesis even though the comparisons of choline acetyltransferase activities were made to younger (1-2 month old) animals. These results combined with a report of decreased QNB binding for striatum in aged rats and mice (32) suggest that the cholinergic system may be undergoing partial degeneration with age in this region.

Estimates of glucose utilization from $^{14}CO_2$ production indicated little or no change with age for all regions. Other attempts to investigate glucose metabolism in vitro have not provided consistent results but in those studies where changes were found these have been small (8, 9,20,21,34). Estimates of glucose utilization in vivo also indicate little change in most regions beyond 12-16 months (15,30). Some regions show changes at ages younger than this which were greater than any found in vitro, suggesting that these may be reflecting reduced functional activity rather than changes in the ability of the brain tissue to respond.

The results from the examination of aging effects in either humans or rats would not seem to provide evidence that the large changes in ^{14}C-acetylcholine synthesis in Alzheimer's disease represent an exacerbation of the normal aging process. The decrease in markers of the cholinergic system has been found to relate to changes in mental function in patients with Alzheimer's disease (24,28) consistent with an involvement of the neurotransmitter defect in the disease symptoms. Following the successes associated with neurotransmitter replacement therapy using L-DOPA in Parkinsonism, similar attempts have been made to reverse the cholinergic deficiency in Alzheimer's disease, particularly with precursors such as choline or lecithin (3,7,26,36). Although any attempts at rational therapy should not be discouraged, the analogy between dopaminergic neurons in the nigro-striatal pathway and cholinergic neurons involved in memory and cognition may be oversimplistic. Presumably cognitive function requires the activation of specific complex neuronal circuits in a programmed fashion. The results presented here indicate that the tissue has lost a large proportion of its capacity for synthesis of acetylcholine and provides some evidence (from the parallel loss of choline acetyltransferase) that this may be the result of a reduction in the number of functional cholinergic nerve endings. As the remaining acetylcholine synthesis still responds normally (at least to K^+ stimulation), increasing the acetylcholine synthesis non-specifically in this reduced pool of synaptic endings may be ineffective in the absence of many of the normal neuronal connections.

REFERENCES

1. Bowen, D.M., Smith, C.B., White, P., and Davison, A.N. (1976): Brain, 99: 459-496.
2. Bowen, D.M., White, P., Spillane, J.A., Goodhardt, M.J., Curzon, G., Iwangoff, P., Meier-Ruge, W., and Davison, A.N. (1979): Lancet, i: 11-14.
3. Boyd, W.D., Graham-White, J., Blackwood, G., Glen, I., and McQueen, J. (1977): Lancet, ii: 711.
4. Davies, P. (1979): Brain Res., 171: 319-327.
5. Davies, P., and Maloney, A.J.F. (1976): Lancet, ii: 1403.
6. Drachman, D.A., and Sahakian, B.J. (1980): In: The Psychobiology of Aging: Problems and Perspectives, edited by D.G.Stein, pp.347-368. Elsevier/North Holland, New York.
7. Etienne, P., Gauthier, S., Johnson, G., Collier, B., Mendis, T., Dastoor, D., Cole, M., and Muller, H.F. (1978): Lancet, i: 508-509.
8. Fox, J.H., Parmacek, M.S., and Patel-Mandlick, K. (1975): Gerontologia, 21: 224-230.
9. Garbus, J. (1955): Am.J.Physiol., 183: 618-619.
10. Gibson, G.E., and Blass, J.P. (1976): J.Neurochem., 26: 1073-1078.
11. Gibson, G.E., and Blass, J.P. (1976): J.Neurochem., 27: 37-46.
12. Gibson, G.E., Jope, R., and Blass, J.P. (1975): Biochem.J., 148: 17-23.
13. Lai, J.C.K., Leung, T.K.C., and Lim, L. (1981): J.Neurochem., 36: 1443-1448.
14. Lippa, A.S., Pelham, R.W., Beer, B., Critchett, D.J., Dean, R.L., and Bartus, R.T. (1980): Neurobiol.of aging, 1: 13-19.
15. London, E.D., Nespor, S.M., Ohata, M., and Rapoport, S.I. (1981): J.Neurochem., 37: 217-221.

16. Marchbanks, R.M., and Wonnacott, S. (1979): Prog.Brain Res., 49: 77-88
17. McGeer, E.G., Fibiger, H.C., McGeer, P.L., and Wickson, V. (1971): Exp.Gerontol., 6: 391-396.
18. McGeer, E., and McGeer, P.L. (1976): In: Neurobiology of Aging, edited by R.D.Terry and S.Gershon, pp.389-403, Raven Press, New York.
19. Meek, J.L., Bertilson, L., Cheney, D.L., Zsilla, G., and Costa, E. (1977): J.Gerontol., 32: 129-131.
20. Parmacek, M.S., Fox, J.H., Harrison, W.H., Garron, D.C., and Swenie, D. (1979): Gerontol., 25: 185-191.
21. Peng, M.-T., Peng, Y.-I, and Chen, F.-N (1977): J.Gerontol., 32: 517-522.
22. Perry, E.K., Perry, R.H., Blessed, G., and Tomlinson, B.E. (1977): J.Neurol.Sci., 34: 247-265.
23. Perry, E.K., Perry, R.H., Gibson, P.H., Blessed, G., and Tomlinson, B.E. (1977): Neurosci.Lett., 6: 85-89.
24. Perry, E.K., Tomlinson, B.E., Blessed, G., Bergmann, K., Gibson, P.H., and Perry, R.H. (1978): Brit.Med.J., ii: 1457-1459.
25. Reisine, T.D., Yamamura, H., Bird, E.D., Spokes, E., and Enna, S.J. (1978): Brain Res., 159: 477-482.
26. Signoret, J.L., Whiteley, A., and Lhermitte, F. (1978): Lancet, ii: 837.
27. Sims, N.R., Bowen, D.M., and Davison, A.N. (1981): Biochem.J., 196: 867-876.
28. Sims, N.R., Bowen, D.M., Smith, C.C.T., Flack, R.H.A., Davison, A.N., Snowden, J.S., and Neary, D. (1980): Lancet, i: 333-336.
29. Sims, N.R., Marek, K.L., Bowen, D.M., and Davison, A.N. (1981): J.Neurochem., (in press).
30. Smith, C.B., Goochee, C., Rapaport, S.L., and Sokoloff, L. (1980): Brain, 103: 351-365.
31. Spokes, E.G.S. (1979): Brain, 102: 333-346.
32. Strong, R., Hicks, P., Hsu, L., Bartus, R.T., and Enna, S.J. (1980): Neurobiol.of aging, i: 59-63.
33. Tucek, S. (1978): Acetylcholine synthesis in Neurones, Chapman and Hall, London
34. Weinbach, E.C., and Garbus, J. (1956): Nature, 178: 1226-1227.
35. White, P., Hiley, C.R., Goodhardt, M.J., Carrasco, L.H., Keet, J.P., Williams, I.E.I., and Bowen, D.M. (1977): Lancet, i: 668-671.
36. Yates, C.M., Blackburn, I.A., Christie, J.E., Glen, A.I.M., Shering, A., Simpson, J., Whalley, L.J., and Zeisel, S. (1980): In: Biochemistry of Dementia, edited by P.J.Roberts, pp.185-212, John Wiley and Sons, Chichester.

The Aging Brain: Cellular and Molecular Mechanisms of Aging in the Nervous System, edited by E. Giacobini et al., Raven Press, New York © 1982.

Microspectrofluorimetric Quantitation of Histochemically Demonstrable Catecholamines in Peripheral and Brain Catecholamine-Containing Neurons in Male Fischer-344 Rats at Different Ages

Matti Partanen, *Antti Hervonen, and Stanley I. Rapoport

*Laboratory of Neurosciences, Gerontology Research Center, National Institute of Aging, Baltimore City Hospitals, Baltimore, Maryland 21224; *Department of Biomedical Sciences, University of Tampere, SF 33101 Tampere 10, Finland*

The age-related changes in the perikaryonal catecholamine stores of both peripheral and central catecholamine-containing neurons were mapped using microspectrofluorimetry of formaldehyde-induced catecholamine fluorescence in 3-, 12-, 24- and 32-month-old Fischer-344 male rats. The catecholamine fluorescence was measured in two peripheral ganglia (superior cervical ganglion and hypogastric ganglion) and in the brain regions known to contain dopamine ($A_{8-10,12}$) norepinephrine (A_{6-7}) and epinephrine neurons (A_{1-2}). To ascertain the real changes in catecholamine content the nonspecific fluorescence of lipofuscin pigment was subtracted from the total fluorescence.

The two peripheral sympathetic ganglia were different in relation to age and transmitter stores. The catecholamine fluorescence decreased significantly with age in the hypogastric ganglion but not in the superior cervical ganglion. The changes in the different brain regions were only slight and a statistically significant decrease in catecholamine fluorescence was detected only in the A_{12} dopamine-containing neurons.

While the biochemical data from the brain indicates a clear decrease in the catecholamine stores, the perikaryonal concentrations can remain unchanged. Microspectrofluorimetry provides advantages in comparison with the biochemical methods when the location of the fluorescent catecholamine is known. The total amine figures at different ages may cover several degenerative and/or compensatory changes.

Abbreviations:

BAF = background autofluorescence
CMGC = coeliac-mesenteric ganglion complex
FIF = formaldehyde-induced fluorescence
HGL = hypogastric ganglion
SCG = superior cervical ganglion

INTRODUCTION

The formaldehyde-induced fluorescence of catecholamines has been used with different experimental conditions in both peripheral and central monoamine-containing neurons (21; 31; 38). Functional changes have been observed in enzyme activities (2), catecholamine content at the terminal neuroeffector level (40) and in neuronal perikarya (1). Age-related changes in activities of catecholamine-synthesizing enzymes and in formaldehyde-induced fluorescence have also been characterized in peripheral sympathetic ganglia (15; 31; 37; 38) and in the brain (16; 37) of the rat. In addition to the histochemical studies, abundant data on agerelated changes in the neurotransmitter content of different brain regions have been obtained using biochemical methods (see 35).

In addition to the developmental studies (13; 14; 22; 29), the few studies which describe the changes in formaldehyde-induced fluorescence with age have been made either on one peripheral sympathetic ganglion (15; 31; 32; 38; 39) or on single brain region (16). So far an overview of age-related changes in the entire catecholamine-containing system is missing. In the present study we therefore examine the relation of aging to histochemically demonstrable catecholamines in two peripheral ganglia and in neurons containing dopamine, norepinephrine and epinephrine in the brain. The Fischer-344 rat was selected for investigation because of its frequent use in aging studies and its availability from a barrier-reared colony. The maximal lifespan of this strain approximates 36 months (6).

MATERIALS AND METHODS

Sixteen male Fischer-344 rats were obtained from Charles River Breeding laboratories (NIA breeding program, Wilmington, Mass.). The rats were 3-, 12-, 24- and 32-months of age, four in each group. After delivery, the rats were housed in an animal cage for 1 to 2 weeks. The rats were anesthetized with sodium pentobarbital (40 mg kg^{-1}, ip). The hypogastric ganglon (HGL), and superior cervical ganglion (SCG) were removed. In addition, the skull was opened and the brain removed and cut immediately into 1 mm-thick coronal sections. The samples were frozen in Freon cooled by liquid nitrogen.

The formaldehyde-induced fluorescence (FIF) method was used to demonstrate catecholamines (9). Samples were freeze-dried for 10 days at -45°C under a vacuum of 10^{-5} Torr, and then were warmed under vacuum. After breaking the vacuum, the samples were treated for 1 h at 80°C with paraformaldehyde vapor equilibrated to 75% relative humidity, and then vacuum-embedded in paraffin. Small pieces of muscle, and 4% gelatin samples with different norepinephrine concentrations (0, 10, 50, 100, 500 and 1000 µg/ml) served as internal standards and were processed in the same way as were the experimental tissues. Tissue samples from two animals in each of four age groups were processed simultaneously with the standards.

The samples were sectioned serially at 10 µm. Peripheral sympathetic ganglia as well as regions in the CNS with catecholamine neurons were identified on the basis of the specific catecholamine fluorescence (FIF). Each sample was sectioned separately and measured immediately thereafter. Sections, 80 to 120 µm apart, were subjected to microspectrofluorimetric measurement. The intensity of FIF was recorded in the SCG and in HGL, and in brain neurons which contained epinephrine (A_1, A_2), norepinephrine (A_6, A_7) and dopamine (A_8, A_9, A_{10}, A_{12}) according to classification based on catecholamine histofluorescence (7) and immunohistochemical mapping. In the brain, the FIF of A_1 and A_2 neurons, which contain epinephrine (19), was pooled (A_{1-2}). Neurons containing norepinephrine (10; 11; 28) in A_6 and A_7 groups were handled separately, as well as neurons containing dopamine in A_8, A_9, A_{10} and A_{12} (20). For further references see Moore and Bloom, (26; 27). In each group, 30 to 150 recordings were made per animal. The numbers of recordings in the HGL, SCG, A_6 and A_9 neurons are given with fluorescence profiles (Figs. 3, 4, 5, 6).

A Leitz MPV-2 microscope equipped with a photomultiplier (S-20) and with PLOEM-II type epi-illuminator was used. Filter block D, which contained specific filters (BG 3, KP 425, TK 455, K 460) for demonstration of FIF, was used for microscopy as well as for FIF intensity measurements. Measurements were made with a 40 x oil objective (Leitz). The diameter of the measuring spot, 10 μm, allowed intracytoplasmic measurements from the perikarya. During measurement the field iris diaphragm was used to avoid fading of fluorescence in surrounding neurons.

After registration of the FIF, the section was treated with 2% sodium borohydride in aqueous solution to disperse the FIF due to the catecholamine, and the catecholamine-containing neurons were remeasured, as described above, to map background autofluorescence (BAF). In each region (HGL, SCG, pooled BAF in A_{1-7}, pooled BAF in A_{8-12}), 20 to 40 measurements were made per animal and mean BAF was substracted from mean FIF to give FIF-BAF, which represent the real catecholamine fluorescence. This was important because the emission curve of lipofuscin autofluorescence partly overlaps with that of catecholamine fluorescence and may affect results. Furthermore it should be pointed out that the BAF values do not represent the overall change of lipofuscin autofluorescence with age, because the filters used were for catecholamine fluorescence and the exication and emission curves are different for lipofuscin and catecholamines. FIF, BAF and FIF-BAF are illustrated in Fig. 2. The intensities of FIF and BAF in HGL, SCG, A_6 and A_9 were divided into intensity classes and are given as fluorescence profiles (Figs. 3, 4, 5, 6). FIF, BAF and FIF-BAF were tested for significance at the $p < 0.05$ level with the Duncan one-way variance test (8). Means $\pm$ S.D. and significant age-related differences in each region are given in Fig. 2.

Norepinephrine standards were recorded (30-40 measurements/per standard) as the samples described above. The intensity of catecholamine fluorescence was found to be related linearly to the norepinephrine concentration (Fig. 1.).

RESULTS

Peripheral Sympathetic Ganglia

The formaldehyde-induced fluorescence after subtraction of the nonspecific background fluorescence, FIF-BAF, which represents the actual catecholamine fluorescence, showed a significant decrease in the hypogastric ganglion (Fig. 2) but not in the superior cervical ganglion. The decrease of FIF-BAF in the hypogastric ganglion was statistically significant ($p<0.05$) between 3 and 12 months.

Brain

The brain areas were divided into groups according the catecholamine presumably responsible for the histofluorescence. Thus the possible

differences in the fate of dopamine, norepinephrine and epinephrine could
be studied. However, no major differences with age were seen. Statistically insignificant changes were seen in most of the regions
mapped (Fig. 2). Only in A_{12} dopamine-containing neurons did FIF-BAF
decrease significantly with age between 24 and 32 months (Fig. 2).

Fluorescence Profiles

Each group of catecholamine neurons consists of neuronal perikarya
emitting different intensities of formaldehyde-induced fluorescence. To
describe this variation of FIF from cell to cell and to detect even
smaller functional shifts in the cellular catecholamine stores, the
measurements from certain regions are also given as fluorescence profiles
(Figs 3-6). The fluorescence profile of FIF in the HGL shifted to the
left, indicating an increase of the weakly fluorescent neurons with age.
In SCG, fluorescence profiles of FIF showed only minimal changes.
(Fig. 4).

In the A_6 group of norepinephrine neurons of the brain, the profile of
FIF betrayed a small shift to the left. In the A_9 group of dopamine
neurons there was a slight tendency of the major fluorescence profile to
shift leftwards (Fig. 6).

The profiles of background autofluorescence are seen as inverted
columns in the same figures (Fig. 3-6). They showed a clear shift to the
right in each region studied, indicating an increase in autofluorescence
material, mostly in lipofuscin.

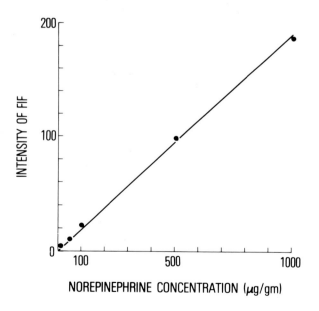

Fig. 1. The intensity of formaldehyde-induced catecholamine fluorescence
is linear with norepinephrine concentration of gelatin standards. Fluorescence intensity is expressed as working units.

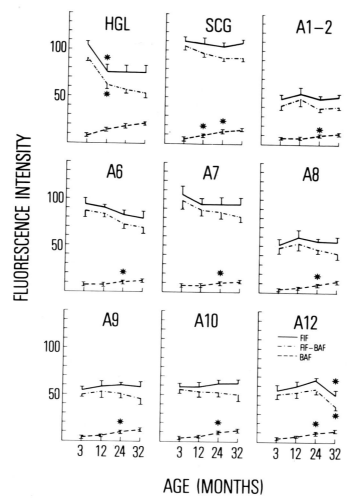

AGE (MONTHS)

Fig. 2. Age-dependent changes for total fluorescence after formal-dehyde-induced fluorescence (FIF), background fluorescence (BAF) and substraction of FIF-BAF are given in four different age groups in both peripheral and central catecholamine neurons. The curve explanations are given in the right lower corner. Each point represents the mean of four animals; ± S.D. is given with BAF and 1/2 S.D. with FIF and FIF-BAF. Stars indicate significant difference from the preceding age group at the $p < 0.05$ level.

Fig. 3-6. The fluorescence intensities of total (FIF) and backkground fluorescence (BAF) of the hypogastric ganglion (HGL) (Fig. 3), superior cervical ganglion (SCG) (Fig. 4), brain A_6 norepinephrine neurons (Fig. 5) and brain A_9 dopamine neurons in four different age groups were divided into intensity classes (1-9; 10-19; etc.) and are given as fluorescence profiles. The profiles for background fluorescence are inverted. The number of measurements for FIF are given within the profile. For BAF, the percentage of neurons within one intensity class is given beside the profile if exceeding 50%.

PERCENT (%)
HGL 3 months
456
HGL 12 months
432
64
HGL 24 months
419
HGL 32 months
368
FLUORESCENCE INTENSITY

Fig. 3

PERCENT (%)
SCG 3 months
451
100
SCG 12 months
545
SCG 24 months
434
SCG 32 months
542
FLUORESCENCE INTENSITY

Fig. 4

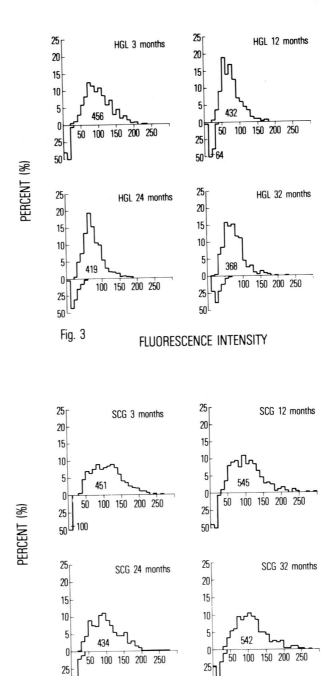

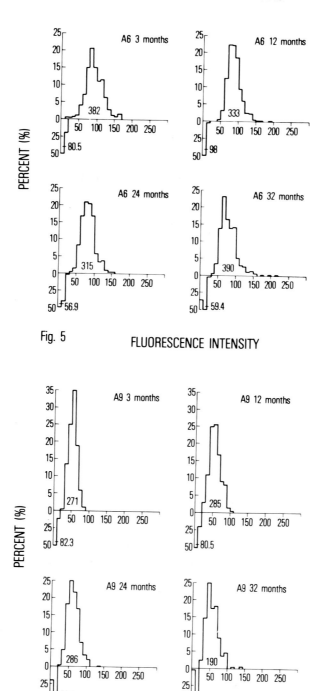

PERCENT (%)
A6 3 months
382
80.5
A6 12 months
333
98
A6 24 months
315
56.9
A6 32 months
390
59.4
FLUORESCENCE INTENSITY

Fig. 5

PERCENT (%)
A9 3 months
271
82.3
A9 12 months
285
80.5
A9 24 months
286
79.4
A9 32 months
190
97.4
FLUORESCENCE INTENSITY

Fig. 6

<u>Comparison of Peripheral and Brain Catecholamine-containing Neurons</u>

In both peripheral sympathetic ganglia of 3-month old rats the mean intensity of FIF was almost the same, and comparable to intensity in norepinephrine-containing neurons in brain regions A_6 and A_7. The intensity of FIF was lower in epinephrine (A_{1-2})- and in dopamine (A_8, A_9, A_{10}, A_{12})-containing neurons (Fig. 2). Although mean FIF intensity was almost the same in the HGL, SCG and A_6 neurons, their fluorescence profiles of FIF were different. The profile was wide in the HGL and SCG but narrow in the A_6 neurons (Fig. 5) and neurons of other brain regions (Fig. 6).

BAF intensity also varied among regions. It was highest in the HGL in every age group and increased less with age in the brain neurons than in the peripheral sympathetic ganglia (Fig. 2).

DISCUSSION

The biochemical data on the age-related changes in different trans- mitters usually describe a sum effect of certain developments in a given region of the brain. A histochemical approach is needed to characterize and localize the possible underlying processes. Due to the high speci- ficity and sensitivity of the formaldehyde-induced fluorescence method, microspectrofluorimetry provides a reliable mean of measuring cellular catecholamine content. In the present study, we relate the catecholamine fluorescence to age in peripheral and central catecholamine neurons. The results indicate that catecholamine concentrations change with age only in selected groups of peripheral and central catecholamine-containing neurons. The fluorescence decreases significantly only in the hypo- gastric ganglion and in the brain in A_{12} dopamine neurons.

Catecholamine concentrations have been shown to decrease with age in the HGL (31) and in the coeliac-mesenteric ganglion complex (CMGC) (38) of rats. The present finding for HGL agrees with these earlier results. Neuronal density also decreases with age in the HGL (30). These age- dependent changes may be related to age-dependent changes in respective target organs. The target tissue of sympathetic neurons can affect their neuronal number and size, catecholamine content and the activity of catecholamine-synthesizing enzymes in peripheral sympathetic neurons (2).

Although the catecholamine concentration does not change significantly with age in the SCG, the activity of tyrosine hydroxylase and choline acetyltransferase, rate-limiting enzymes in catecholamine and acetyl- choline synthesis respectively, increases (37). Glucose utilization (a measure of functional activity) also increases with age (30). These observations, together with increased plasma catecholamines in older Fischer-344 rats (4) suggest that overall sympathetic activity might increase with age in the SCG.

Age-dependent changes in catecholamine content and synthetizing enzymes may be regulated by changes in electrical input but also intrinsic senescence of the neuron itself may also play a role. The activity of monoamine oxidase, an intracytoplasmic degradative enzyme for catecholamines, increases with age in the rat (36). Also the norepinephrine uptake changes with age in the chicken iris (17).

In brain catecholamine neurons, catecholamine fluorescence decreases significantly in A_{12} dopamine neurons, but not in the other neurons. In the rat hypothalamus, the dopamine concentration and dopamine turnover decreases with age (25; 34; 41). However, tyrosine hydroxylase activity increases in the hypothalamus (37). The activity of monoamine oxidase, an enzyme responsible for intracellular degradation of catecholamines, increases in the whole brain of the rat (3; 18; 42). Despite the earlier evidence for decreased dopamine concentration, dopamine fluorescence did not change in the dopamine neurons of groups A_8, A_9 and A_{10}. The discrepancy may be due to the fact that in the present study the measurements were made on neuronal perikarya, whereas in earlier studies catecholamine concentrations were measured per organ weight, and may reflected changes in surrounding tissues.

A_{12} dopamine neurons are located at the arcuate nucleus and innervate the median eminence, and are important factors in the feedback regulation of secretion of pituitary hormones. They are a target for peripherally-secreted testosterone, whereas A_8, A_9 and A_{10} dopamine neurons do not concentrate tritiated testosterone (12). A_{12} neurons regulate secretion of prolaction, growth hormone, melanocyte-stimulating hormone and gonadotropin (5; 23; 24; 33). We found that dopamine fluorescence does not change significantly in A_{12} neurons between 3 and 24 months but decreases significantly between 24 and 32 months of age. These changes might be related to possible changes in hormonal patterns with age and/or also to hypothalamic aging. It should be noted, however, that Hoffman and Sladek (16) reported an increae in dopamine fluorescence and number of fluorescent neurons in the arcuate nucleus between 3 and 28 months. The discrepancy may be due to differences between age group.

In norepinephrine neurons (A_6, A_7) and epinephrine neurons (A_{1-2}) no significant changes were observed in catecholamine fluorescence. Previous reports indicate that norepinephrine concentration decreases (25; 41), norepinephrine turnover decreases or is constant (34; 41) and tyrosine hydroxylase and monoamine oxidase activities increase (37) with age in some or all of these neurons.

Although A_6 and A_7 neurons can concentrate tritiated testosterone as can A_{12} neurons in arcuate nucleus (12), A_6 and A_7 neurons show no changes in catecholamine fluorescence, whereas in A_{12} neurons catecholamine fluorescence decreases significantly between 24 and 32 months. This difference may reflect anatomical and functional differences between the neuron groups. A_{12} neurons contain dopamine as a neurotransmitter (20), are located in the arcuate nucleus, send short axons to the median eminence and pituitary, and mainly regulate secretion of pituitary hormones. A_6 and A_7 neurons contain norepinephrine (10), are located in the pons in the locus coeruleus (A_6) and near of the lemiscus lateralis (A_7), and project to the di- and telencephalon including the cerebral cortex and brain stem, the cerebellum and spinal cord and as the basis of anatomical distribution regulate the function of the brain at different levels.

REFERENCES

1. Alho, H., and Hervonen, A. (1982): Histochem. J. in press.
2. Black, I.B., and Reis, D.J. (1975): Brain Res., 84:29-278.
3. Broch, O.J. Jr. (1973): J. Neurochem., 20:847-852.
4. Chiueh, C.C., Nespor, S.M., and Rapoport, S.I. (1980): Neurobiol. of Aging, 1:157-163.
5. Celemens, J.A., Shaar, C.J., and Smalstig, B. (1980): Fed. Proc., 39,11:2907-2911.
6. Coleman, G.L., Barthold, S.W., Osbaldiston, G.W., Foster, S.J., and Jonas, A.M. (1977): J. Gerontol., 32:258-278.

7. Dahlström, A., and Fuxe, K. (1964): Acta Physiol. Scand. Suppl., 232(62):1-55.
8. Duncan, D.B. (1957): Biometrics., 13:164-169.
9. Eränkö, O. (1967): J. roy. micr. soc., 87:259-276.
10. Grzanna, R., and Molliver, M.E. (1980): Neurosci., 5:21-40.
11. Grzanna, R., Morrison, J.H., Coyle, J.T., and Molliver, M.E. (1977): Neurosci. Lett, 4:127-134.
12. Heritage, A.S., Stumpf, W.E., Sar, M., and Grant, L.D. (1980): Science, 207:1377-1379.
13. Hervonen, A. (1971): Acta Physiol. Scand., Suppl. 368:1-94.
14. Hervonen, A., and Kanerva, L. (1972): Z. Anat. Entwickl-Gesch., 137:257-269.
15. Hervonen, A., Vaalasti, A., Partanen, M., Kanerva, L., and Hervonen, H. (1978): J. Neurocytol., 7:11-23.
16. Hoffman, G.E., and Sladek, J.R. Jr. (1980): Neurobiol. of Aging, 1:27-37.
17. Hoffman, D.W., Marchi, M., Giacobini, E. (1980): Neurobiol. of Aging, 1:65-68.
18. Horita, A. (1968): Biochem. Pharmacol., 17:2091-2096.
19. Hökfelt, T., Fuxe, K., Goldstein, M., and Johansson, O. (1974): Brain Res., 66:235-251.
20. Hökfelt, T., Johansson, O., Fuxe, K., Goldstein, M., and Park, D. (1976): Med. Biol., 54:427-453.
21. Jonsson, G., Einarsson, P., Fuxe, K., and Hallman, H. (1975): Med. Biol., 53:25-39.
22. Kanerva, L., Hervonen, A., Hervonen, H. (1974): Med. Biol., 52:144-153.
23. Kastin, A.J., Schally, A.V., and Kostrzewa, R.M. (1980): Fed. Proc., 39(11):2931-2936.
24. Martin, J.B. (1980): Fed. Proc., 39(11):2902-2906.
25. Miller, A.E., Shaar, C.J., and Riegle, G.D. (1976): Exp. Aging Res., 2:475-480.
26. Moore, R.Y., and Bloom, F.E. (1978): Ann. Rev. Neurosci., 1:129-169.
27. Moore, R.Y., and Bloom, F.E. (1979): Ann. Rev. Neurosci., 2:113-168.
28. Nagatsu, I., Inagaki, S., Kondo, Y., Karasawa, N., and Nagatsu, T. (1979): Acta Histochem. Cytochem., 12(1):20-37.
29. Partanen, M., Hervonen, A. (1979): Histochemistry, 62:249-258.
30. Partanen, M., Rapoport, S.I., and London, E.D. (1981): Auton. Nerv. Syst., in press.
31. Partanen, M., Santer, R.M., and Hervonen, A. (1980): Histochem. J., 12:527-535.
32. Partanen, M., Santer, R.M., and Hervonen, A.: In preparation.
33. Porter, J.C., Nansel, D.D., Gudelsky, A.A., Foreman, M.M., Pilotte, N.S., Parker, C.R., Burrows, G.H. Jr., Bates, G.W., and Madden, J.D. (1980): Fed. Proc., 39(11):2896-2901.
34. Ponzio, F., Brunello, N., and Algeri, S. (1978): J. Neurochem., 30:1617-1620.
35. Pradhan, S.N. (1980): Life Sci., 26:1643-1656.
36. Prange, A.J. Jr., White, J.E., Lipton, M.A., and Kinkead, A.M. (1967): Life Sci., 6:581-586.
37. Reis, D.J., Ross, R.A., and Joh, T.A. (1977): Brain Res., 136:465-474.
38. Santer, R.M. (1979): Neurosci. Lett., 15:177-180.
39. Santer, R.M., Partanen, M., and Hervonen, A. (1980): Cell Tissue Res., 211:475-485.

40. Schipper, J., Tilders, F.J.H., and Ploem, J.S. (1980): Brain
    Res., 190:459-472.
41. Simpkins, J.W., Mueller, G.P., Huang, H.H., and Meites, J. (1977):
    Endocrinology, 100(6):1672-1678.
42. Stramentinoli, G., Gualano, M., Catto, E., and Algeri, S. (1977):
    J. Gerontol., 32:392-394.

The Aging Brain: Cellular and Molecular
Mechanisms of Aging in the Nervous System,
edited by E. Giacobini et al., Raven Press, New
York © 1982.

Developing and Aging Brain Serotonergic Systems

P. S. Timiras, D. B. Hudson, and C. Miller

Department of Physiology-Anatomy, University of California, Berkeley, California 94720

A causal link between age-related changes in neurotransmission and aging of the central nervous system (CNS), although eagerly sought by several laboratories, remains elusive. In view of the crucial role that neural controls play in regulating all body functions particularly homeostasis, the discovery of this link is of prime importance for understanding the major events of the lifespan, including aging. Despite support for CNS alterations with advancing age in structure (e.g. reduced number of selected neurons, dendrites or synapses), biochemistry (e.g. regional neurotransmitter alterations), and function (e.g. neurologic and behavioral deficits), the available evidence is sufficient only to construct several theories of aging which await further verification (25, 27, 30, 34). Some of the reasons for our failure to establish unequivocally both the central role of the CNS in the aging process, and that of the neurotransmitters in the aging of the CNS, reflect practical and theoretical difficulties inherent to neurotransmitter identification and measurement of their brain levels, turnover and functional implications. Until our knowledge is more solidly established in this respect, the observed phenomena-- including those presented in this chapter-- will continue to represent "descriptive" rather than "conceptual" or "mechanistic" models. Yet, even the descriptive approach may provide useful information especially when coupled with pharmacological manipulations and clinical correlations.

In this chapter, our primary interest is directed to the serotonergic system, well-known for its role in neuroendocrine regulation and often implicated as "pacemaker" of growth, development, and aging (34). In addition to reporting serotonin levels in discrete brain areas throughout the lifespan and the activity of its metabolizing enzymes at selected ages, we have investigated the effects of pharmacologic and dietary interventions capable of altering brain serotonin levels and modifying the timetable of physiological events associated with the sequential phases of the lifespan. With the increasing number of candidates for neurotransmitters and knowledge of their chemistry and function, new avenues are opened to unravel thus far unanswered questions on CNS aging. We will discuss, briefly, some new concepts within the context of serotonin to point out to the reader profitable approaches to be explored in the search for this important link between the aging of the CNS and that of the entire organism.

In general, systematic studies of neurotransmitter levels in the CNS have disclosed only minor change under conditions of normal aging (i.e. free of overt pathology), whereas clear-cut regional neurotransmitter deficits have been associated with characteristic neurologic (Parkinson) and mental (Alzheimer) diseases of old age. To explain the relative

constancy of classical neurotransmission in old age despite progressive
functional detriments, one consideration is the possibility that transmitters may be released not only in synaptic but also in non-synaptic
areas: for example, axonal varicosities for the serotonergic system (6)
and dendrites for the dopaminergic nerves of the substantia nigra (2).
With aging, the structural disappearance of the synapse would entrain
the decrease in neurotransmitters at this site but this decrease could
be compensated by the release of greater amounts from non-synaptic regions. Glial cells also have been implicated in uptake and metabolism
of neurotransmitters under special demand conditions, and the gliosis,
which is usually found in old brains, may contribute to maintaining levels of neural transmitters comparable to those of the adult (32). However, this compensation, while leaving regional amine content unchanged,
may not maintain functional integrity. Another current concept underlies the coexistence of more than one transmitter in a single neuron, for
example serotonin and substance P (49). Thus, an imbalance may occur
with aging, not only among neurotransmitters from specific neuronal systems, as we have repeatedly suggested (28), but also within the same
neuron. It has been hypothesized that each neuron is supplied with the
complete set of genes and has the potential to syntehsize the complete
enzymatic machinery for all transmitter substances (18). Suppression
and derepression may be programmed on a life continuum so that the neurotransmitter which signals passage from one life-period to the next might
act as a pacemaker (34). Finally, although incompletely developed, the
concept of neuromodulation has been proposed to parallel neurotransmission. Neuromodulators may operate in a hormone-like fashion to affect
neurotransmitter metabolism, release and re-uptake, and receptor interaction. (1, 7). One such example is the interrelation between serotonin
and suckling-induced prolactin release (19) and another example is the
role of thyroid hormones in regulating normal development of serotonin
cyclicity in the hypothalamus and pineal (33).

It emerges from the foregoing that the effects of aging on neural
transmission should be viewed as multi-factorial and their causal role
in aging of the whole organism may depend not on one but on a cascade of
decrements or excesses leading to an imbalance of neural interactions.
In the endocrines, the function of one gland generally leads to dysfunction of several others; similarly looking at only one transmitter system
might give only an one-sided glimpse-- albeit an important one-- of the
entire picture. Therefore, while the focus of this chapter is on the
serotonergic system, relation to the other neural transmitters will be
emphasized within the limits of the allotted space.

1. Regional Serotonin Levels in Developing and Aging Brain

Developmental and aging patterns of serotonin levels show definite
regional and age specificity (Table 1). In the cerebral hemispheres,
levels are highest at 8 days of age, subsequently, as a probable consequence of the continuing addition of non-serotonergic elements with
brain maturation, levels fall to slightly reduced values which remain
essentially constant throughout young adulthood. At later ages, from
six months on, levels increase moderately. In the mesodiencephalon,
levels are low during early development and increase to adult values at
40 days: they remain constant throughout adulthood but are increased at
two years of age. In the pons medulla, levels are already high at birth
and remain constant with some temporary fluctuation until and including

TABLE 1. Serotonin Levels in Selected Brain Areas of Female Rats from Birth to Two Years of Age

	Development: Days				Adulthood: Months				Senescence: Years
	8	12	22	40	2	4	6	12	2
Cerebral Hemispheres [a]	680 ± 30 [b] 146% (34) [c]	430 ± 10 92% (7)	470 ± 10 101% (4)	446 ± 19 96% (6)	425 ± 16 91% (9)	465 ± 33 100% (8)	528 ± 28 113% (10)	598 ± 40 129% (7)	568 ± 40 122% (7)
Corpus Striatum [a]	------	------	------	1138 ± 22 95% (2)	922 ± 47 78% (10)	1179 ± 60 100% (8)	1003 ± 39 85% (10)	1249 ± 78 106% (6)	1052 ± 50 89% (10)
Hypothalamus [a]	------	------	------	------	1994 ± 68 107% (11)	1898 ± 92 100% (8)	1861 ± 117 98% (10)	------	1812 ± 112 95% (13)
Mesodiencephalon	907 ± 58 75% (36)	870 ± 5 72% (8)	------	1242 ± 52 102% (8)	1193 ± 79 99% (10)	1202 ± 45 100% (8)	1194 ± 53 99% (10)	1245 ± 31 103% (10)	1437 ± 91 119% (13)
Pons Medulla	1105 ± 72 105% (20)	1450 ± 130 138% (7)	1145 ± 55 109% (8)	------	1081 ± 95 103% (11)	1051 ± 98 100% (9)	1103 ± 39 105% (10)	1303 ± 56 124% (9)	1252 ± 61 119% (10)

a. In development, cerebral hemispheres include corpus striatum, mesodiencephalon includes hypothalamus.
b. Mean ± S.E.; values represent ng/g wet tissue of serotonin measured by fluorometry.
c. Percent change compared to 4-month-old adults taken as 100%: number in ( ) represents numbers of animals.

TABLE 2. Ratio of Serotonin to Norepinephrine Levels in Selected
          Brain Areas in the Adult and Senescent Female Rat

	Adulthood: Months			Senescence: Years
2	4	6	12	2
Cerebral Hemispheres				
1.85 425/229[a]	1.95 465/238	1.93 528/273	2.33 598/257	2.46 568/231
Hypothalamus				
0.83 1994/2395	1.07 1898/1771	1.07 1861/1846	------	1.35 1812/1346
Mesodiencephalon				
2.21 1193/539	2.73 1202/440	2.96 1194/403	2.33 1245/533	3.21 1437/448
Pons Medulla				
2.42 1081/447	2.25 1051/466	2.96 1103/373	2.50 1330/521	2.54 1252/492

a. Mean value for serotonin (ng/g)/norepinephrine (ng/g)
   measured by fluorometry-- the values of serotonin are
   presented in detail in Table 1, those for norepinephrine
   are reported elsewhere (28).

old age. In the hypothalamus and corpus striatum, only adult and senescent values are recorded and these remain unchanged through old age.
In the hypothalamus, despite the steady-state of serotonin in old animals, turnover is increased (23). These data taken alone underline the
constancy of the serotonergic system in several brain areas once adult
values have been reached. They also reveal a progressive, age-related
increase in serotonin levels in some areas such as cerebral hemisphere
and, particularly, mesodiencephalon. When these data are examined in
relation to the changes which occur with aging in other neurotransmitter
systems (but not reported here and only partially in 28), then significant changes in the balance of serotonin to other neural transmitters,
especially catecholamines, become apparent.

2. Correlated Changes of Monoamines in Developing and Aging Brain

From our observations and those of other investigators, catecholamine
levels in several brain areas decrease with aging (28). This decrease,
associated with the unchanged or increased levels of serotonin (Table 1),
implies that the balance between catecholaminergic and serotonergic
systems is altered with aging (26). Such alteration is well demonstrated
when the ratio of serotonin to norepinephrine is measured in terms of
age and brain area (Table 2). As expected from the respective regional
distribution of the two monoamines, serotonin to norepinephrine ratio
is higher in mesodiencephalon and pons medulla than in cerebral hemispheres and hypothalamus. In all areas, except the pons medulla, the

TABLE 3.   Ratio of Serotonin to Dopamine Levels in Selected Brain
           Areas in the Adult and Senescent Female Rat

	Adulthood: Months			Senescence: Years
2	4	6	12	2
Cerebral Hemispheres				
0.63 [a] 425/674	0.55 465/837	0.65 528/806	1.41 598/423	1.28 568/442
Corpus Striatum				
0.088 922/10,520	0.086 1,179/13,666	0.082 1,003/12,274	0.134 1,249/9,304	0.120 1,052/8,737

a. Mean value for serotonin (ng/g)/dopamine (ng/g) measured
    by fluorometry-- the values of serotonin are presented
    in detail in Table 2, those for dopamine are reported
    elsewhere (28).

ratio increases progressively with age, particularly at 12 and 24 months.
Similarly, the ratio of serotonin to dopamine, low in the corpus striatum, increases significantly with aging in both the cerebral hemispheres
and the corpus striatum (Table 3).

3. Changes in Activity of Metabolic Enzymes for Serotonin in the Aging Brain

Changes in the activity of tryptophan hydroxylase, the synthesizing
enzyme of serotonin, in selected brain areas with development has been
reported in rats. In the midbrain, for example, low activity at birth
is followed by a peak at twelve days and then, with progressive brain
maturation, a drop to lower values which remain unchanged in adulthood
(24). Our studies carried out in adult and senescent rats show a differential between cerebral hemispheres and mesodiencephalon, the activity in the latter area being double of that in the former (Table 4).
Differences in activity between adult and senescent rats were not
observed in the cerebral hemisphere and were small in the mesodiencephalon, the increased activity probably paralleling the high serotonin
levels with old age in this area (Table 1).

Developmental changes in the activity of monoamine oxydase, the catabolizing enzyme of serotonin, have been observed in rats and reported
(31). Monoamine oxydase activity was similar in both brain areas
studied and remained unaffected with aging.

4. Age-Related Physiopathologic Consequences of Experimentally-Induced Changes in Brain Serotonin

Although the above presented data are indicative of a predominance of
brain serotoninergic over catecholaminergic input with aging, they do
not by themselves constitute adequate proof for a mechanistic role of
serotonin in aging (5). Therefore, we undertook a series of experiments
wherein brain serotonin was manipulated by dietary and pharmacologic

TABLE 4. Activity of Serotonin Synthesizing (Tryptophan Hydroxylase) and Catabolizing (Monoamine Oxidase) Enzymes in Two Brain Areas of Adult and Senescent Female Rats

| Enzyme | Adulthood: Months | | | | Senescence: Years |
	2	4	6	12	2
	Cerebral Hemispheres				
Tryptophan Hydroxylase (n moles/hr/ mg protein)	-----	-----	-----	0.59[a] ±0.07 (5)	0.49 ±0.03 (7)
	Mesodiencephalon				
	-----	-----	-----	1.09 ±0.23 (4)	1.44 ±0.09 (7)
	Cerebral Hemispheres				
Monoamine Oxidase (n moles/hr/ mg protein)	107.1 ±8.0 (2)	93.9 ±8.8 (2)	93.2 ±0.4 (2)	-----	82.1 ±1.5 (7)
	Mesodiencephalon				
	93.7 ±9.8 (2)	101.4 ±4.9 (3)	105.0 ±6.2 (2)	-----	95.9 ±2.8 (7)

a. Mean ± S.E.: number in ( ) represents numbers of animals.

means. Some of the results are summarized briefly here, however, inasmuch as the work is still in progress, our conclusions can only be tentative.

Reduction of tryptophan in the diet, initiated at weaning and continued for various period of time from one to two years, markedly reduced serotonin levels in the brain (36) and delayed growth and maturation as well as some aspects of aging (15, 20-22). As shown in Figure 1, whole body growth of the rats was markedly inhibited while the rats were on the tryptophan-deficient diet, the degree of inhibition being proportional to the severity of the dietary restriction. During this period, the mortality of deficient animals was higher than that of the controls. (With respect to the latter no differences were seen in any of the parameters studied whether in animals receiving standard Purina rat chow or in those receiving the experimental Teklad diet supplemented with adequate tryptophan.) When the animals were returned to a control diet containing optimal levels of tryptophan the rats showed a rapid catch-up growth. In addition, these animals appeared to be physiologically younger than their age-matched controls; they were capable of establishing their body temperature faster and better after cold water emersion; they produced litters at 28 months of age, well beyond the age of reproduction in the controls; they showed a lesser incidence of neoplasia and a slightly longer lifespan (Fig. 1). Similar effects

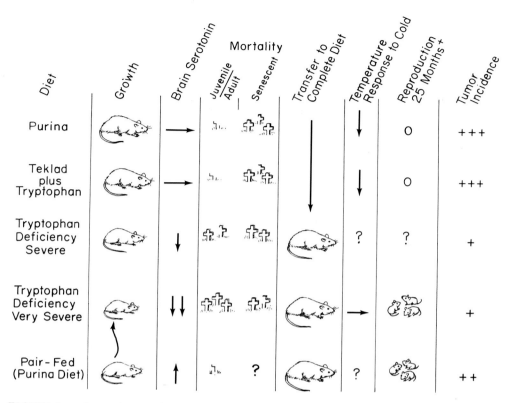

FIGURE 1. Somatic, Endocrine, Neurochemical and Pathologic Consequences of Prolonged Dietary Tryptophan Restriction in Female Rats and Effects of Rehabilitation.

although generally less beneficial, were observed in the pair-fed, caloric-restricted animals in which, however, serotonin levels were not decreased. Animal experiments, several years ago, demonstrated that reduced caloric intake early in life was associated with reduced body size and prolonged lifespan. More recent studies show that dietary restriction delays, without inhibiting, puberty in both male and female rats but extends the length of the reproductive period in females only (10, 14). Exercise, alteration in energy and amino acid metabolism, alteration in the function of the immune system and a variety of endocrine changes have all been implicated in the organism's adaptation to low caloric intake. Each of these variables has been shown to affect growth and aging processes in predictable ways. Our experiments show that restriction of a single dietary component, tryptophan, which is also the precursor of serotonin, will induce similar effects as food restriction.

Because serotonin is an important signal for the hypothalamic control of several endocrine functions (33), the possibility is raised that alteration in this signal triggers the change in growth and aging. This possibility was investigated in another series of experiments in which brain serotonin levels, and perhaps more importantly brain serotonin

TABLE 5. Pharmacologic or Endocrine Depression of Brain Serotonin: Effects on Growth and Reproductive Function in Female Rats

Treatment	Growth	Brain Serotonin	Aging of Reproductive Function[a] Estrous Cyclicity	Serum LH
PCPA[b] (intra-hypothalamic)		↓	early constant estrus	LH surge blocked
PCPA (systemic, 1 injection neonatally)		↓	precocious puberty and onset of constant estrus	LH surge blocked
PCPA (systemic, from weaning to adulthood)		↓↓	delayed puberty, early prolonged diestrus	LH surge blocked
Hypothyroid-ism[c] (peri-natally)		↓	?	?
Testosterone[d] (1 injection neonatally)		↓	precocious puberty and onset of constant estrus	LH surge blocked

    a. Estrous cyclicity is based on daily vaginal smears; serum LH is measured by radioimmunoassay.
    b. PCPA = parachlorophenylalamine--doses ranged from 35 to 300 mg/kg.
    c. Hypothyroidism was induced by adding 0.2% propylthiouracil to the maternal diet from day 18 of gestation to day 15 post-partum.
    d. Testosterone doses ranged from 10 µg to 1.25 mg/kg.

circadian cyclicity (33) were altered by the administration of pharmacologic (parachlorophenylalamine, PCPA) or endocrine (testosterone) inhibitors of serotonin. Topical administration of PCPA in the suprachiasmatic nucleus of the hypothalamus, a nucleus well-known for its control of several cyclic functions, blocks the afternoon proestrus LH-surge necessary for ovulation in rats undergoing regular estrous cycles; cyclicity in these animals is interrupted and the animals enter a period of constant estrus reminiscent of what occurs in aged female rats (Table 5) (34). Neonatal administration of a single injection of PCPA, or of testosterone, significantly affects the early postnatal development of serotonergic systems and this induces long-term effects on reproductive function, which seems to be shifted in time--with an earlier onset of puberty and early onset of aging (Fig. 5). The stage of brain maturation at the time of serotonin inhibition is important in producing the above cited effects: if PCPA is administered at weaning, at the time when brain maturation is well advanced, multiple injections are necessary to modify reproductive function (Table 5) (29). If brain maturation is delayed, as in hypothyroidism, then the effectiveness of PCPA is evident at a later age (33).

Declining cognitive function in humans has been associated most frequently with impaired cholinergic function, particularly in pathological
cases such as senile dementia (8, 11, 13, 17, 35); yet the traditional
view that senile dementia is a disease exclusively of cholinergic systems and neocortex is challenged by reports of variant forms, such as
loss in the nucleus locus ceruleus with a noradrenergic deficit and the
lowering of brain neuropeptides (3, 16). Our observations, reported
here and elsewhere, in support of a key role for serotonin as a pacemaker of aging stem not only from some of the available (but still con-
troversial) evidence in the aged organism but also, by analogy, of the
role of this transmitter as a timing mechanism for neurogenesis (12).
As stated in the introduction, the complexity of the nervous system
cannot, perhaps, be resolved to a single factor. Rather, there is adequate strong inference for the role of serotonin to warrant further
studies of the mechanisms by which serotonergic alterations might occur:
for example, whether there is a genetic timetable for serotonin synthesis or whether serotonin, like other neurotransmitters, is vulnerable
over time to age-associated deteriorative changes such as oxidative
damage. These efforts, taken collectively, will provide the appropriate
physiological basis for the identification of those interventions, e.g.,
parmacologic, which may maintain homeostasis and delay aging.

ACKNOWLEDGMENTS

The original research presented in this paper was supported by NIH
grant AG00043.

REFERENCES

1. Barchas, J.D., Akil, H., Elliott, G.R., Holman, R.B., and Watson, S.J.
    (1978): Behavioral neurochemistry: Neuroregulators and behavioral
    states. Science, 200:964-973.

2. Björklund, A. and Lindwall, O. (1975): Dopamine in dendrites of sub-
    stantia nigra neurons: suggestions for a role in dendritic
    terminals. Brain Res., 83:531-537.

3. Bondareff, W., Mountjoy, C.Q., and Roth, M. (1981): Noradrenergic
    denervation of cerebral cortex in senile dementia. XII International
    Congress of Gerontology, Hamburg, FRG, July 12-17, Abstracts, p. 230.

4. Chan-Palay, V., Jonsson, G., and Palay, S.L. (1978): Serotonin and
    substance--P coexist in neurons of the rat's central nervous system.
    Proc. Nat. Acad. Sci., 75:1582-1586.

5. Dilman, V.M., Lapin, I.P., and Oxenkrug, G.F. (1979): Serotonin and
    Aging. In: Serotonin in Health and Disease. Vol. V: Clinical
    Applications, edited by W.B. Essman, pp. 111-212. SP Medical
    and Scientific Books, New York.

6. Dismukes, R.K. (1979): New concepts of molecular communication
    among neurons. Behav. Brain Sci., 2:409-448.

7. Florey, E. (1967): Neurotransmitters and modulators in the animal
    kingdom. Fed. Proc., 26:1164-1178.

8. Gibson, G.E., Peterson, C., and Jenden, D.J. (1981): Brain acetyl-
    choline synthesis declines with senescence. Science, 213:674-676.

9. Hökfelt, T., Ljungdahl, H., Steinbusch, H., Verhofstad, A., Nilsson, G., Brodin, E., Pernow, B., and Goldstein, M. (1978): Immunohistochemical evidence for substance-P like immunoreactivity in some 5-hydroxytryptamine-containing neurons in the central nervous system. Neuroscience, 3:517-538.

10. Holehan, A.M. and Merry, B.J. (1981): Reproductive potential and temporal hormonal profiles of puberty and the oestrous cycle in the female dietary restricted long-lived rat. XII International Congress of Gerontology, Hamburg, FRG, July 12-17, Abstracts, p. 112.

11. Kolata, G.B. (1981): Clues to the cause of senile dementia. Science, 211:1032-1033.

12. Lauder, J.M., Wallace, J.A., Krebs, H., and Petrusz, P. (1980): Serotonin as a Timing Mechanism in Neuroembryogenesis. In: Progress in Psychoneuroendocrinology, edited by F. Brambilla, G. Racagni, and D. de Wied, pp. 539-556. Elsevier/North Holland Biomedical Press, Amsterdam.

13. Lehmann, H.E. (1979): Psychopharmacotherapy in psychogeriatric disorders. In: Brain Function in Old Age, Bayer-Symposium VII, Grosse Ledder, Germany, edited by F. Hoffmeister and C. Muller, pp. 456-479. Springer-Verlag, Berlin and New York.

14. Merry, B.J. and Holehan, A.M. (1981): Modification of serum hormone profiles associated with sexual maturation and ageing in male rats in which lifespan is extended through dietary intervention. XII International Congress of Gerontology, Hamburg, FRG, July 12-17. Abstracts, p. 113.

15. Ooka, H., Segall, P.E., and Timiras, P.S. (1978): Neural and endocrine development after chronic tryptophan deficiency in rats; II. Pituitary-thyroid axis. Mech. Ageing Dev., 7:19-24.

16. Oram, J.J., Edwardson, J.A., and Millard, P.H. (1981): Investigation of cerebrospinal fluid neuropeptides in idiopathic senile dementia. XII International Congress of Gerontology, Hamburg, FRG, July 12-17. Abstracts, p. 232.

17. Ordy, J.M. (1979): Geriatric psychopharmacology: Drug modification of memory and emotionality in relation to aging in human and nonhuman primate brain. In: Brain Function in Old Age, Bayer-Symposium VII, Grosse Ledder, Germany, edited by F. Hoffmeister and C. Muller, pp. 435-455. Springer-Verlag, Berlin and New York.

18. Osborne, N.N. (1981): Communication between neurons; current concepts. Neurochemistry International, 3:3-16.

19. Rotsztejn, N.H. (1980): Neuromodulation in neuroendocrinology. Trends in Neurosci., 3:67-70.

20. Segall, P.E., Ooka, H., Rose, K., and Timiras, P.S. (1978): Neural and endocrine development after chronic tryptophan deficiency in rats: I. Brain monoamine and pituitary responses. Mech. Ageing Dev., 7:1-17.

21. Segall, P.E. and Timiras, P.S. (1974): Age-related changes in thermoregulatory capacity of tryptophan-deficient rats. Fed. Proc., 33(3):1404.

22. Segall, P.E. and Timiras, P.S. (1976): Pathophysiologic findings after chronic tryptophan deficiency in rats: A model for delayed growth and aging. Mech. Ageing Dev., 5:109-124.

23. Simpkins, J.W., Mueller, G.P., Huang, H.H., and Meites, J. (1977): Evidence for depressed catecholamine and enhanced serotonin metabolism in aging male rats: possible relation to gonadotropin secretion. Endocrinology, 100:1672-1678.

24. Sze, P. (1981): Developmental-regulatory aspects of brain trypto-phan hydroxylase. In: Serotonin-Neurochemistry and Function. Advances in Experimental Biology and Medicine, edited by B. Haber, S. Gabay, M.R. Issidorides, and S.G.A. Alivisatos, pp. 507-524. Plenum Press, New York.

25. Timiras, P.S. (1978): Biological perspectives on aging: In search of a masterplan. Am. Sci., 66:605-613.

26. Timiras, P.S. (1975): Neurophysiological factors in aging: Recent advances. Presented at X International Congress of Gerontology, June 22-27, Vol. I., pp. 50-52. Jerusalem, Israel.

27. Timiras, P.S. and Bignami, A. (1976): Pathophysiology of the aging brain. In: Special Review of Exp. Aging Research. Progress in Biology, edited by M.F. Elias, B.E. Eleftheriou, and P.K. Elias, pp. 351-378. EAR, Inc., Bar Harbor.

28. Timiras, P.S. and Hudson, D.B. (1980): Changes in neurohumoral transmission during aging of the central nervous system. In: Neural Regulatory Mechanisms During Aging, edited by R.C. Adelman, J. Roberts, G.T. Baker III, S.I. Baskin, and V.J. Cristofalo, pp. 25-51. Alan R. Liss, Inc., New York.

29. Timiras, P.S., Hudson, D.B., and Jones, S.L. (1980): Pharmacolog-ically induced changes in serotonin and aging. In: Progress in Psychoneuroendocrinology, edited by F. Brambilla, G. Racagni, and D. de Wied, pp. 571-578. Elsevier/North Holland Biomedical Press, Amsterdam.

30. Timiras, P.S., Segall, P.E., and Walker, R.F. (1979): Physiological aging in the central nervous system: perspectives on "interventive" gerontology. In: Aging--Its Chemistry, Proceedings of the Third Arnold O. Beckman Conference in Clinical Chemistry, edited by A.A. Dietz, pp. 46-63. American Association for Clinical Chemistry, Inc., Washington, D.C.

31. Vaccari, A., Brotmann, S., Cimino, J., and Timiras, P.S. (1977): Sex differences of neurotransmitter enzymes in central and peri-pheral nervous systems. Brain Res., 132;176-185.

32. Vernadakis, A. (1975): Neuronal-glial interactions during devel-opment and aging. In: Biology of Aging and Development, edited by G.J. Thorbecke, pp. 173-188. Plenum Press, New York.

33. Walker, R.F. and Timiras, P.S. (1981): Serotonin in Development of Cyclic Reproductive Function. In: Serotonin Neurochemistry and Function. Advances in Experimental Biology and Medicine, edited by B. Haber, S. Gabay, M.R. Issidorides, and S.G.A. Alivisatos, pp. 525-542. Plenum Press, New York.

34. Walker, R.F. and Timiras, P.S. (1981): Pacemaker insufficiency and the onset of aging. In: Cellular Pacemakers II, edited by D. Carpenter, pp. 396-425. Wiley Interscience, New York.

35. Wisniewski, H.M. and Iqbal, K. (1980): Ageing of the brain and dementia. Trends in Neurosciences, October:226-228.

36. Wurtman, R.J., Hefti, F., and Melamed, E. (1980): Precursor control of neurotransmitter synthesis. Pharmacol. Rev., 32:315-336.

The Aging Brain: Cellular and Molecular
Mechanisms of Aging in the Nervous System,
edited by E. Giacobini et al., Raven Press, New
York © 1982.

Age-Related Change of Binding Regulation in Dopamine and α_2-Adrenergic Receptors in the Brain

Y. Nomura, K. Oki, I. Yotsumoto, and T. Segawa

*Department of Pharmacology, Institute of Pharmaceutical Sciences,
Hiroshima University School of Medicine, Hiroshima 734, Japan*

It has been reported from our laboratory that the central dopamine (DA) and noradrenaline (NA) nervous system functionally changes with increasing age. (9-14). Specific [^{3}H]spiperone binding to synaptic membranes is highly selectively inhibited by (d)-enantiomer of butaclamol (18) and agonist binding to DA receptors is regulated by guanine nucleotides (1-3, 22). In contrast, from findings regarding effects of GTP and isoproterenol on [^{3}H]clonidine binding, binding regulation in α_2-adrenoceptors has been suggested in the rat brain (5, 7, 17, 19, 20). However, no detail of age-related change in the regulation of DA and α_2-adrenergic receptors has been documented in the brain.

The present study was designed to examine age-related change in binding characterization and regulation of striatal [^{3}H]spiperone binding and cerebral cortical [^{3}H]-clonidine binding to crude synaptic membranes in the rat brain.

MATERIALS AND METHODS

[^{3}H]Spiperone binding was performed using homogenates of the striatum by the method of Seeman et al. (18). The fresh tissues from developing Wistar rats were suspended in 15 vol. of 15 mM Tris-HCl buffer (pH 7.4) containing 5 mM Na$_2$-EDTA, 1.1 mM ascorbate and 13.3 µM pheniprazine, crudely homogenized with a glass-teflon homogenizer, preincubated at 37 °C for 60 min. The sample was centrifuged at 39,000 x g for 15 min, resuspended in 14 ml of buffer and finally homogenized with a Polytron homogenizer (setting No. 6) for 20 sec. A 0.8 ml of portion of homogenates (0.25 - 0.4 mg protein) was transferred into polyethylene tubes, 0.1 ml of buffer or (d)-butaclamol (final concentration, 1 µM) and 0.1 ml of [^{3}H]spiperone (final concentration, 0.095 nM to 0.899 nM). After 30 min incubation at 23 °C, an aliquot of 1.0 ml was filtered through a Whatman GF/B filter. The filter was washed with 10 ml of buffer and then placed into a liquid scintillator vial, 10 ml of scintillator (ACS II, Amersham) was added and radioactivity was measured. Specific

binding was defined as that inhibited by 1 μM of (d)-buta-
clamol. In order to know the stereoselective inhibition of
butaclamol on [³H]spiperone binding, incubation was carried
out in the presence of [³H]spiperone (final concentration,
i nM to 0.1 mM) with striatal membranes. Another competition experiments was carried out by the method of Usdin et
al. (21). [³H]Spiperone (final concentration, 0.47 or 0.5
nM) with or without NaCl 100 mM and/or GTP 50 μM were added
to a 50 mM Tris-HCl buffer (pH 7.1) containing 1.1 mM ascorbate and various concentration of apomorphine (final concentration , 10 nM to 0.1 mM) to detect change of binding
affinity (IC50) of apomorphine.

[³H]Clonidine binding was carried out using crude synaptic membranes from the cerebral cortex. Crude mitochondrial P2 fractions were dispersed with a Polytron
(setting No. 6) for 30 sec and centrifuged at 48,000 X g for
20 min. After adding distilled water, samples were stood
for 30 min at room temperature and centrifuged at 48,000 X g
for 20 min. Resulting pellets were suspended in 50 mM Tris-
HCl buffer (pH 7.7). Binding experiments were carried out
by the method of U'Prichard et al. (10). Reaction mixture
which was composed of 0.8 ml of membrane suspension (0.2 -
0.4 mg protein), 0.1 ml of GTP solution (final concentration
10 μM), 0.02 ml of [³H]clonidine (final concentration, 0.05
- 4 nM) together with 0.1 ml of non-radioactive clonidine
(final concentration, 1 μM) or buffer were incubated at 25°C
for 30 min. Specific binding was defined as the excess over
blank containing 1 μM clonidine.

To examine the effect of isoproterenol treatment on [³H]-
clonidine binding, cerebral cortical slices suspended in
modified Krebs-Ringer solution containing 0.1 % ascorbate
(40 mg wet tissue weight/ml) were incubated with isoproterenol (final concentration, 200 μM) at 37 °C for 40 min.
The suspension was then centrifuged at 17,000 X g for 30
sec. The washing was performed three times. [³H]Clonidine
binding was performed by the method described above.

Estimation of protein was carried out by the Folin
reagent method of Lowry et al. (6). Differences between
experimental values were analysed by Student's t-test.

AGE-RELATED CHANGE IN STRIATAL DOPAMINE RECEPTORS

1. Effects of (d)- and (l)-butaclamol on [³H]spiperone
   binding

Total binding of [³H]spiperone to crude synaptic membranes was examined in the presence of various concentrations of (d)- or (l)-butaclamol in the striatum at various
ages. Table 1 shows IC50 of (d)- and (l)-butaclamol for
[³H]spiperone binding. (d)-Butaclamol inhibited [³H]-
spiperone binding 210.9-, 238.0- and 221.7-fold greater than
(l)-butaclamol in 1-, 7- and 70-day-old rats, respectively.
The ratio of inhibitory activity of (d)- and (l)-butaclamol

TABLE 1. <u>IC_{50} of (d)- and (l)-butaclamol for total $[^3H]$-spiperone binding in the developing striatum</u>

Days	IC_{50} (μM)		Ratio
	(d)-Butaclamol	(l)-Butaclamol	$\dfrac{IC_{50} \text{ of (l)-butaclamol}}{IC_{50} \text{ of (d)-butaclamol}}$
1	0.055 ± 0.007 (3)	11.6 ± 0.2 (3)	210.9
7	0.050 ± 0.009 (3)	11.9 ± 0.3 (3)	238.0
70	0.060 ± 0.002 (3)	13.3 ± 0.1 (3)	221.7

IC_{50} values are the mean + S.E. with the number of independent experiments in parenthesis. Each experiment was carried out in triplicate.

for $[^3H]$spiperone binding was not different in developing animals between days 1 and 70, suggesting the ablity by which binding sites could recognize (d)-enantiomer of butaclamol does not change with age.

2. K_D and Bmax in $[^3H]$spiperone binding

A Scatchard plot of specific binding on day 70 indicated the existence of two binding sites : one with high affinity

TABLE 2. <u>Aging in K_D and Bmax of striatal $[^3H]$spiperone binding</u>

Days	Low		High	
	K_D (nM)	Bmax (pmol/mg)	K_D (nM)	Bmax (pmol/mg)
1	-	-	0.075 + 0.001 (2)	0.073 + 0.003 (2)
7	-	-	0.073 + 0.017 (2)	0.075 + 0.012 (2)
15	1.35 + 0.24 (6)	0.46 + 0.03 (6)	0.069 + 0.009 (6)	0.062 + 0.010 (6)
30	1.70 + 0.19 * (4)	0.88 + 0.04 *** (4)	0.084 + 0.019 (4)	0.160 + 0.031 ** (4)
70	1.51 + 0.27 (3)	0.55 + 0.05 * (3)	0.090 + 0.037 (3)	0.083 + 0.033 (3)
360	0.95 + 0.26 (3)	0.43 + 0.03 (3)	0.060 + 0.007 (3)	0.098 + 0.012 (3)

K_D and Bmax were determined by Scatchard plots. Each value is the mean + S.E. with the number of independent experiments in parenthesis. Significance, * $P < 0.05$, ** $P < 0.01$, *** $P < 0.001$ vs. value on a preceding day examined.

(K_D = 0.090 nM) and the other with low affinity (K_D = 1.51 nM). Table 2 shows the age-realted change in K_D and Bmax of [^{3}H]spiperone binding. Both types of the high and low affinity binding were detected on days 1 and 7. K_D and Bmax in low affinity significantly increased between days 15 and 70 and K_D decreased between days 30 and 70. Bmax in high affinity binding reached a peak on day 30. In the case of mouse brain, total protein as well as water- and detergent-soluble protein markedly increase during the first four weeks of the postnatal life, after which it continued to increase at a reduced rate (4). Therefore, the reduction of the number of DA receptors from day 30 to day 70 may not be due to the increase of the protein content between days 30 and 70. A developmental study on striatal [^{3}H]haloperidol binding expressed as fmol/mg tissue weight also indicates to be a peak on day 28 and the small decrease from day 28 to adult and to be closely parallel to the change in specific activity of DA-stimulated adenylate cyclase (15).

3. Effects of Na$^+$ and GTP on competition by apomorphine for striatal [^{3}H]spiperone binding

The addition of sodium chloride 100 mM to a 50 mM Tris-HCl buffer (pH 7.1) significantly increased specific [^{3}H]-spiperone binding on days 1, 7, 15 and 70. The increasing effect of sodium chloride may be due to the protection of receptor complex from degradation by cations such as Na$^+$. Sodium chloride 100 mM shifted twice a concentration-inhibition curve of apomorphine for [^{3}H]spiperone binding to a left and significantly decreased IC$_{50}$ of apomorphine on days 15 and 70 but not on day 7 (Table 3). Sodium bromide 100 mM caused the same

TABLE 3. Effects of sodium chloride and GTP on competition by apomorphine for striatal [^{3}H]spiperone binding in the developing striatum

Days	IC$_{50}$ of apomorphine			NaCl 100 mM plus GTP 50 μM
	Control	NaCl 100 mM	GTP 50 μM	
7	1.72 + 0.15 (3)	1.70 + 0.42 (3)	1.33 + 0.06 (3)	1.46 + 0.20 (2)
15	0.84 + 0.08 (3)	0.48 + 0.07 (3) *	0.81 + 0.08 (3)	0.84 + 0.03[++] (3)
70	1.10 + 0.10 (6)	0.53 + 0.02 (7) **	1.17 + 0.09 (3)	1.29 + 0.08[+++] (5)

Each value shows the mean + S.E. with the number of experiments in the parenthesis. Significance, * $P < 0.05$, ** $P < 0.01$ vs. control. ++ $P < 0.01$, +++ $P < 0.001$ vs. NaCl alone.

effect as sodium chloride. Sodium chloride did not affect
IC_{50} of α-flupenthixol. Therefore, Na^+ affecting agonist
affinity for DA receptors reaches maturity between days 7 and
15. GTP 50 μM reversed sodium chloride-induced decrease of
IC_{50} of apomorphine but GTP did not affect inhibitory activity of apomorphine in the absence of sodium chloride. GTP
50 μM produced the reversal of Na^+-induced decrease in IC_{50}
of apomorphine on day 15 but not on day 7. The regulation by
both Na^+ and GTP in agonist binding for DA receptors could
reach functional maturity between days 7 and 15. If the
regulation by GTP in agonist binding is related to the negative heterotropic effect of GTP (16), GTP regulatory protein
which controls agonist binding would not exist on day 7. Na^+
and guanine nucleotide may interact with the physiological
effectors and regulate ligand binding to several receptors.
    Recently we found that IC_{50} of sulpiride, a specific DA_2
receptor antagonist, for [³H]spiperone binding was 31-fold
decreased by Na^+ 100 mM compared to that in control in 70-
day-old rats but not by GTP 50 μM. The Na^+ effect was high
in fetuses at 18 days of gestation and gradually decreased
with increasing age. Thus, Na^+-dependent binding of
sulpiride to DA_2 receptors probably reaches functional maturity in fetuses at 18 days of gestation and Na^+-dependency of
the effect decreases during postnatal development.

4. Correlation between [³H]spiperone binding and other DA-
   nergic function in the striatum

    Bmax of [³H]GTP binding also reached a peak on day 30 in
the striatum, subsequently declined on days 70 and 360 (Fig.
1B). There is a significant correlation (r = 0.867, P< 0.02)
between the developmental change of [³H]spiperone binding
and that of [³H]GTP binding, suggesting that GTP regulatory
protein functionally couples DA receptors in the developing
striatum. With regard to the biological function of DA
receptors, behavioral responses to methamphetamine which is
indicated by methamphetamine-induced increase of locomotor
activity was observed to be a maximum in 30-day-old rats (13)
as well as spontaneous activity, although apomorphine-induced
increase reached a peak on day 20 (Fig. 1C). The maximum
effect of methamphetamine on day 30 is partially due to the
maximum density in striatal [³H]spiperone binding on day 30.
It is probable that postsynaptic DA receptor system is most
functional around 30 days and rapidly decreases by around 70
days. On the other hand, DA and 3',4'-dihydroxyphenylacetic
acid contents continued to increase at 70 days (Fig. 1A),
suggesting that presynaptic elements in DAnergic synapses are
still maturing even on day 70. Therefore, functional aging in
the striatal DAnergic synapses seems to begin in postsynaptic
sites ealier than in presynaptic sites.

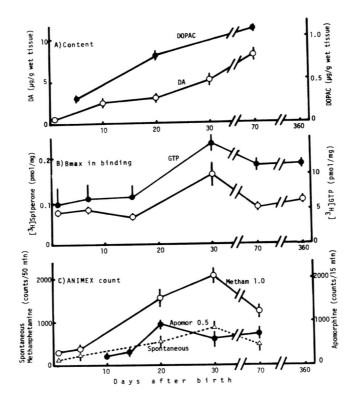

Fig. 1. Age-related change of striatal DAnergic activity in postnatal rats. A) DA and 3',4'-dihydroxyphenyl-acetic acid (DOPAC) content, B) Bmax in [^{3}H]spiperone binding and [^{3}H]GTP binding to crude synaptic membranes, C) ANIMEX counts following an i.p. injection of metham-phetamine (1.0 mg/kg) or apomorphine (0.5 mg/kg). ○——○, Methamphetamine ; ●——●, apomorphine ; △······△, control (spontaneous activity).

AGE-RELATED CHANGE IN CORTICAL α₂-ADRENOCEPTORS

1. Effect of GTP on K_D and Bmax in [^{3}H]clonidine binding

To identify age-related change in cerebral cortical α₂-adrenoceptors, specific [^{3}H]clonidine binding to synaptic membranes was examined. Scatchard analysis of [^{3}H]clonidine binding indicated that K_D and Bmax rapidly increased between days 1 and 70 (Table 4). Ligand affinity to cortical α₂-adrenoceptors seems to decrease and the density of the receptors increases with increasing age at earlier stage of postnatal development. A similar finding regarding the developmental change in Bmax has been reported by Morris et al. (8). There was no significant difference in both K_D and Bmax between days 70 and 360. Age-related change perhaps

does not proceed during 1 year of postnatal life in rats.
The addition of GTP 10 μM increased K_D on days 7, 70 and 360
and reduced Bmax on days 7, 30 and 70. Influence of GTP on
K_D and Bmax suggests the presence of GTP regulatory protein
as a coupling factor in the α_2-adrenoceptor-effector system.
Since GTP did not change K_D and Bmax on day 1, a functional
link between binding site and GTP unit reaches maturity
within a week after birth. It is unclear whether α_2-adreno-
ceptors locate pre- and/or postsynaptically in the cerebral
cortex (Fig. 2), although 6-hydroxydopamine-induced increase
of [³H]clonidine binding suggests that α_2-adrenoceptors are
predominantly postsynaptic (19). In contrast, a finding from

TABLE 4. Aging in effect of GTP on K_D and Bmax in [³H]-
          clonidine binding

Days	Control		GTP 10 μM	
	K_D (nM)	Bmax (pmol/mg)	K_D (nM)	Bmax (pmol/mg)
1	0.27 + 0.04*** (3)	0.047 + 0.005*** (5)	0.29 + 0.06 (3)	0.039 + 0.009 (4)
7	1.14 + 0.07* (5)	0.140 + 0.023* (3)	2.57 + 0.33+++ (3)	0.115 + 0.016+ (3)
30	2.06 + 0.26 (5)	0.251 + 0.021 (5)	1.95 + 0.13 (3)	0.170 + 0.009+ (3)
70	1.62 + 0.01 (3)	0.239 + 0.010 (3)	2.45 + 0.12+++ (3)	0.169 + 0.015+ (3)
360	1.45 + 0.09 (3)	0.221 + 0.018 (3)	2.03 + 0.14+ (3)	0.164 + 0.010 (3)

Each value shows the mean + S.E. with the number of
separate experiments, each of which was performed in triplicate. Significance, * $P < 0.05$, *** $P < 0.001$ vs. 70-day-old
rats. + $P < 0.01$, +++ $P < 0.001$ vs. control.

our laboratory shows that the inhibitory effect of clonidine
on 20 mM K⁺-evoked release of L-[³H]NA from cerebral cortical
slices becomes functional between day 1 and day 7 (14), suggesting presynaptic localization of α_2-adrenoceptors which
regulate NA release. Since the inhibitory effect of GTP on
[³H]clonidine binding and that of clonidine on depolariza-
tion-induced L-[³H]NA release synchronize at early postnatal stage, possible existence of a link between recognition
binding sites and GTP units in α_2-adrenoceptors is further
suggested. On day 360, there was a tendency of low K_D and
Bmax and of low effect of GTP on both parameters, compared to
those on day 70, indicating the tendency of aging in α_2-
adrenoceptors during a year. This is in contrast with a
tendency of the reduction in DA receptor density in the
striatum between days 70 and 360 (Table 2).

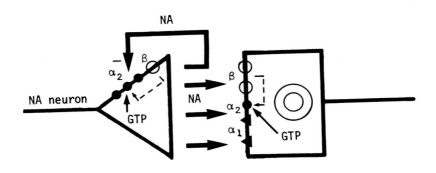

Fig. 2.   Regulation mechanism in α_2-adrenoceptor binding by GTP and β-adrenoceptors in cortical NAnergic synapses. α_2-adrenoceptor function seems to be regulated by GTP and β-adrenoceptors in both pre- and postsynaptic sites.

2. Effects of isoproterenol on K_D and Bmax in [³H]clonidine binding

After preincubation of cortical slices with isoproterenol 200 μM in Krebs-Ringer solution at 37 °C for 40 min, specific [³H]clonidine binding to crude synaptic membranes were examined, to know α_2-β-receptor interaction in the cortex. The treatment with isoproterenol significantly increased Bmax in [³H]clonidine binding without changing K_D (Table 5). The same alteration was observed on days 7 and 360 as that on day 70

TABLE 5.   Aging in effect of isoproterenol on K_D and Bmax in cortical [³H]clonidine binding

| Days | Control | | Isoproterenol 200 μM | |
	K_D (nM)	Bmax (pmol/mg)	K_D (nM)	Bmax (pmol/mg)
7	1.15 + 0.25 (4)	0.138 + 0.020 (4)	1.35 + 0.54 (3)	0.264 + 0.005 (3) **
70	0.98 + 0.07 (4)	0.123 + 0.012 (4)	1.01 + 0.03 (4)	0.222 + 0.038 (4) *
360	1.37 + 0.26 (4)	0.138 + 0.019 (4)	1.49 + 0.22 (4)	0.208 + 0.011 (4) *

Each value shows the mean + S.E. with the number of experiments in parenthesis. Each experiment was performed in triplicate. Significance, * $P < 0.05$, ** $P < 0.01$, *** $P < 0.001$ vs. control.

(Table 5). The increase in Bmax of [^{3}H]clonidine binding probably is not due to residual isoproterenol because of following facts : 1) after three times washings with cold Krebs-Ringer solution, isoproterenol in the slices was not detectable by a high-pressure liquid chromatography (Waters, TSK-GEL LS-410, ODS column) and a fluorescence detector (shimadzu, FLD-2A), 2) in vitro addition of isoproterenol did not increase but reduced [^{3}H]clonidine binding (IC_{50} = 3.4 µM). Bmax in [^{3}H]clonidine binding was increased by isoproterenol at 7 and 360 days, suggesting that a close interrelatioship between α_2- and β-receptors presumably reaches functional maturity by day 7 and continues at least until one year.

The molecular mechanism concerning interrelationship between α_2- and β-adrenoceptors in view of GTP unit and adenylate cyclase in pre- and/or postsynaptic sites is an interesting subject in the future study.

ACKNOWLEDGEMENTS

We are grateful to Mr. M. Kawai, Miss Y. Kinoshita and Miss E. Motomori for their valuable technical assistance. This work has been supported in part by Grant-in-Aid for Scientific Research No. 457552 from the Ministry of Education, Science and Culture, Japan.

REFERENCES

1. Creese, I., and Snyder, S. H. (1978): Eur. J. Pharmacol., 50: 459-461.
2. Creese, I., Usdin, T., and Snyder, S. H. (1978): Nature London, 278: 577-578.
3. Creese, I., Usdin, T., and Snyder, S. H. (1979): Mol. Pharmacol. , 16: 69-76.
4. Grossfeld, R. M., and Shooter, E. M. (1971): J. Neurochem. 18: 2265-2277.
5. Johnson, R. W., Reisine, T., Sponitz, S., Wiech, N., Ursillo, R., and Yamamura, H. I. (1980): Eur. J. Pharmacol., 67: 123-127.
6. Lowry, O. H., Rosebrough, J. N., Farr, A. L., and Randall, R. J. (1951): J. biol. Chem., 193: 265-275.
7. Maggi, M. J., U'Prichard, D. C., and Enna, S. J. (1980): Science, 207: 645-647.
8. Morris, M. J., Dausse, J.-P., Devynck, M.-A., and Meyer, P. (1980): Brain Res., 190: 268-271.
9. Nomura, Y., Naitoh, F., and Segawa, T. (1976): Brain Res., 101: 305-315.
10. Nomura, Y., and Segawa, T. (1978): Eur. J. Pharmacol., 50: 153-156.

11. Nomura, Y., and Segawa, T. (1979): <u>Br. J. Pharmacol.</u>, 66: 531-535.
12. Nomura, Y. (1980): <u>Naunyn-Schmiedeberg's Arch. Pharmacol.</u>, 313: 33-37.
13. Nomura, Y., Yotsumoto, I., and Oki, K. (1981): <u>J. Pharm. Pharmacol.</u>, 33: 264-266.
14. Nomura, Y., Yotsumoto, I. (1981): <u>Develop. Neurosci.</u>, (in press).
15 Pardo, J. V., Creese, I., Burt, D. R., and Snyder, S. H. (1980): <u>Brain Res.</u>, 125: 376-382.
16. Rodbell, M. (1980): <u>Nature London</u>, 284: 17-22.
17. Rouot, B. M., U'Prichard, D. C., and Snyder, S. H. (1980): <u>J. Neurochem.</u>, 34: 374-384.
18. Seeman, P., Westman, K., Protiva, M., Jirek, J., Jain, P. C., Saxena, A. K., Anad, N., Humbern, L., and Philipp, A. (1979): <u>Eur. J. Pharmacol.</u>, 56: 247-251.
19. U'Prichard, D. C., Bechtel, W. D., Rouot, B. M., and Snyder, S. H. (1979): <u>Mol. Pharmacol.</u>, 16: 47-60.
20. U'Prichard, D. C., and Snyder, S. H. (1980): <u>J. Neurochem.</u>, 34: 385-394.
21. Usdin, T. B., Creese, I., and Snyder, S. H. (1980): <u>J. Neurochem.</u>, 34: 669-676.
22. Zahniser, N. R., and Molinoff, P. B. (1978): <u>Nature London</u>, 275: 453-455.

The Aging Brain: Cellular and Molecular Mechanisms of Aging in the Nervous System, edited by E. Giacobini et al., Raven Press, New York © 1982.

Dopaminergic Function During Aging in Rat Brain

M. Trabucchi, *P. F. Spano, *S. Govoni, *F. Riccardi, and A. Bosio

*Department of Pharmacology, University of Brescia, Brescia and *Department of Pharmacology and Pharmacognosy, University of Milan, Milan, Italy*

A number of studies indicates the existence of degenerative phenomena in the aging brain. Anatomically, changes in neurons size, number and intraneuronal accumulation of lipofuscin have been described. The biosynthesis, the catabolism and the receptors for various neurotransmitters are altered in the aging nervous system (4,6,10). Among the various compounds, catecholamines have been the most studied in relation to the aging process. Tyrosine hydroxylase and dopa decarboxylase show a significant decline with aging in various brain regions both in animals and man (15).

The dopaminergic system, in particular, seems to be affected by the aging process. Decreased dopamine (DA) synthesis (17), dopamine sensitive adenylyl cyclase (DA-AC) activity and DA receptor function have been reported by us as well as by other investigators (4,19). DA-AC activity is decreased in striatum, t. olfactorium, n. accumbens and substantia nigra of old rats (4). Similarly in these animals the density of DA receptors as labelled by ^{3}(H)-spiroperidol is decreased in striatum and t. olfactorium (5). On the other hand, the impairement of the neuronal mechanisms regulating dopaminergic activity is confirmed by the fact that the acute haloperidol treatment elicits a less pronounced increase of striatal DA turnover in old rats (Fig. 1). This fact suggests that a decline in the capacity of DA system in adapting to environmental changes is part of the aging process in the brain.

Other observations (9,16) indicate that also in the case of noradrenergic transmission the functional impairement in old animals is worsened by stress, a condition normally requiring an acute activation of the system. This lack of capability of the aging brain to adapt to environmental changes or pharmacological manipulations has been observed in particular at receptor level. Greenberg and Weiss (6) in fact showed that 24 months old rats have an impaired ability to increase the β-adrenergic receptor density in response to reserpine treatment.

Another interesting aspect of the problem is the existence of different receptors for a given neurotransmitter which may be differentially affected by the aging process.

A number of evidences (7,13,20) indicates that DA receptors

FIG. 1

Effect of haloperidol treatment (1 mg/kg i.p.) on striatal DOPAC levels in adult (4 months) and aged (24 months) rats.

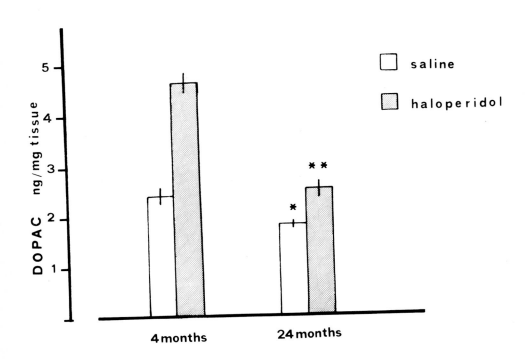

DOPAC concentrations were measured according to the radioenzimatic method of Argiolas et al. (1). Animals were killed 1 hr after haloperidol injection. Values are the mean ± S.E.M. of three experiments with four animals in each group.

[+]p < 0.01 in respect to saline treated adult rats
[++]p < 0.01 in respect to haloperidol treated adult rats

may be classified according to their association to (D$_1$) or independence from (D$_2$) an adenylate cyclase. The aim of our study is to investigate whether the different classes of DA receptors are equally affected by aging. The results indicate that D$_1$ receptors number is significantly reduced in 23 months old rats while D$_2$ receptors sites are increased.

MATERIALS AND METHODS

Mature (3-4 months) or senescent (23-24 months) male Sprague-Dawley rats (Charles River, Calco, Italy) were used in our study. The animals were randomly caged to avoid environmental differences, housed at constant temperature and humidity and exposed to a daily cycle of 12 hours of light, from 8 a.m. to 8 p.m. Animals had free access to food and water.

FIG. 2

Apomorphine displacement of (^{3}H)spiroperidol binding in striatal membranes preparations of adult (4 months) and aged (24 months) rats.

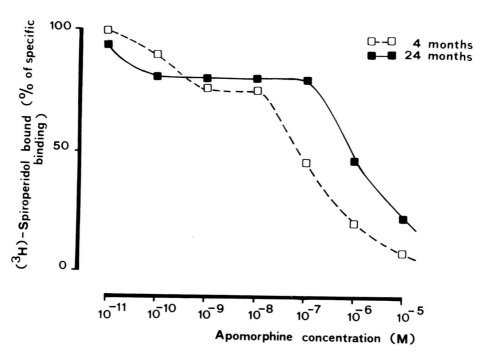

Values represent the mean of three experiments run in triplicate.

TABLE 1

Kinetic parameters of (^{3}H)spiroperidol and (^{3}H)domperidone binding in striatal membranes preparations of adult (4 months) and aged (24 months) rats.

	(^{3}H)Spiroperidol binding		(^{3}H)Domperidone binding	
	K_d	B_{max}	K_d	B_{max}
Adult	1.32 ± 0.11	198 ± 7	2.9 ± 0.3	145 ± 16
Aged	1.21 ± 0.13	$125 \pm 6^+$	2.8 ± 0.2	$287 \pm 22^+$

$^+p < 0.01$ respect to adult.
K_d values are expressed as nM, B_{max} values as f.mol/mg protein $\pm$ S.E.M. Values are extrapolated from 3 binding studies performed using five concentrations of the radioligand.

Senescent rats with pathological affections (tumors, respiratory
infections, etc.) were excluded from our study.

(^{3}H)-spiroperidol and (^{3}H)-domperidone binding. Dopaminergic
receptors labelled by (^{3}H)-spiroperidol (Amersham, 23 Ci/mmol)
and by (^{3}H)-domperidone (NEN 60 Ci/mmole) were studied in accord
with the method of Burt et al. (3) and Waitling et al. (21) respectively. Briefly P_2 brain tissue suspension was incubated at
37°C for ten minutes in the presence of various concentrations of
ligand. Samples were filtered under vacuum through Whatman GF/B
filters. Specific (^{3}H)-spiroperidol binding was measured as the
difference in binding obtained with incubation in the presence or
in absence of 10^{-6}M haloperidol. Specific (^{3}H)-domperidone binding
was determined as the difference in binding obtained with incubation in absence or presence of 1 mM dopamine. Protein content was
measured according to Lowry et al. (8).

RESULTS

In Fig. 2 is presented the displacement curve of ^{3}H-spiroperi
dol by apomorphine in striatal membranes preparations of adult
(3-4 months) and aged (23-24 months) rats. In adult animals the
curve is biphasic with a plateau between 10^{-9}M and 10^{-8}M apomorphine. This type of curve indicates the existence of multiple
binding sites. Very preliminary lesion experiments suggest that
the first portion of the curve (between 10^{-11} and 10^{-9}M apomorphi
ne) is associated with dopamine receptors located at least in part
on nigrostriatal dopaminergic afferents. In old animals the plateau
is extended from 10^{-10}M to 10^{-7}M apomorphine. The second component of the curve is also different. In this case the IC_{50} for
apomorphine is about 2×10^{-6}M in old rats compared to 2×10^{-7}M in
the young ones. However this displacement curves are difficult to
interpret since apomorphine and spiroperidol are not selective
for one population of DA receptors, but in different concentrations they may interact with the various binding sites. In addition, in this type of study it is difficult to assess the contribution of one class of binding sites to the others in determining
the final displacement curve. For this reason we decided to use
specific labelled ligands for studying the different populations
of DA receptors. In Table 1 are reported the kinetic parameters
of (^{3}H)spiroperidol and (^{3}H)domperidone binding in the striatum
of adult and aged rats. As previously reported we confirmed a
decrease in the number of binding sites for (^{3}H)spiroperidol. On
the contrary, the number of binding sites for (^{3}H)domperidone is
increased by 100% in the 24 months group. No age-dependent modifi
cations in the Kd for the different ligands were observed.

DISCUSSION

The results indicate that the previously described (4,5) age
dependent decrease of DA receptor function may be ascribed to DA
recognition sites coupled to adenylyl cyclase activity. In fact,
when we used a ligand specific for the dopaminergic receptors

not linked to a cyclase activity (i.e. domperidone, 1,21) we observed an increase in the number of binding sites. In a previous report (12) it has been shown that the number of binding sites for (^{3}H)sulpiride, ligand for D_2 receptors, is not modified in aged rats. Among the different hypothesis, the discrepancy between the results obtained with (^{3}H)domperidone and (^{3}H)Sulpiride may be explained on the basis of a greater selectivity of (^{3}H)-domperidone for the D_2 receptor sites. It is possible that the loss of D_1 receptors concomitantly to an increase of D_2 sites reflects a different cellular localization of D_1 and D_2 dopaminer gic recognition sites. In the aged brain a reduction of neuron number associated with gliosis has been reported (2). The data showing a diminished content of DOPAC in striatum of aged animals may indirectly suggest a decrease of DA neurons. It is possible that D_1 and D_2 receptors are located in different neurons or that glial cells contain a certain amount of D_2 receptors. The loss in D_1 binding sites would therefore reflect a neuronal loss, while the increase in D_2 sites a supersensitive reaction to a decrease availability of DA or an increase in glial cells containing D_2 receptors. This view is in part supported by the fact that in the striatum of aged rats we found an increase (+140%) of the glutamine synthetase activity (Fig. 3), a marker enzyme for glial cells (11).

FIG. 3

Glutamine synthetase activity (GS) in striatum of adult (4 months) and aged (24 months) rats.

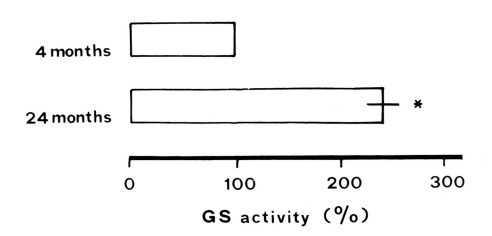

$^+$p 0.01 respect to adult
Glutamine synthetase activity was measured using the radioisotopic assay described by Pishak and Phillips (4).The results reported are expressed as % of the specific activity of the enzyme in adult animals.

In support of a different cellular localization of D_1 and D_2 receptors is the fact that the intrastriatal injection of kainic acid induces a decrease in the number of (^{3}H)spiroperidol binding sites while the kinetic parameters of (^{3}H)sulpiride binding are not modified (13).

The intrastriatal injection of kainic acid is known to induce a cell loss within the area of injection accompanied by a reactive gliosis (18). The ultimate physiological meaning of the selective changes in DA receptors observed in the brain of aged rats is still unclear.

Tentatively, it may be suggested that cyclic AMP formed following the interaction of DA with D_1 sites might regulate long term intracellular events. On the other hand, the ionic neuronal mechanisms, important for the DA transmission, would be supported by D_2 receptors, that are fully operant in the aging brain.

ACKNOWLEDGEMENTS

The animals have been kindly gifted by the Italian Study group on Brain Aging.

REFERENCES

1. Argiolas A., Fadda F., Stefanini E. and Gessa G.L. (1977) J. Neurochem. 29:599-603

2. Brizzle K.K., Ordy J.M., Hanscke J. and Kaack B. (1976) Aging 3:229-242

3. Burt D.R., Creese I. and Snyder S.H. (1977) Science 196:326-328

4. Govoni S., Loddo P., Spano P.F., Trabucchi M. (1977) Brain Res. 138:565-570

5. Govoni S., Memo M., Saiani L., Spano P.F. and Trabucchi M. (1980) Mechanisms of Ageing and Development 12:39-46

6. Greenberg L.H. and Weiss B. (1979) J. Pharm. Expt. Ther. 211:309-316

7. Laduron P.M. and Leysen J.E. (1979) Biochem. Pharmacol. 28:2161-2165.

8. Lowry O.H., Rosebrough H.J., Farr A.H. and Randall R.J. (1951) J. Biol. Chem. 193:265-275

9. McNamara, Coheen M., Miner A.T., Vernon A., Davis J.N. (1977) Brain Res. 131:313-320

10. Maggi A., Schmidt M.J., Ghetti B., Enna S.J. (1979) Life Sciences 24:367-374

11. Martinez-Hernandez A., Bell K.P. and Worenberg M.D. (1977) Science 195:1356-1358

12. Memo M., Lucchi L., Spano P.F. Trabucchi M. (1980) Brain Res. 202:488-492

13. Memo M., Spano P.F. and Trabucchi M. (1980) British J. Pharmacol. 72:124P-125P

14. Pishak M.R. and Phillips (1979) Analytical Biochem. 94:82-88

15. Reis D.J., Ross R.A. and Joh T.H. (1977) Brain Res. 136:465-474

16. Ritter S., Pelzer N.L. (1978) Brain Res. 152:170-175

17. Samorajski T. (1975) in:Aging, vol. 1, edited by Brody A., Hartman D. and Ordy J.M., pp. 199-214, Raven Press, New York

18. Schwarcz R. and Coyle J.T. (1977) Brain Res. 127:235-249

19. Severson J.A. and Finch L.E. (1980) Brain Res. 192:147-162

20. Spano P.F., Memo M., Stefanini E., Fresia P. and Trabucchi M. (1980) in:Receptors for neurotransmitters and peptide hormones, edited by Pepeu G., Kuhar M.J. and Enna S.J., pp. 243-251, Raven Press, New York

21. Waitling K.J., Dowling J.E. and Iversen L.L. (1979) Nature 281:578-580

The Aging Brain: Cellular and Molecular Mechanisms of Aging in the Nervous System, edited by E. Giacobini et al., Raven Press, New York © 1982.

Altered Mechanisms of Opiate and Dopaminergic Action During Aging

George S. Roth

Endocrinology Section, Clinical Physiology Branch, Gerontology Research Center, National Institute on Aging, National Institutes of Health at Baltimore City Hospitals, Baltimore, Maryland 21224

The ability of organisms to respond to various hormones, neurotransmitters, drugs and related agents is altered during the aging process (35, 36). Since such substances play important roles in regulating physiological functions, it is vitally important to understand the changes which occur in the mechanisms of their actions. These mechanisms are both diverse and complex, depending on the type of agent, and may involve many cellular components as well as neurohumoral factors which serve to modulate cellular responsiveness. This report will focus on two classes of neurotransmitters, the opiates and dopaminergics, and the mechanisms by which their actions become altered with aging.

The initial event in the actions of both opiate and dopaminergic agents is attachment to specific cellular receptors. These are protein molecules located on the cell membrane and can be further subdivided on the basis of pre- or post-synaptic location, pharmacological specificity and biological actions (10, 16, 42). In the case of dopamine agonists, binding to so called D1 (believed to be post-synaptic) receptors results in stimulation of adenylate cyclase and elevation of cyclic AMP levels (16). D2 receptors are believed to be primarily presynaptic and their particular actions are not mediated through cyclic AMP (16). The relative specificity of various agonists and antagonists for the different receptor classes is still somewhat confusing, however, both from a pharmacological and biochemical perspective.

Opiate receptors can also be divided into various classes, based on pharmacological and ligand specificity (10, 42). The distinctions here are equally as confusing as for the dopaminergic system and many different ligands are currently being evaluated for measurement of the opiate receptors.

Little is known about other intermediate steps in the mechanism of action of opiate and dopaminergic substances, but ultimately binding of these agents to their respective receptors results in particular biological effects. These may be tissue dependent. For example, dopaminergic effects in the corpus striatum include regulation of stereotypic behavior (6, 7), while in uterus dopamine may inhibit contractility (3). Dopaminergics may even serve to regulate immunological responsiveness of lymphocytes (43). Opiate receptors are also found to be present in many organs, and in addition to regulating pain perception and behavior through the central nervous system (2, 32) may regulate reproductive system function (12), as well as dietary intake (20) and body core temperature (21).

Because of their important physiological roles, and since many other hormone and neurotransmitter controlled functions exhibit altered responsiveness during aging (35, 36), both dopaminergic and opiate actions have become the subject of recent interest for gerontologists.

Opiate Action During Aging

Most studies of opiate action during aging have focused on sensitivity to pain. Although in general, pain thresholds appear to increase with increasing age, some controvery exists. For example Nicàk (29) and Parè (31) suggest that sensitivity of rats to electrical shock decreases with age. Similar findings have been reported for mice by Nilsen (30). In contrast, Gorden et al. (8) observed increased sensitivity to electrical shock in older rats, while Lippa et al. (18) could detect no age differences. In humans, post operative administration of morphine appears to result in greater pain relief in older individuals (1), and older subjects tend to respond to an opiate placebo in greater frequency than do young counterparts (17).

In our own laboratory, we have observed that sensitivity to both thermal and electrical pain stimulation decreases as rats age from 2 to 24 months of age (11). These age differences are at least partially eliminated by naloxone administration, suggesting that changes may occur in the endogenous opiod system during aging (11).

We are aware of only one other type of analysis for opiate action during aging. McDougal et al. (23) reported that older rats were more resistant than young to the acquisition of tolerance to the thermic effects of morphine. Older rats also exhibit a smaller hypothermic response to high morphine doses than young (21). In constrast, however, at low morphine doses older rats display a greater hyperthermic response.

Both sensitivity to pain and thermoregulation are extremely complex processes. Age changes could occur at various levels, ranging from the opioid receptors, to endogenous opioid levels, to the various neural pathways and end organs involved. Nevertheless, it has become important to attempt to elucidate the precise mechanisms by which such opiate mediated functions become altered during the aging process.

Several laboratories have now, in fact, examined opiate receptors during aging. Messing et al. (26, 27) used ^{3}H- dihydromorphine specific binding for this purpose and reported decreased opiate receptor concentrations in frontal poles, anterior cortex and striatum of senescent male Fisher 344 rats and thalamus and midbrain of senescent female rats. No significant differences between senescent (26 mo.) and mature (5 mo.) male rats were observed in amygdala, thalamus and midbrain, although amygdala exhibited a trend toward a possible reduction with age. Only frontal poles exhibited an age difference in affinity, being about twice as high in the older rats.

Our own group has examined these receptors by means of ^{3}H-etorphine specific binding. In reasonable agreement with Messing et al. (26, 27), we have observed decreased concentrations of opiate receptors in the frontal poles, striatum and hippocampus of aged male Wistar rats (11). Amygdala and anterior cortex exhibited a trend toward decrease with increasing age, but this was not significant. We could detect no significant age changes in binding affinity in any brain regions examined (11).

Finally, McDougal et al. (23) employed ^{3}H-naloxone and found a progressive decrease in specific binding in the hypothalamus of male Fisher 344 rats between 3 and 27 months of age. No significant age differences were observed in other regions. These investigators suggest that loss of hypothalamic opiate receptors might explain their previously observed age differences in morphine thermo-regulation and development of tolerance (21, 22).

In contrast, none of the observed decreases in opiate receptor concentrations can explain the increase in pain threshold observed with age in our own (11) and other laboratories (1, 17, 29, 30, 31). Although the increased affinity reported for frontal poles in aged male rats by Messing et al. (26) might be consistant with age related increases in pain threshold, they observed a concommitant decrease in this opiate receptor concentration. Moreover, we also observed loss of opiate receptors in senescent frontal poles (11), but without any change in binding affinity. Thus, possible explanations for the apparent discrepancy between altered receptors and pain response include: higher endogenous opioid levels in aged rats, mediation of pain sensitivity by brain regions other than those examined, difficulties inherent in attempting to localize age changes at a single step in such a complex process, and possible differential spinal pathways mediating the various types of pain.

Dopaminergic Action During Aging

A number of studies have suggested that dopaminergic functions may be impaired during senescence (13, 33, 37, 44). These include reduced dopamine uptake (13), reduced dopamine synthesis (37), and decreased dopamine sensitive adenylate cyclase activity (33, 44) in various brain areas. In an effort to elucidate the mechanisms by which such dopaminergic functions become altered with age, several laboratories have examined dopamine receptors in particular brain regions.

Makman's group (41) have reported that dopamine receptors measured by ^{3}H-spiroperidol specific binding are lost from striatum, frontal cortex and anterior limbic cortex as rabbits aged from 5 to 65 months. The relative reductions are approximately 30%, 30% and 20% for the three regions, respectively. Binding affinity remains constant over this period. Since spiroperidol is a dopaminergic antagonist, receptors were also measured using ^{3}H-2-amino, 6, 7-dihydroxyl-1, 2, 3, 4 tetrahydronaphthalene (ADTN). ADTN binding sites were reduced by more than 50% in stiatum. It has been suggested that the binding sites in striatum are primarily post-synaptic while 2/3 of the spiroperidol binding sites may exist at other loci (24). Moreover, the 50% loss of ADTN sites during aging closely parallels the loss of dopamine stimulated adenylate cyclase which is also believed to be post-synaptic (19).

Although possible loss of speicifc neurons might be an explanation for decreases in receptors in aged rat brain, Makman et al. (19) find no evidence for neuronal loss of striatum, anterior limbic cortex, or frontal cortex as assessed by dopamine and norepinephrine concentrations as well as choline acetylase activity with ^{3}H-quinuclindinyl-benzilate binding. Thus, age related loss of dopamine receptors would appear to be due to intrinsic or extrinsic cellular changes rather than simple cell loss.

In this laboratory we have observed a 33% reduction in specific binding sites for haloperidol in corpora striata of Wistar rats between 6 and 24 months of age (14). No change in binding affinity was detected. Preliminary studies suggest a comparable decrease in ^{3}H-spiroperidol (15) as well as a greater reduction in ^{3}H-ADTN specific binding (unpublished data). In contrast, binding affinities do not change with age.

Misra et al. (28) also observed at 40% reduction in spiroperidol specific binding sties in the striata of aged rats of an unspecified strain. In addition, they likewise found no age change in binding affinity.

Similar observations have already been made by Severson and Finch (39) in striata of C57BL/6J mice. ^{3}H-spiroperidol specific binding sites progressively decreased about 50% between 3 and 28 months of age, while binding affinity remained unaltered. ^{3}H-spiroperidol binding sites also decreased about 35% in hypothalamus between 8 and 28 months of age while no change was observed in olfactory bulbs. ADTN binding sites decreased about twice as much as spiroperidol sites over comparable age ranges. This finding is in close agreement with that of Makman et al. (41).

A possible difference between the two groups arises from interpretation of data. Severson and Finch (39) suggest that unlike the situation in rabbits there is some evidence for decreased choline acetyltransferase in rat striatum. They, therefore, postulated an age-related loss of striatal interneurons as a possibel cause of decreased dopamine sensitive adenylate cyclase receptors. More recently, however, the same group (34) has pointed out that dopamine sensitive adenylate cyclase in striatum is substantially decreased before 12 months in rats (38), an age when supersensitization responses to chronic haloperidol are not altered in mice (see below). Thus, subsequent impairments in supersensitization may derive from loss of different striatal cells or may require more extensive loss.

These investigators have also recently examined dopamine receptors in caudate nucleus, substantia migra, putamen, and nucleus accumbans obtained from different aged humans post morten (40). Significant age-related decreases in receptor concentration as measured by both ^{3}H-ADTN and ^{3}H-spiroperidol binding were observed in both caudate nucleus and substantia nigra. No age differences in binding affinity were observed in any brain regions.

In contrast to most of the above observations, Govoni et al. (9) reported that striatal ^{3}H-spiroperidol binding sites did not change in concentration between 3 and 30 months in Sprague-Dawley rats. Instead, binding affinity was reduced by a factor of 5. Reduced spiroperidol binding was also detected in the aged tuberculum olfactorium. The reason(s) for the discrepancy between this latter study and those of the other four laboratories is not clear at this time. However, again it is conceivable that species/strain differences may be involved. Also likely is the possibility of complications arising from the multiple forms of dopamine receptor, since the specificity of various ligands may vary under different assay and preparation conditions. More recently, experiments from the same laboratory using ^{3}H-spiroperidol for D1 receptors and ^{3}H-sulpiride for D2 receptors have suggested that age related decreases in concentration do occur for the former but not the latter sites (25). Binding affinity was not altered with age at either site.

Attention has also been focused on the ability to regulate dopamine receptor levels in response to various manipulations. Severson et al. observed that senescent C57BL/6J mice were unable to proliferate striatal dopamine receptors following chronic haloperidol treatment even though young counterparts increased receptors by 25-30%. In contrast, we have employed 6-hydroxydopamine to induce denervation of Wistar rats and detected no age difference in the relative ability to develop receptor supersensitivity. Both mature and senescent animals showed receptor increases of about 50%.

Conceivably differences between these two studies are due to the type of manipulation used to attempt induction of supersensitivity. Snyder's group (4, 5) has reported that 6-hydroxydopamine may be more effective than haloperidol in causing supersensitivity. Possibly older animals require a more severe challenge to enable them to proliferate striatal dopamine receptors.

Conclusions and Significance

Certain effects of both opiate and dopaminergic agents are altered during aging. Many investigators have attempted to elucidate the mechanisms responsible for such changes. Since the initial sites of action for these agents are specific cellular receptors, much attention has been focused at this level.

There is now reasonably good agreement that loss of dopamine receptors from the corpus striatum occurs in mice, rats, rabbits and humans with aging. Such loss may be responsible for age related decreases in ability to stimulate adenylate cyclase and certain stereotypic behavior patterns.

Loss of opiate receptors has also been observed during aging in rats but disagreement exists as to which brain regions are most affected. In any case, loss of these receptors cannot account for the increased pain threshold observed by several laboratories in aged rodents (11, 29, 30, 31) and humans (1, 17). However, receptor loss may account, at least partially, for the decreased ability of senescent rats to develop morphine tolerance and to produce hypothermic responses to this drug (21, 22).

Further studies will certainly be necessary in several key areas. These include mechanisms by which receptor levels may be altered with age, examination of factors other than receptors which might result in altered responsiveness during aging, and better understanding of the different neurotransmitter subtypes and their roles in regulating particular physiological processes.

References

1. Bellville, J.W., Forrest, W.H., Miller, E., and Brown, B.W. (1971): J. Am. Med. Assoc. 217:1836-1841.
2. Bloom, F., Segal, D., Ling, N., and Guillemin, R. (1976): Science 194:630-632.
3. Burns, J.K. (1980): J. Physiol (London) 310:47P.
4. Burt, D.R., Creese, I., and Snyder, S.H. (1977): Science 196:326-328.
5. Creese, I., Burt, D.R., and Snyder, S.H. (1977): Science 197:596-598.
6. Ernst, A.M., and Smelik, P.G. (1966): Experienta 22:837-838.

7. Fogg, R., and Pakkenberg, H. (1971): Exp. Neurol. 31:75-86.
8. Gorden, W.C., Scobie, S.R., and Franese, S.E. (1978): Exp. Aging Res. 4:23-35.
9. Govoni, S., Memo, M., Saiani, L., Spano, P.F., and Trabucchi, M. (1980): Mech. Ageing and Devel. 12:39-46.
10. Hazum, E., Chang, K-J., and Cuatrecasas, P. (1980): Proc. Nat. Acad. Sci. U.S. 77:3038-3041.
11. Hess, G.D., Joseph, J.A., and Roth, G.S. (1981): Neurobiology of Aging 2:49-55.
12. Jacquet, Y.F. (1980): Science 210:95-97.
13. Jonec, V., and Finch, C.E. (1975): Brain Res. 91:197-215.
14. Joseph, J.A., Berger, R.E., Engel, B.T., and Roth, G.S. (1978): J. Gerontology 33:643-649.
15. Joseph, J. A., Filburn, C.R., and Roth, G.S.: Life Sciences (in press).
16. Kebabian, J.W., and Calne, D.B. (1979): Nature 277:93-96.
17. Kenshalo, D.R. (1977): In: Handbook of the Psychology of Aging, edited by J. Birren, and W. Schaie, pp. 562-579. Van Nostranal Reinhold Co., New York.
18. Lippa, A.S., Pelham, R.W., Beer, B., Critchett, D.J., Dean, R.L., and Bartus, R.T. (1980): Neurobiology of Aging 1:13-19.
19. Makman, M.H., Ahn, H.S., Thal, L.J., Sharpless, N.S., Dvorkin, B., Horowitz, S.G., and Rosenfeld, M. (1980): Brain Res. 192:177-183.
20. Margules, D.L., Moisset, B., Lewis, H.J., Shibuya, H., and Pert, C.B. (1978): Science 202:988-991.
21. McDougal, J.N., Marques, P.R., and Burks, T.F. (1980): Life Sciences 27:2679-2685.
22. McDougal, J.N., Marques, P.R., and Burks, T.F. (1981): Life Sciences 28:137-145.
23. McDougal, J.N., Pedigo, N.W., Marques, P.R., Vamamura, H.I., and Burks, T.F. (1980): Abstracts of the Society for Neuroscience 6:78.
24. McGeer, D.L., McGeer, E.G., Fibiger, H.C., and Wickson, V. (1971): Exp. Gerontology 6:391-396.
25. Memo, M., Lucchi, L., Spano, P.F., and Trabucchi, M. (1980): Brain Res. 202:488-492.
26. Messing, R.B., Vasquez, B.J., Samaniego, B., Jensen, R.A., Martinez, J.L., and McGaugh, J.L. (1981): J. Neurochem. 36:784-790.
27. Messing, R.B., Vasquez, B.J., Spiehler, V.R., Martinez, J.L., Jensen, R.A., Rigter, H., and McGaugh, J.L. (1980): Life Sciences 26:921-927.
28. Misra, C.H., Shelat, H., and Smith, R.C. (1979): Abstracts of the Society for Neuroscience 5:30.
29. Nicák, A. (1971): Exp. Gerontol. 6:111-114.
30. Nilsen, P.L. (1961): Acta Pharmacol. et Toxicol. 18:10-22.
31. Paré, W.P. (1969): J. Comparative and Physiol. Psychol. 69:214-218.
32. Pert, C.B., and Snyder, S.H. (1973): Proc. Nat. Acad. Sci. U.S. 70:2243-2247.
33. Puri, S.K., and Volicer, L. (1976): Mech. Ageing and Devel. 6:53-58.
34. Randall, P.K., Severson, J.A., and Finch, C.E.: J. Pharmacol. and Exp. Therapeutics (in press).
35. Roth, G.S. (1979): Fed. Proc. 38:1910-1914.
36. Roth, G.S. (1979): Mech. Ageing and Devel. 9:497-514.

37. Samorajski, T. (1975): In: Ageing Vol. 1, edited by H. Brody, D. Harman, and J.M. Ordy, pp. 199-214. Raven Press, New York.
38. Schmidt, M.J., and Thornberry, J.F. (1978): Brain Res. 139:169-177.
39. Severson, J.A., and Finch, C.E. (1980): Brain Res. 192:147-162.
40. Severson, J.A., Marcusson, J., Winblad, B., and Finch, C.E.: J. Neurochem. (in press).
41. Thal, L.J., Horowitz, S.G., Dvorkin, B., and Makman, M.H. (1980): Brain Res. 192:185-194.
42. Tyers, M.B. (1980): Br. J. Pharmacol. 69:503-512.
43. Uzan, A., Phan, T., LeFur, G. (1981): J. Pharm. Pharmacol. 33:102-103.
44. Walker, J.P., and Boas-Walker, J. (1973): Brain Res. 54:391-396.

The Aging Brain: Cellular and Molecular Mechanisms of Aging in the Nervous System, edited by E. Giacobini et al., Raven Press, New York © 1982.

Modifications in Rat Brain GABA Receptor Binding as a Function of Age

D. A. Kendall, R. Strong, and S. J. Enna

Departments of Pharmacology and of Neurobiology and Anatomy, University of Texas Medical School, Houston, Texas 77025

Alterations in central nervous system function are responsible for many of the debilities associated with aging. Among the more obvious infirmities that may be traced to changes in brain function include incoordination, memory loss, apathy and depression. Numerous studies have been undertaken to define the morphological, biochemical and physiological changes that occur in the central nervous system as a function of age in order to understand the biological basis for these behavioral and motor impairments (6). These studies have revealed that there is a significant amount of neuronal degeneration associated with the aging process and that certain neurons, such as cerebellar Purkinje cells, are particularly vulnerable in this regard (14,16). Furthermore, brain function is also compromised because of age-related alterations in neurotransmitter synthesis, storage and release (17,22,25). Finally, more recent work has revealed a number of region and transmitter selective modifications in brain neurotransmitter receptor recognition sites (2,8,11, 20,23,24,27,28). It is unclear at present whether these neurochemical changes are simply secondary to neuronal degeneration or whether, in some cases, they may be a primary manifestation of the aging process.

In recent years particular emphasis has been placed on examining the involvement of γ-aminobutyric acid (GABA) neurotransmission in the etiology and symptomatology of a variety of neuropsychiatric disorders, as well as with respect to the disabilities associated with the normal aging process. The reason for this interest is that GABA is one of the most widely distributed neurotransmitters in brain and therefore, alterations in GABAergic function would be expected to modify the activity of a variety of other transmitter systems (3,4). Alterations in GABA transmission have been found to be present in numerous disorders, including Huntington's and Parkinson's diseases, and tardive dyskinesia (5). Since the symptoms of these disorders resemble, superficially at least, many of the dysfunctions associated with senility, it seems likely that modifications in the GABA system may occur as a consequence of aging. Surprisingly however, from a neurochemical standpoint, the GABA system appears to be somewhat less affected by age than other neurotransmitter

systems (8,20). Thus, although the activity of glutamic
acid decarboxylase, the enzyme chiefly responsible for the
synthesis of GABA, is reportedly reduced in older animals,
this reduction has been found in only certain brain regions
and is species specific (8). In contrast, decreases in
choline acetyltransferase activity, a measure of acetylcholine synthesis, are much more widespread (8,28). In addition, while age-related changes in β-adrenergic, dopamine,
cholinergic muscarinic and opiate receptor binding sites
have been found, GABA receptor binding is reportedly unchanged (15,20,23,28). This latter finding is particularly
intriguing given the recent data indicating that the electrophysiological responses to GABA are altered in the hippocampus of aged rats (18).

Over the past few years, studies have indicated that
there may be kinetically, and possibly pharmacologically
and functionally, distinct subsets of GABA receptors (1,7,
12). Whereas 3H-GABA binding to brain membranes normally
appears to be associated with a single, relatively low
affinity (∿300 nM) site, pretreatment of membranes with the
nonionic detergent Triton X-100 reveals a second, higher
affinity (∿10 nM), lower capacity, binding component. While
both the high and low affinity sites appear to have similar
pharmacological characteristics, it has been suggested that
they may be functionally independent (1). These data have
been interpreted to indicate that Triton removes an endogenous modulator (GABAmodulin) of the higher affinity component, enabling the detection of this site using a ligand
binding assay. Since GABA receptor binding was examined
in earlier studies using brain membranes not exposed to the
detergent, it is conceivable that an age-related modification in the high affinity binding component may not have
been detected.

In the present study, the influence of aging on GABA
receptor binding to membranes treated with Triton X-100 was
examined. The results indicate that there is a significant
age-related decline in high affinity GABA binding in most
brain regions and that, in some areas, low affinity binding
is reduced as well. These findings suggest that modifications in GABA receptor recognition sites may account for
some of the motor and mental impairments associated with
the aging process.

MATERIALS AND METHODS

Male Sprague-Dawley rats, aged 5-6 months (mature) and
26-27 months (aged) were used in all studies. The animals
were obtained from the aging colony maintained for the
National Institute of Aging at Charles Rivers Laboratories
in Wilmington, Mass.

The animals were killed by decapitation and the brains
rapidly removed, dissected on ice and stored at -20°C until
assayed. GABA receptor binding using 3H-GABA (57 Ci/mmole)
as a ligand was performed as previously described (7).
Briefly, the frozen tissue was homogenized with a Brinkman

Polytron in 20 vol of distilled water, centrifuged at 48,000 x g for 10 min and then washed two times by resuspending and centrifuging as above. Following the final centrifugation the tissue was resuspended in 100 vol of 0.05 M Tris-citrate buffer (pH 7.1 at 4oC) containing Triton X-100 (0.05 or 0.1%, v/v) and this suspension was incubated for 30 min at 37oC. Subsequent to this incubation the homogenate was centrifuged at 48,000 x g for 10 min at 4oC, and the pellet resuspended and centrifuged twice more to rid the tissue of detergent. The resultant pellet was resuspended a final time in 100 vol of Tris buffer. Portions (0.5 - 1.0 mg protein) of this homogenate were added to 12 ml Sorvall centrifuge tubes containing ^{3}H-GABA (7 nM). In some cases the tubes contained the radioisotope and one of various concentrations (1-500 nM) of unlabeled GABA. The samples were incubated at 4oC for 5 min and the binding reaction terminated by centrifugation at 48,000 x g for 10 min. The resultant supernatant was decanted and the pellet rinsed rapidly and superficially with 15 ml of ice-cold distilled water. Membrane bound radioactivity was extracted into 1 ml of Protosol (New England Nuclear) tissue solubilizer, after which 10 ml of Econoflour scintillation cocktail were added and radioactivity monitored using a Searle Mark III scintillation spectrometer. Specific ^{3}H-GABA receptor binding was defined as the amount of radioligand displaced by 1 mM unlabeled GABA. In some cases, complete displacement curves were generated and the data was converted to determine the receptor site affinity (K_d) and concentration (B_{max}) using the method of Scatchard. Protein was analysed by the method of Lowry et al (19). A two-tailed t-test was used to calculate the level of significance for any differences between means. A $p \leq 0.05$ was considered statistically significant.

Unlabeled GABA was purchased from Sigma Chemical Co. (St. Louis, MO) and ^{3}H-GABA from New England Nuclear (Boston Mass.). All other chemicals and reagents were obtained from commercial suppliers.

RESULTS

The influence of Triton X-100 treatment on the specific binding of ^{3}H-GABA to rat cerebellar membranes was analysed using tissue obtained from mature and aged rats (Fig. 1). While no significant difference was noted in binding between the two age groups in control tissue, ^{3}H-GABA receptor binding was markedly lower in the older age group when the membranes had been treated with either 0.05 or 0.1% Triton X-100. Although Triton enhanced binding in both age groups, the enhancement was much less in the older animals, with specific binding being 20-30% less in the older animals after exposure to 0.05% Triton and approximately 20% less than the younger group in tissue exposed to a 0.1% concentration of detergent.

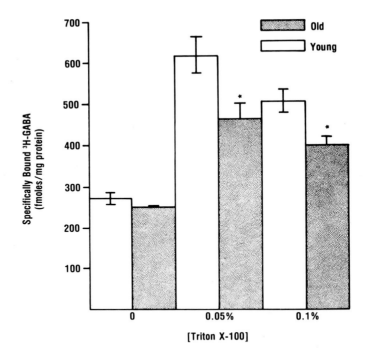

FIG. 1. Effect of Triton X-100 on ^{3}H-GABA receptor binding
in cerebellar membranes of mature and aged rats. Prior to
the GABA receptor binding assay, the membranes were incubated for 30 min at 37° in Tris-citrate buffer containing
either 0.05% of 0.1% (v/v) Triton X-100. Control animals
were preincubated with buffer in the absence of detergent.
After several rinses to rid the tissue of Triton, the membranes were analysed for GABA receptor binding using the
standard procedure as described in Methods. The height of
each bar represents the mean $\pm$ s.e.m. of 4-5 separate
experiments, each of which was performed in triplicate.

*$p < 0.05$ compared to corresponding mature value.

To determine whether the reduced ^{3}H-GABA binding
was restricted to the cerebellum, receptor binding was
analysed in three other brain regions following treatment
with Triton (0.05%). The results indicated that, like the
cerebellum, GABA receptor binding was reduced over 29% in

the cerebral cortex, midbrain and forebrain in the older animals, though the difference was not statistically significant in the latter region (Table 1). Receptor binding site saturation analysis in cerebral cortex revealed two components for GABA binding; a low affinity having a K_d of approximately 100 nM and a higher affinity site with a K_d of 30 nM (Fig. 2). These results also indicated that the differences in receptor binding between mature and aged animals was due to a decrease in the binding site concentrations in both the high and low affinity sites (Fig. 2 and Table 2). Similar results were obtained with midbrain, where both the high and low affinity B_{max} values were some 20-30% less in the aged animals than in the 6 mongh old group (Table 2). In cerebellum, however, only the high affinity component was reduced in the aged brain, with the B_{max} for the low affinity site being identical in the two age groups (Table 2). In no case were any significant differences noted in GABA receptor affinity between the mature and the aged animals following Triton treatment.

TABLE 1. ^{3}H-GABA binding in mature and aged rat brain regions[a]

| Brain Region | Specifically Bound ^{3}H-GABA [a] (fmol/mg protein) | |
	Mature	Aged
Forebrain	329 + 36	236 + 46
Cortex	632 + 42	484 + 19 [b] (-23%)
Midbrain	343 + 7	260 + 10 [b] (-24%)
Cerebellum	640 + 48	513 + 28[b] (-20%)

[a] Each value represents the mean + s.e.m of 4-5 separate experiments, each of which was performed in triplicate.

[b] $p < 0.05$ compared to corresponding mature value.

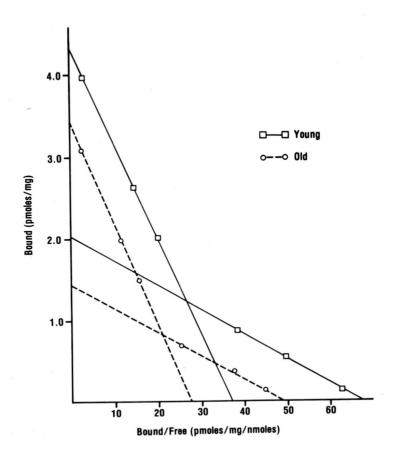

FIG. 2. Scathard analysis of 3H-GABA binding in rat brain cerebral cortex in mature and aged animals. Prior to the 3H-GABA binding assay the tissue was preincubated for 30 min at 37° in a 0.05% Triton X-100 (v/v) Tris-citrate buffer system. After several rinses to rid the tissue of detergent, the membranes were analysed for GABA recepror binding using saturation analysis as described in Methods. Each point represents the mean of 4-5 separate experiments, each of which was analysed in triplicate.

_____ Mature

- - - - - - - - - - - - Aged

TABLE 2. 3H-GABA binding in mature and aged rat brain regions [a]

Brain Region	Mature		Aged	
	High Affinity[b]	Low Affinity	High Affinity	Low Affinity
	2.02+0.08 30.2+2.1	4.35+0.09 117.9+10.0	1.48+0.16[c] 30.2+3.7	3.40+0.09[c] 123.0+12.5
Midbrain	1.61+0.06 41.7+1.7	3.07+0.1 134.2+9.7	1.26+0.05[c] 40.0+1.5	2.24+0.09 126.4+11.9
Cerebellum	2.65+0.1 33.8+1.7	3.3+0.2 128.9+6.4	2.10+0.1[c] 36.8+4.7	3.10+0.3 160.0+19.2

a Each value represents the mean $\pm$ of 4-5 separate experiments, each of which was performed in triplicate.

b B_{max} values are pmol/mg protein and K_d is nM.

c $p < 0.05$ compared with mature value.

DISCUSSION

        It is likely that many of the motor and mental abnor-
malities associated with normal aging are due to disruptions
in neurotransmission at the synaptic level. In addition to
age-related modifications in transmitter synthesis, uptake
and metabolism, investigators have found that postsynaptic
processes, such as transmitter-stimulated cyclic AMP accumulation, are also reduced in the aged brain (12, 26). Furthermore, alterations in postsynaptic receptor recognition
site binding for a number of neurotransmitters have been reported, with the present data indicating that the GABA receptor binding system may also be affected in this manner.
        As for many neurotransmitters, there appear to be at
least two kinetically distinct classes of GABA receptor
binding sites. However it is unknown whether these sites
represent different states of the same receptor or whether
they are anatomically and functionally distinct. Although
early studies suggested that these sites are pharmacologically identical (7), more recent data indicate that only
the lower affinity component may be linked to the benzodiazepine receptor system (1), suggesting a dissimilarity in
their functional capacity.
        Unlike other neurotransmitter receptor sites however,
the number and affinity of GABA binding sites appear to be
regulated by an endogenous protein termed GABAmodulin (13).
Binding assays performed in the presence of GABAmodulin detect only a single, low affinity, receptor binding component.
However, after removal of GABAmodulin, either by extensively
washing or by treating the membranes with Triton, a higher
affinity binding site is revealed. The results of the present study indicate that the GABAmodulin component of the
receptor is intact in aged animals since there was no significant difference in binding between the two age groups
using membranes that had not been treated with detergent.
In fact, the presence of GABAmodulin masks the loss of GABA
receptors that appears to take place during the aging process. Since the precise in vivo role of this modulator in
regulating the activity of GABA receptors is unknown, it
could be argued that the binding data obtained in the presence of this substance is a better reflection of the biological state of the receptor. If this is the case, then it
may be concluded that aging has little effect on GABA receptor function, at least as measured by binding assays. On
the other hand, if the receptor binding sites regulated by
GABAmodulin are crucial for normal activity, then the present
data suggests that there may be an alteration in GABA neurotransmission with age because of the decline in recognition
site binding. In this regard it is notable that recent
studies have been able to localize the high affinity GABA
receptor binding component to postsynaptic densities (21).
However, studies aimed at examining the functional activity
of GABA receptors in the aged brain must be undertaken in
order to more conclusively determine the manner in which

this change in receptor binding expresses itself with regard to neuronal activity.

While the reason for the loss of GABA receptors in aged rats is unknown, several possibilites exist. A decrease in GABA receptor binding could result from an overstimulation of the receptor system (9,10) which, in the present case, would imply that GABAergic neurons are hyperactive in these brain regions. Alternatively, the receptor loss could be secondary to an age-related degeneration in GABA-receptive cells. Moreover, a decrease in GABA binding could ensue as a consequence of a decrease in receptor synthesis that may be independent of synaptic activity. Clearly, the functional expression of this receptor loss will be dependent, to some extent, on which of these possibilities account for the change.

In summary, an age-related decline in the number, but not affinity, of GABA receptor binding sites in several regions of the rat brain has been detected. Since it is possible that this change in GABA receptor binding is an adaptive phenomenon, it is conceivable that there may be no net change in GABAergic function. On the other hand, if the loss is due to neuronal dropout or to an uncompensated change in GABA receptor synthesis or degradation, the decline in receptor binding most likely represents a diminution in GABAergic activity. Because of the importance of GABA in maintaining normal central nervous system activity, a decrease in GABA tone would undoubtedly contribute to many of the abnormalities associated with aging.

ACKNOWLEDGEMENTS

Supported in part by USPHS grants NS-13803, a Research Career Development Award NS-00335 (S.J.E.) and a National Institute of Aging Predoctoral Award (R.S.).

REFERENCES

1. Browner, M., Ferkany, J.W. and Enna, S.J. (1981): J. Neurosci., 1:514-518.

2. Cubells, J.F., and Joseph, J.A. (1981): Life Sci., 28: 1215-1218.

3. Enna, S.J. (1981): Biochem. Pharmacol., 30:907-913.

4. Enna, S.J. (1981): Trends in Pharmacol. Sci., 2:62-64.

5. Enna, S.J. (1981): IN: Neuropharmacology of Central Disorders, edited by G.C. Palmer, pp. 507-537, Academic Press, New York.

6. Enna, S.J., Samorjski, T., and Beer, B., editors (1981): IN: Brain Neurotransmitters and Receptors in Aging and Age Related Disorders. Raven Press, New York.

7. Enna, S.J. and Snyder, S.H. (1977): Mol. Pharmacol. 13: 442-453.

8. Enna, S.J. and Strong, R. (1981): IN: Brain Neurotransmitters and Receptors in Aging and Age Related Disorders, edited by S.J. Enna, T. Samorajski, and B. Beer, pp. 133-142, Raven Press, New York.

9. Ferkany, J.W., and Enna, S.J. (1980): Life Sci., 27:143-149.

10. Ferkany, J.W., Strong, R., and Enna, S.J. (1980): J. Neurochem., 34:247-249.

11. Freund, G. (1980): Life Sci., 26:371-375.

12. Govoni, S., Loddo, P., Spano, P.F., and Trabucchi, M. (1977): Brain Res., 138:565-570.

13. Guidotti, A., Toffano, G., and Costa, E. (1978): Nature, 275:353-355.

14. Hall, T. C., Miller, A.K., and Corsellis, J. (1975): Neuropath. Appl. Neurol., 1:267-292.

15. Hess, G. D., Joseph, J.A., and Roth, G.S. (1981): Neurobiol. Aging, 2:49-55.

16. Inukai, T., (1928): J. Comp. Neurol., 45:1-28.

17. Jonec, V., and Finch, C.E. (1975): Brain Res., 91:197-215.

18. Lippa, A.S., Critchett, D.J., Ehlert, F., Yamamura, H.I., Enna, S.J. and Bartus, R.T. (1981): Neurobiol. Aging, 2:3-8.

19. Lowry, O.H., Rosenbrough, J.J., Farr, A.L. and Randall, R.J. (1951): J. Biol. Chem., 193:265-275.

20. Maggi, A., Schmidt, M.J., Ghetti, B., and Enna, S.J. (1979): Life Sci., 24:367-374.

21. Matus, A. (1981): Trends in Neurosci., 2:51-53.

22. McGeer, P.L., and McGeer, E.G. (1976): J. Neurochem., 26:65-76.

23. Misra, C.H., Shelat, H.S. and Smith, R.C. (1980): Life Sci., 27:521-526.

24. Pittman, R.N., Minneman, K.P., and Molinoff, P. (1980): J. Neurochem., 35:273-275.

25. Ponzio, F., Brunello, N. and Algeri, S. (1978): J. Neurochem., 30:1617-1620.

26. Schmidt, M.J. and Thornberry, J.F. (1978): Brain Res., 139:169-177.

27. Shih, J.C., and Young, H. (1978): Life Sci., 23:1441-1448.

28. Strong, R., Hicks, P., Hsu, L., Bartus, R.T., and Enna, S.J. (1980): Neurobiol. Aging, 1:59-63.

The Aging Brain: Cellular and Molecular Mechanisms of Aging in the Nervous System, edited by E. Giacobini et al., Raven Press, New York © 1982.

Pyruvate Dehydrogenase Complex and Choline Acetyltransferase in Aging and Dementia

S. Sorbi, *L. Amaducci, J. P. Blass, and **E. D. Bird

*Dementia Research Service, Division of Chronic and Degenerative Diseases, Department of Neurology, Cornell University Medical College, Burke Rehabilitation Center, White Plains, New York 10605; *Department of Neurology, University of Florence, Florence 50134, Italy; **Department of Neurology-Neuropathology, Harvard Medical School, McLean Hospital, Boston, Massachusetts 02178*

Two abnormalities are well known in dementias: abnormalities in the cholinergic system (1,2,8,9,12,22) and decreases in cerebral metabolic rate (4,5,6,8,19).

For Alzheimer brain at autopsy, marked reductions have been found by several groups in choline acetyltransferase (CAT) activity, a marker of the cholinergic system (2,9,12,31,33). They are related to the degree of pathological damage (23) and to the degree of dementia (30). CAT activity is reduced in frontal cortex, in hippocampus and in several basal ganglia--caudate, accumbens, putamen, and globus pallidus (1,2,9, 12,31,33). In addition to the reduction in this cholinergic marker in postmortem brain specimens, a significant decrease in enzyme activity has been observed in biopsy brain specimens from Alzheimer patients where acetylcholine synthesis is also reduced (30). The decrease in the neurotransmitter acetylcholine seems to be related to the duration of illness and to the degree of mental deterioration (30). Involvement of the cholinergic system is not specific for Alzheimer-type dementias since a decrease in CAT activity has been found as well in alcoholic dementia (2), in Huntington's disease (3), and in Creutzfeldt-Jakob disease (32) but not in multi-infarct dementia (33). The major cholinergic projections to the cerebral cortex originate from the nucleus basalis of Meynert (13). The decrease in the cholinergic marker in paleocortical fields may be related to a primary lesion of subcortical structures (1,31,39).

Decreases in cerebral blood flow, cerebral glucose utilization and cerebral oxygen consumption typically occur in patients with dementia (5,6). They do not appear to be specific for any particular type of dementia (6). They occur in Alzheimer-type and multi-infarct dementias as well as in toxic and deficiency states associated with dementia (5,6). Even mild impairment of carbohydrate oxidation impairs cognitive functions (6).

Ochoa and Nachmanson (21) demonstrated in 1940 that the neurotransmitter acetylcholine was made by the condensation of acetyl-coenzyme-A (acetyl-CoA) with choline. The normal source of acetyl-CoA is from the oxidation of pyruvate derived from the glucose by glycolysis (21). Recently, a close correlation has been observed between activity of the pyruvate dehydrogenase complex (PDHC) and CAT in cat (27), rat (36), and human (24) brains. Furthermore, cholinergic function is exquisitely sensitive to impairments of pyruvate oxidation (6,38). We now report decreases in PDHC activity (34) accompanying the deficiencies in CAT (14,15) in Alzheimer and Huntington brains.

The brain specimens from Alzheimer's disease, Huntington's chorea patients, and age-matched controls were obtained from the brain bank of McLean Hospital, Belmont, Mass. (USA) and were studied double-blind.

In all brains examined, pathological or normal, we found a significant correlation between PDHC and CAT activities (r=0.97; P<0.0001; PDHC=6.50CAT + 1.59). However, in two brain regions, hippocampus and frontal cortex (Brodman's area 10), activities of these two enzymes did not correlate as well. PDHC in control hippocampus and frontal cortex was 9 and 18% of putamen activity, whereas CAT activity was 6 and 3% (Table 1). Without these two regions the CAT-PDHC correlation rose to r=0.99 (P<0.0001, PDHC=7.19CAT + 0.11).

TABLE 1.   CAT and PDHC activities in control brains[a]

	CAT	PDHC
Putamen	100 ± 7	100 ± 6
Caudate	74 ± 6	74 ± 6
Amygdala	20 ± 3	21 ± 2
Hippocampus	6 ± 1	9 ± 1
Cerebellar cortex	3 ± 1	4 ± 1
Frontal cortex	3 ± 1	18 ± 1

[a]CAT and PDHC activities are expressed as percent of putamen ± SEM.

Fumarase (26) correlated with neither CAT nor PDHC activities in any of the regions examined.

In Alzheimer brains, PDHC activity was markedly reduced (P<0.05) in the frontal cortex. The expected reduction in CAT occurred as well (Table 2). These studies confirm those of Perry et al (24); their assay for PDHC gave activites about 40% of those reported here. Fumerase activity was, however, normal in Alzheimer brain frontal cortex.

TABLE 2.   Enzyme activities in Alzheimer frontal cortex[a]

	Control (12)	Alzheimer (5)
CAT	0.063 ± 0.004	0.037 ± 0.005[b]
PDHC	3.3 ± 0.4	2.3 ± 0.2[c]
FUMARASE	181 ± 4	180 ± 7

[a]Activity expressed as nmoles/min/mg prot (mean ± SEM).
[b]P<0.005; [c]P<0.05.

CAT and PDHC activities were also both markedly decreased in affected areas of Huntington's chorea brains where, again, fumarase was normal (Table 3).

TABLE 3. Enzyme activities in Huntington brains[a]

	PDHC	CAT	FUMARASE
Caudate	40[b]	40[b]	100
Putamen	50[c]	50[c]	94
Amygdala	88	80	96
Frontal cortex	95	103	99

[a]Values are percent of control activities. At least 12 subjects were studied for each region. [b]P<0.001; [c]P<0.005.

To investigate a potential genetic basis for the decreases in PDHC in Huntington and Alzheimer brains, we examined PDHC activity in cultured skin fibroblasts. Alzheimer line GM 0364, Huntington proband line GM 1169, Huntington at risk GM 2077, and control cells lines GM 1960, GM 2185, GM 2037, GM 0288 were obtained from The Mutant Genetic Repository, Copewood, NJ (USA). No differences in PDHC activity were detected before or after activation (dephosphorylation) with dichloroacetate (DCA) (29) in the Huntington or Alzheimer cell lines (Table 4).

TABLE 4. PDHC in cultured human fibroblasts[a]

	Original	Activated[b]
Controls (4)	1.51 ± 0.02	2.68 ± 0.07
Alzheimer (1)	1.42	2.86
Huntington (2)	1.46 ± 0.01	2.79 ± 0.01

[a]PDHC activity is expressed as nmoles/min/mg prot (mean ± SEM). Each cell line was studied in at least three separate experiments. [b]PDHC was assayed before (original) and after (activated) incubation at 37° C for 30 minutes with dichloroacetate (29). Numbers in parentheses are numbers of subjects studied.

We have also investigated CAT activity in another dementing syndrome, Creutzfeldt-Jakob disease. Brains of three Creutzfeldt-Jakob autopsy proven patients and 10 age-matched controls were studied. A diffuse decrease of this cholinergic marker occurred in cortical areas as well as in the basal ganglia. In particular, frontal (Brodman area 10) and temporal (Brodman area 22) cortices showed a significant (P<0.001) decrease in CAT activity as did caudate, accumbens, putamen and hippo-campus (Table 5). Measurements of PDHC or other metabolic enzymes are not yet available for these brains.

TABLE 5. CAT activity in Creutzfeldt-Jakob disease[a]

	CAT	P<
Frontal cortex	23	0.001
Temporal cortex	24	0.001
Caudate	17	0.001
Putamen	4	0.001
Accumbens	7	0.001
Thalamus	17	0.001
Hippocampus	6	0.001

[a]CAT activity is expressed as percent of controls.

DISCUSSION

Two biochemical changes occur in a number of disorders which cause dementia: decreases in cerebral carbohydrate oxidation and decreases in cerebral CAT activity. Reductions in cerebral metabolic rate, manifested in reduced CMR-O_2, CMR-glu, and cerebral blood flow, characteristically occur not only in Alzheimer disease and in multi-infarct dementia but also in several less common dementing disorders. Reductions in cerebral CAT occur in Alzheimer disease (1,2,9,12,31,33), Huntington disease (3), alcoholic dementia (2), and Creutzfeldt-Jakob disease (32), but not in multi-infarct dementia (33). Indirect evidence suggests that there may be a cholinergic deficiency in other systems degenerations which also often lead to dementia (35). Generally, these two changes have been looked on as independent. The decreased cerebral metabolic rate is conventionally attributed to a loss of rapidly-metabolizing neuronal structures (including nerve endings) and to a decreased metabolic demand on the structures remaining, due to a decreased firing rate which reflects the impairment in processing information (19). The decrease in CAT appears to be due to a more or less selective loss of cholinergic neuronal structures, probably including both cell bodies and nerve endings. The data presented above and other information suggest the possibility that these two sets of changes may be linked mechanistically.

There is an intimate link between cerebral carbohydrate oxidation and cholinergic function (6,16,17,38). The synthesis of acetylcholine is exquisitely sensitive to conditions which impair brain carbohydrate catabolism, and the resulting decrements in acetylcholine synthesis are functionally significant (6,38). Oxidation of pyruvate by the pyruvate dehydrogenase complex has at least four critical functions in cholinergic neurones. It is the major source of the acetyl group of acetylcholine (6,38). Indeed, there appears to be a specific pool of pyruvate in brain for acetylcholine synthesis (17). The distribution of PDHC generally parallels that of CAT, in feline (27,28), rat (36), and human (24) brains (Table 1). CAT itself is not rate limiting for acetylcholine synthesis, and data have been presented to suggest that regional PDHC activity correlates with regional acetylcholine synthesis even better than does the distribution of CAT (10,24). Our data on frontal cortex are consistent with that assumption. The activity of PDHC in human frontal cortex was 18% of that for putamen (Table 1), and Cheney and Costa (10) reported that acetylcholine turnover in rat frontal cortex was 19% of that in putamen (10). A second function of PDHC in cholinergic neurones is to provide other biosynthetic intermediates, notably active acetate for lipid biosynthesis. A third function is in energy metabolism. Oxidation of pyruvate by PDHC appears to be normally the rate-limiting step in the oxidation of pyruvate by the Krebs cycle (11,18). Pyruvate derived from glucose is quantitatively the major oxidative substrate of brain and therefore the major source of electrons for the electron transport chain. Impairment of oxidative metabolism severe enough to reduce ATP levels kills neurones (25). Recently, Morgan and Routtenberg (20) reported that the phosphorylation state of a 41,000 delton α-peptide of PDHC plays an important role in synaptic plasticity and can be influenced by learning and training. These and other studies suggest that PDHC may plan an important role in behaviors classified as "memory and learning." Thus, mild reductions of PDHC in cholinergic neurones can be expected to reduce the synthesis of their major neurotransmitter and perhaps their ability to repair and renew their membranes and other cellular constituents. Severe reductions of PDHC can be expected to destroy these neurones. In fact, severe hereditary defects in PDHC typically impair higher function and lead to more or less widespread loss of nerve cells, sometimes even to microcephaly (7).

The deficiencies of PDHC reported here, whatever their importance ultimately turns out to be, are probably not primary. They do not occur in all areas of the brain of affected subjects and have not been found in cultured skin fibroblasts. On the other hand, ultrastructural studies suggest that damage to the oxidative machinery of neurones may have a role in the pathophysiology of dementias. For instance, abnormal mitochondria are prominent in the earliest stages of Alzheimer lesions (37). If loss of PDHC plays a role in the loss of cholinergic neurones, one might expect to find decreases of PDHC activities in areas of demented brain where CAT activity is still relatively normal. This possibility is relatively easy to test experimentally. The limited data available now are consistent with the idea that intrinsic derangements in the oxidative machinery of the brain--and specifically in PDHC--contribute to the brain damage in some dementias.

Acknowledgement

Support was from the NIH (grants NS15125, NS16994, and AA03883), the Will Rogers Institute, and The Winifred Masterson Burke Relief Foundation.

REFERENCES

1. Amaducci,L., Bracco,L., Sorbi,S. (1981): In: Neuronal Aging and Its Implications in Human Neurological Diseases, edited by R. Terry, L. Bolis, G. Toffano (in press). Raven Press, New York.
2. Antuono,P., Sorbi,S., Bracco,L., Fusco,T., Amaducci,L. (1980): In: Aging of the Brain and Dementia, edited by L. Amaducci, P. Antuono, A.N. Davison, pp. 151-158. Raven Press, New York.
3. Bird,E.D., Iversen,L.L. (1974): Brain, 97: 457-472.
4. Blass,J.P., Gibson,G.E. (1979): In: Advances in Neurology, edited by S. Fahn, pp. 229-253. Raven Press, New York.

5. Blass,J.P. (1980): In: Aging of the Brain and Dementia, edited by
    L. Amaducci, P. Antuono, A.N. Davision, pp. 261-270. Raven Press,
    New York.
6. Blass,J.P., Gibson,G.E. (1980): In: Biochemistry of Dementia,
    edited by P.J. Roberts, pp. 121-134. John Wiley & Sons, New York.
7. Blass,J.P. (1981): In: Metabolic Basis of Inherited Disease, edited
    by J.B. Stanbury, J. Wyngaarden, D.S. Fredrickson, J. Goldstein,
    and M. Brown, (in press). McGraw-Hill, Cambridge.
8. Bowen,D.M., Smith,C.B., White,P., and Davison,A.N. (1976): Brain,
    99: 459-496.
9. Bowen,D.M., Smith,C.B., White,P., Flack,R.H.A., Carrasco,L.H.,
    Gedye,J.L., and Davison,A.N. (1977): Brain, 100:427-53.
10. Cheney,D.L., Costa,E. (1978): In: Cholinergic-Monoaminergic Inter-
    actions in Brains, edited by L.L. Butcher, pp. 229-245. Academic
    Press, New York.
11. Cremer,J.E., Teal,H.M. (1974): FEBS Lett., 39:17-20.
12. Davies,P., Maloney,A.J. (1976): Lancet, 2:1403.
13. Emson,P.C., Lindvall,O. (1979): Neuroscience, 4:1-30.
14. Fonnum,F. (1966): Biochem. J., 100:479-484.
15. Fonnum,F. (1975): J. Neurochem., 24:407-409.
16. Gibson,G.E., Shimada,M. (1978): J. Neurochem., 31:757-760.
17. Gibson,G.E., Blass,J.P., Jenden,D.J. (1978): J. Neurochem., 30:
    71-76.
18. Ksiezak-Reding,H., Blass,J.P., Gibson,G.E. (1981): Trans. Am. Soc.
    Neurochem., 12:265.
19. Lassen,N.A., Ingvar,D.H. (1980): In: Aging of the Brain and
    Dementia, edited by L. Amaducci, P. Antuono, and A.N. Davison,
    pp. 91-98, Raven Press, New York.
20. Morgan, D.G., Routtenberg,A. (1981): Science, (in press).
21. Nachmansohn,D.. (1959): Chemical and Molecular Basis of Nerve
    Activity. Academic Press, New York.
22. Perry,E.K., Gibson,P.H., Blessed,G., Perry,R.H., Tomlinson,B.E.
    (1977): J. Neurol. Sci., 34:247-265.
23. Perry,E.K., Tomlinson,B.E., Blessed,G., Bergmann,K., Gibson,P.H.,
    Perry,R.H. (1978): Br. Med. J., 1:1457-59.
24. Perry,E.K., Perry,R.H., Tomlinson,B.E., Blessed,G., Gibson,P.H.
    (1980): Neurosci. Lett., 18:105-110.
25. Pulsinelli,W., Brierley,J., Duffy,T., Levy,D., Plum,F. (1981):
    J. CBF Metab., 1(suppl):166-167.
26. Racker,E. (1950): Biochem. Biophys. Acta., 4:211-214.
27. Reynolds,S.F. (1974): The Distribution of Pyruvate Dehydrogenase
    in the Cat CNS in Relation to Normal and Abnormal Neural Function.
    Ph.D. Dissertation. University of California, Los Angeles.
28. Reynolds,S.F., Blass,J.P. (1976): Neurology, 26:625-628.
29. Sheu,K.F.R., Hu,C.W.C., Utter,M.F. (1981): J. Clin. Invest.,
    67:1463-1471.
30. Sims,N.R., Bowen,D.M., Smith,C.C.T., Flack,R.H.A., Davison,A.N.,
    Snowden,J.S., and Neary,D. (1980): Lancet, 1:333-336.
31. Sorbi,S., Amaducci,L. (1979): Riv. Pat. Nerv. Ment., 4:171-179.
32. Sorbi,S., Amaducci,L. (1980): Arch. Sui. Neurol. Neuroch. Psych.,
    127:253-254.
33. Sorbi,S., Antuono,R., Amaducci,L. (1980): It. J. Neurol. Sci.,
    2:75-83.
34. Sorbi,S., Blass,J.P. (1981): J. Biochem. Biophys. Meth., (in press).

35. Sorbi,S., Blass,J.P. (1981): In: Current Neurology, edited by S.H. Appel, (in press). John Wiley & Sons Ltd., New York.
36. Sterry,S.H., Fonnum,F. (1980): J. Neurochem., 35:249-254.
37. Terry,R.D., Wisniewski,H.M. (1972): In: Aging and the Brain, edited by C. M. Gaitz, pp. 89-116. Plenum Press, New York.
38. Tucek,S. (1978): Acetylcholine Synthesis in Neurones. Chapman and Hall, London.
39. Whitehouse,P.J., Price,D.L., Clark,A.W., Coyle,J.T., DeLong,M.R. (1981): Ann. Neurol. 10:122-126.

The Aging Brain: Cellular and Molecular Mechanisms of Aging in the Nervous System, edited by E. Giacobini et al., Raven Press, New York © 1982.

Cholinergic Receptors in the Hippocampus in Normal Aging and Dementia of Alzheimer Type

A. Nordberg, *R. Adolfsson, *J. Marcusson, and *B. Winblad

*Department of Pharmacology, University of Uppsala, S-751 23 Uppsala, Sweden; *Umeå Dementia Research Group, Departments of Pathology and Psychiatry, University of Umeå, S-901 87 Umeå, Sweden*

Both normal and pathological ageing of the brain are associated with degenerative changes and regional or generalized losses of synapses, dendrites or nerve cells. In Alzheimer's disease senile plaques and neurofibrillary tangles are found in the brain especially in the hippocampus and cortex. In addition, severe defects in the cholinergic system of these brain areas can be measured (37). Since both direct and indirect evidence (15) indicate that cholinergic mechanisms play a role in memory function, the changes observed in Alzheimer's disease might represent severe and accelerated forms of age-related memory decline. These findings may also focus the interest on the life span of cholinergic enzymes and receptors.

Studies on the ontogenesis of cholinergic receptors in rat brain has shown that the number of muscarinic receptor binding sites increases linearly from birth up to day 15-20 of age when it reaches the mature level (4, 18). The nicotine-like cholinergic receptor binding sites (measured by α-bungarotoxin), on the other hand, seem to be higher in specific activity during the first postnatal days than at maturity (4). Studies in chick embryo brain have shown that the cholinergic enzymes choline acetyltransferase (CAT) and acetylcholinesterase (AChE) commence activity at the same time as the muscarinic receptor binding sites (16) although the activity of CAT develops at a slower rate in comparison to AChE and the number of muscarinic binding sites (16).

Brooksbank et al. (9) studied the development of the cholinergic system in human brain at different age periods; fetal period 18-22 weeks; perinatal period 26-44 weeks; early postnatal period 2-15 months and adult life 58-70 years. They found that in the cerebral cortex the highest number of muscarinic receptor binding sites and the highest activity of CAT were attained at the perinatal period. In the cerebellum, on the other hand, the highest number of muscarinic binding sites was found in the fetal period and then there was a fall in number of binding sites with age. The activity of CAT in the cerebellum was highest during gestation. This study by Brooksbank et al. (9) is, as far as we know, the only study on ontogenesis of cholinergic receptors in human.

Table 1 summarizes data from the literature on changes in cholinergic enzymes and receptors with ageing in the brain. Data from both animal and human are given. In rodents, both unchanged and decreased activity of CAT with age have been reported in the cortex, hippocampus

TABLE 1. Published value on choline acetyltransferase (CAT) and acetylcholine esterase (AChE) activity and number of muscarinic receptors in different parts of the brain at normal ageing and Alzheimer's disease.

	HUMAN		Mb Alzheimer	ANIMALS	
Brain region	Normal ageing			Rat	Mouse
CAT					
cortex	▼22,36 ▲8		▼▼7,8,12,13,36,38,45,46,49	▲25,27	▼27
hippocampus	▼11,40		▼▼11,12,13,36,44,46	▲25	▼48
basal ganglia	▲7,24,36 ▼23		▼12,13,38,44 ▲36,46	▲28	▼21,25
AChE					
cortex	▲39		▼▼11,12,13,42	▼29	
hippocampus	▲39		▼▼11,12,13		
basal ganglia	▲7,24,36 ▼23		▼11,12,13,41	▲43	▼28
Muscarinic receptors					
cortex	▼35,49 ▲14		▲8,11,14,38,45,49	▲28	▼17
hippocampus	▼33 ▲14		▲11,14,31 ▼44	▲28 ▼28	
basal ganglia	▲14		▲14,38,44	▲28	

Figures indicate reference number.

and basal ganglia. Also the number of muscarinic receptors seem to remain unchanged or decreased with age in rodents. In human brain most studies have shown a decrease in the activity of CAT in the cortex and hippocampus of normal ageing subjects while the activity of CAT remains unchanged in the basal ganglia. No change in AChE activity with normal ageing has been reported. It is not clear whether the number of muscarinic receptors in brain changes with age. Both unchanged and decreased number of binding sites have been reported in the hippocampus and cortex. In Alzheimer's disease a very marked decrease in CAT activity, in comparison to age-matched controls, is found in the hippocampus, cortex and to a lesser extent in the basal ganglia. The activity of AChE is also reduced in Alzheimer's disease. With one exception, all studies have found no change in muscarinic receptor concentration in Alzheimer's disease when compared to control autopsy cases.

In this study our work was focused on cholinergic receptors in the hippocampus. The antero-posterior distribution of muscarine- and nicotine-like receptors and the effect of normal ageing on receptor properties were studied in the human hippocampus. In addition cholinergic receptors were measured in the hippocampus of Alzheimer's disease and multi-infarct dementia.

The muscarinic antagonist quinuclidinyl benzilate (QNB) was used as labelled ligand for the muscarine-like receptor binding sites. For the nicotine-like receptor binding sites both labelled tubocurarine (TC) and α-bungarotoxin (α-Btx) were used as receptor ligands (19, 32). Previous studies in mouse hippocampus have shown (19, 32) that tubocurarine has two binding sites while α-bungarotoxin has one binding site in the hippocampus.

MATERIAL AND METHODS

Human Brain Tissue

Hippocampus was taken at autopsy from a total of 54 patients; 10 patients with Alzheimer's disease (65-85 years), 13 patients with multi-infarct dementia (67-90 years) and 31 controls (3 days - 93 years). The patients in the control material had no recorded history of neurological or psychiatric illness. The cause of death was heart infarctions or malignant disease. The infants died from respiratory and circulatory insufficiency. In the Alzheimer group the diagnosis was put on clinical grounds (insidious onset, memory loss, intellectual and personality deterioration, typical non-fluctuating progressive down-hill course, absence of hypertension, stroke or other secondary causes of dementia; and in whom other diseases causing dementia could be excluded. All patients were severely demented according to rating scales. Autopsy revealed in these cases non or slight arteriosclerosis and no encephalomalacias. No depigmentation of substantia nigra was observed. The patients who fulfilled the criteria of MID had a Hachinski score of 7 or above and all had had a step-wise mental deterioration and a history of hypertension, transitory ischemic attacks or stroke. At autopsy 10 of these patients had small brain infarctions and the three patients without infarctions showed a more pronounced arteriosclerosis of the basal brain vessels. There were no significant differences in times death - autopsy or brain weight between the different groups. The mean time death - autopsy in the whole material was 34 hours. The bodies were brought to the pathology department 2-4 hours after death and were kept at +4° C until autopsy. At autopsy the hippocampus was cut out in its whole length, put into air-tight plastic tube and frozen at -80° C until analysis. In 11 of the control patients the hippocampus was divided before freezing in five equal parts (1-5) from anterior to posterior.

Measurement of ^{3}H-QNB, ^{3}H-TC and ^{3}H-α-Btx binding sites

The brain tissues were homogenized in 20-30 vol of ice-cold sucrose 0.32 M and centrifuged at 1000 g for 10 minutes. The pellet (Pl) was discarded and the supernatant centrifuged at 17000 g for 15 minutes. The supernatant was discarded and the crude synaptosomal fraction (P2) was resuspended and homogenized in the original volume of ice-cold sucrose 0.32 M. The P2 fractions were kept frozen (-90° C) until receptor binding studies were performed. An aliquote of the crude synaptosomal fraction (P2) (final protein concentration in the incubation media 0.1 mg/ml) was incubated at 25° in 50 ml M NaKPO$_4$ buffer (pH=7.4) containing tritium labelled quinuclidinyl benzilate (^{3}H-QNB SA 16 Ci/mmol; 0.2 nM), tritium labelled tubocurarine (^{3}H-TC 16.5 Ci/mmol; 3 nM) or tritium labelled α-bungarotoxin (^{3}H-α-Btx 63 Ci/mmol; 2.6 nM). In ^{3}H-Btx binding studies the incubation media also contained 0.02 % albumin. ^{3}H-QNB and ^{3}H-α-Btx were incubated with the P2 fraction for 60 minutes while ^{3}H-TC was incubated for 15 minutes. After incubation the samples were immediately centrifuged in a Microfuge^R for 5 minutes. The incubation tubes were then put into a running wheel where the supernatant was slung out into a collecting van leaving a dry pellet left in the incubation tube. The tip of the tubes were cut and the pellet dissolved in 1 ml soluene-toluene (1:3) overnight. After addition of 4 ml Instafluor^R, the radioactivity was measured by liquid scintillation. The specific binding was determined by subtracting non-specific binding in presence of 10^{-4} M unlabelled atropine (for ^{3}H-QNB binding) and 10^{-4} M unlabelled tubocurarine (for ^{3}H-TC, ^{3}H-α-Btx binding). Protein content was measured according to Lowry et al. (20).

In some of the ^{3}H-QNB experiments competition studies with oxotremorine (concentration range 10^{-8} -10^{-2} M) present in the incubation media were performed. The agonist ^{3}H-QNB competition data were fitted to a one or two site model by non-linear least square method (5, 3).

RESULTS

1. Normal ageing

Figure 1 shows the number of muscarinic receptor binding sites in human control hippocampus at different ages (3 days to 87 years). As can be seen from the figure the highest number of muscarinic binding sites were measured at 3 days and 3 weeks of age. From 3 years of age a slight continuous decrease in number of muscarinic binding sites was noticed with increasing age (r=0.48 p < 0.05). A decrease in number of nicotine-like binding sites (determined by ^{3}H-TC) with age (range 57-87 years) was found, as shown in Figure 2.

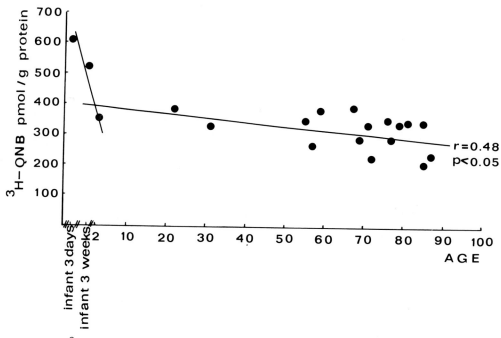

FIG. 1. ^{3}H-QNB binding sites in human hippocampus at different ages (3 days - 93 years). Each point represents data from one individual, r = linear regression analysis.

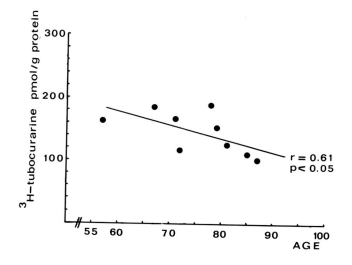

FIG. 2. ^{3}H-TC binding sites in human hippocampus at different ages (57 - 87 years). Each point represents data from one individual, r = linear regression analysis.

In 9 control hippocampus (3 days - 85 years) competition studies with ^{3}H-QNB and different concentrations of unlabelled oxotremorine were performed. The competition data were fitted to a one or two site receptor model using non-linear least square analysis. As can be seen in Figure 3, a two-site receptor model fits the experimental data much better than a one site model. It is also known from studies in rat brain that muscarinic agonists bind to two or even three receptor sites distinguished by their affinity for agonists (6). As shown in Table 2 the proportion of high and low affinity muscarinic binding sites were analysed in human hippocampus at different ages to determine whether increasing age might influence the proportion of agonist binding sites. The results indicate that the proportion of high and low affinity muscarinic binding sites was about the same at all ages investigated.

When the number of ^{3}H-QNB and ^{3}H-TC binding sites were measured in five parts of the hippocampus a rather even distribution was found (Table 3). When the individual data for both ^{3}H-QNB and ^{3}H-TC binding were plotted against age, a negative correlation was found in the anterior parts. A strong positive correlation between number of ^{3}H-QNB and ^{3}H-TC binding sites was obtained in parts 1, 4, 5 (Table 3).

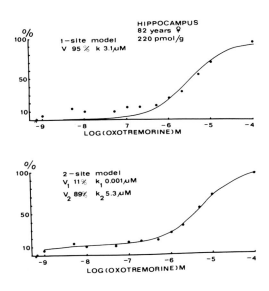

FIG. 3. ^{3}H-QNB-agonist competition studies. ^{3}H-QNB binding was performed with different concentrations of (10^{-9} - 10^{-4}M) oxotremorine present in the incubation media. Per cent of ^{3}H-QNB binding displaced by oxotremorine is given on the Y-axis. The competition data were fitted to a 1-site or 2-site receptor model by non-linear least square analysis. The points represent the experimental data obtained and the solid line the best fit of the experimental data.

TABLE 2. Number of muscarinic binding sites and proportion of high and low affinity binding sites in human hippocampus at different ages.

Age	Total Number of binding sites (B_T) pmol/g protein	High affinity binding sites			Low affinity binding sites		
		Number of binding sites pmol/g protein	in per cent of B_T (V_1%)	Affinity constant 10^{-8} M	Number of binding sites pmol/g protein	in per cent of B_T (V_2%)	Affinity constant 10^{-6} M
3 days	607	79	13 ± 1	9.7 ± 0.7	528	87 ± 1	2.4 ± 0.1
3 weeks	523	136	26 ± 1	6.4 ± 0.6	403	77 ± 2	5.2 ± 0.4
3 years	350	49	14 ± 1	0.2 ± 0.04	305	87 ± 1	2.9 ± 0.1
22	383	42	11 ± 1	3.0 ± 0.3	352	92 ± 1	2.1 ± 0.1
55	345	48	14 ± 1	10.4 ± 1.5	300	37 ± 1	3.4 ± 0.2
59	382	107	28 ± 1	10.5 ± 8.0	275	72 ± 2	4.7 ± 0.2
76	356	78	22 ± 1	11.9 ± 0.9	281	79 ± 1	3.9 ± 0.2
82	220	24	11 ± 1	1.0 ± 0.004	196	89 ± 1	5.3 ± 0.1
85	346	35	10 ± 1	8.6 ± 0.5	315	91 ± 1	3.0 ± 0.1

MV ± S.E.

TABLE 3. Distribution of ^{3}H-QNB and ^{3}H-TC binding sites in five antero-posterior (1-5) parts of hippocampus from 11 individuals. Linear regression (r) was used by analysing number of ^{3}H-QNB, ^{3}H-TC binding sites (pmol/g protein) at different ages (55-84 years) and the interrelationship between these binding sites.

Part	^{3}H-QNB pmol/g protein	^{3}H-TC pmol/g protein	^{3}H-QNB binding sites/age r=(linear regression analysis)	^{3}H-TC binding sites/age r	^{3}H-TC binding sites against ^{3}H-QNB binding sites r=(linear regression analysis)
1	389 ± 36	137 ± 10	-0.42	-0.37	0.62[x]
2	391 ± 45	146 ± 16	-0.26	-0.36	0.14
3	430 ± 41	122 ± 17	-0.40	-0.12	0.53
4	419 ± 32	128 ± 16	-0.27	-0.21	0.67[x]
5	449 ± 62	140 ± 29	+0.16	+0.23	0.66[x]

MV ± S.E.

[x]$p < 0.05$

2. Alzheimer's disease and multi-infarct dementia

As seen in Table 4, no marked difference in number of ^{3}H-QNB, ^{3}H-TC and ^{3}H-α-Btx binding sites was found in the hippocampus of Alzheimer patients in comparison to age-matched controls. In multi-infarct dementia, on the other hand, a reduced number of ^{3}H-QNB binding sites was found in comparison to controls. The absolutely lowest individual number of ^{3}H-QNB binding sites was found in the hippocampus of one patient who happened to be analyzed in parallel and where chronic alcohol abuse had caused the dementia condition (143 pmol/g protein as compared to 300 pmol/g protein for the control group). When the individual ^{3}H-QNB binding data were plotted against age (Figure 4) it was found that the youngest patient with Alzheimer's disease (age 65 years) had a thirty per cent lower number of muscarinic binding sites in comparison to the age matched controls. Figure 5 shows the individual data for ^{3}H-QNB binding in multi-infarct dementia and it can be seen that nearly all values are below the control line.

TABLE 4. Number of cholinergic receptor binding sites in the hippocampus of Alzheimer's disease and multi-infarct dementia.

	Muscarine-like binding sites (^{3}H-QNB)	Nicotine-like binding sites	
		^{3}H-TC	^{3}H-α-Btx
	pmol/g protein		
Controls	300 ± 15 (n=16)	147 ± 10 (n=10)	7 ± 1 (n=10)
Alzheimer's disease	282 ± 17 (n=10)	145 ± 9 (n=10)	8 ± 1 (n=10)
Multi-infarct dementia	264 ± 17[x] (n=13)	155 ± 20 (n=13)	8 ± 1 (n=13)

MV ± S.E. [x]$p < 0.05$

DISCUSSION

From the results of the present study it is evident that the number of muscarinic receptor binding sites in the human hippocampus decrease with age. At an early age there is a marked decrease in muscarinic receptor sites and from 50-60 years of age there seems to be another drop in the number of binding sites although less pronounced. This negative correlation between muscarinic binding sites and increasing age is seen in the anterior part of the hippocampus but not in the posterior part. Brooksbank et al. (9) also found in the human cortex a higher number of muscarinic binding sites during gestation in comparison to adults. These findings are in contrast with the findings in rat brain, where the number of muscarinic binding sites has been shown to increase continuously up to adult age (4).

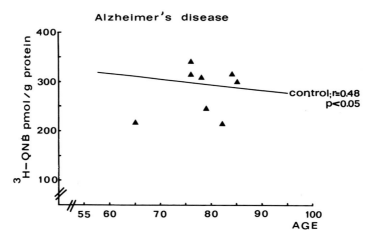

FIG. 4. ^{3}H-QNB binding sites in human hippocampus of
patients with dementia of Alzheimer type (age
65-85). Each point represents data from one
individual. The solid line represents age
matched controls, r = regression analysis.

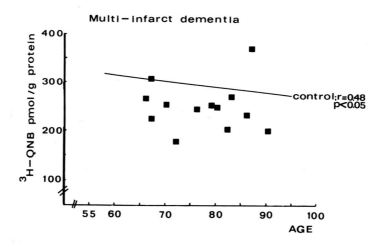

FIG. 5. ^{3}H-QNB receptor binding sites in human hippocampus of multi-infarct dementia patients (age
66-90 years). Each point represents data from
one individual. The solid line represents age-
matched controls, r = regression analysis.

In the present study a negative correlation between number of nicotine-like binding sites (measured by ^{3}H-TC as a ligand) and increasing age was also observed, both in the whole hippocampus and in the anterior part in comparison to the posterior part. As far as we know this is the first study where a decrease in nicotine-like receptor binding sites with normal ageing has been shown.

Studies by Mouritzem Dam (30) have shown that in normal ageing there is an increased cell density of pyramidal cells from the anterior to the posterior part of the hippocampus. Studies by Meldrum and Brierley (26) and Ball (2) indicate a difference in vulnerability between the anterior and posterior part of the hippocampus. These findings could be consistent with the difference in muscarinic and nicotine-like binding sites between the anterior and posterior part of the hippocampus observed in the present study.

Two types of muscarinic agonist binding sites with at least a 100 times difference in affinity constant were demonstrable in human hippocampus. The proportion of high and low affinity binding sites was consistent with previous data for rat brain. No marked difference in proportion of agonist binding sites was found between different ages. One of the oldest patients (82 years) who had the lowest number of muscarinic binding sites (220 pmol/g) had about the same proportion of high and low affinity binding sites as the younger patients. The affinity constant for the high affinity binding sites of this patient, however, was the lowest measured.

Another important finding in the present study is the positive correlation between the number of nicotine-like and muscarine-like binding sites which could be considered to represent a constitutional trait where patients with a low number of cholinergic receptors might constitute a more vulnerable group for disorders concerning memory function than patients with a high number of cholinergic receptors.

As was shown in Table 1 results from different research groups indicate that in Alzheimer's disease there is a marked decrease in brain CAT activity, especially in the hippocampus, indicating abnormalities of the cholinergic system in the brain. Recently Rossor et al. (46) have demonstrated a marked decrease in CAT activity in the posterior but not in the anterior part of the hippocampus of patients with dementia of Alzheimer type. A significant correlation between degree of intellectual impairment and CAT deficit in the cortex has been found as well as a relationship between CAT deficit and number of senile plaques (39). Several explanations for deficits in CAT activity have been given including loss of cholinergic neurons or abnormal nerve terminals. Another possible explanation for reduced CAT activity could be that Alzheimer patients seem to have a deranged glucose metabolism (1) which might lead to a defective acetyl-CoA production and secondarily to a reduced ACh synthesis and a lowering of the CAT activity. A reduced synthesis of ACh in temporal-lobe biopsy samples from patients with Alzheimer's disease was measured by Sims et al. (47).

Alcohol abuse often leads to a dementia condition. It is noticeable that chronic alcoholics have brain transmitter changes similar to those of Alzheimer patients (10). These data suggest that chronic alcohol abuse can accelerate the ageing process, at least in certain neuronal systems. Chronic ethanol treatment of rats has been shown to induce an increase of the number of muscarinic binding sites in the abstinence period (33). In contrast to these findings, a reduced number of muscarinic receptor binding sites has been found in the hippocampus of chronic alcoholics (31). The relationship between our earlier reported changes and those in the present study warrants further investigation.

With one exception (45) all studies (including the present) have found no change in the number of muscarinic binding sites of the hippocampus in Alzheimer's disease compared to age-matched controls. Nevertheless, it is interesting to note that the youngest patient with Alzheimer's disease (age 65 years) in this study had a much lower number of muscarine and nicotine-like receptor binding sites in comparison to the age-matched controls. It is possible that changes in receptor binding sites might be found in the younger population of patients with Alzheimer's disease. We have recently (50) shown that Alzheimer patients with an early onset of the disease show very marked catecholaminergic and cholinergic deficiencies while senile dementia patients with a late onset have brain neurotransmitter and enzyme concentrations close to age-matched controls. Extended studies might give further biochemical evidence for the division between Alzheimer patients and senile dementia patients. It must also be considered of importance to investigate possible changes in receptor properties in discrete areas of the hippocampus. A selective decrease in hippocampal CAT activity in multi-infarct dementia was recently reported (37) and our finding of the decreased number of muscarinic binding sites in patients with multi-infarct dementia indicates a cholinergic involvement also in this type of dementia.

ACKNOWLEDGEMENTS

This study was supported by grants from the Swedish Medical Research Council (No. 12X-5664, 25X-5641, 25X-5817), the Swedish Tobacco Company, Hansson's, Osterman's, Mångberg's, Pfannenstill's and Sundblad's funds and the Medical Faculty, University of Umeå.

REFERENCES

1. Adolfsson, R., Bucht, G., Lithner, F., and Winblad, B. (1980): Acta Med. Scand., 208:387-388.

2. Ball, M.J. (1977): Acta Neuropath. (Berl), 37:111-118.

3. Bartfai, T., and Hedlund, B. (1979): Molecular Pharmacol., 15: 531-544.

4. Ben-Barak, J., and Dudai, Y. (1979): Brain Res., 166:245-257.

5. Birdsall, N.J.M., Burgen, A.S.V., and Hulme, E.C. (1978): Molecular Pharmacol., 14:723-736.

6. Birdsall, N.J.M., Hulme, E.C., and Burgen, A. (1980): Proc. R. Soc. Land. B., 207:1-12.

7. Bowen, D.M., Smith, C.B., White, P., and Davison, A.N. (1976): Brain 99:459-496.

8. Bowen, D.M., Spillane, J.A., Curzon, G., Meier-Ruge, W., White, P., Goodhardt, M.J., Iwangoff, P., and Davison, A.N. (1979): Lancet, I:11-14.

9. Brooksbank, B.W.L., Martinez, M., Atkinson, D.J., and Balazs, R. (1978): Dev. Neurosci., I:267-284.

10. Carlsson, A., Adolfsson, R., Aquilonius, S.-M., Gottfries, C.-G., Oreland, L., Svennerholm, L., and Winblad, B. (1980): In: Ergot Compounds and Brain Function: Neuroendocrine and Neuropsychiatric Aspects, edited by M. Goldstein et al. pp. 295-304. Raven Press, New York.

11. Davies, P. (1978): In: Alzheimer's Disease: Senile Dementia and Related Disorders, edited by R. Katzmann, R.D. Terry and K.L. Blick, pp. 453-459. Raven Press, New York.

12. Davies, P. (1979): Brain Res., 171:319-327.

13. Davies, P., and Maloney, A.J.F. (1976): Lancet, II:1403.

14. Davies, P., and Verth, A.H. (1978): Brain Res., 138:385-392.

15. Drachman, D.A. (1978): In: Alzheimer's Disease: Senile Dementia and Related Disorders, edited by R. Katzmann, R.D. Terry and K.L. Blick, pp. 141-148. Raven Press, New York.

16. Enna, S.J., Yamamura, H.I., and Snyder, S. (1976): Brain Res., 101:177-183.

17. James, T.C., and Kanungo, M.S. (1976): Biochem. Biophys. Res. Commun. 72:170-175.

18. Kuhar, M.J., Birdsall, N.J.M., Burgen, A.S.V., and Hulme, E.C. (1980): Brain Res., 184:375-383.

19. Larsson, C., and Nordberg, A. (1980): In: Neurotransmitters and their Receptors, edited by V.Z. Littauer, Y. Dudai and I. Silman, pp. 297-301. John Wiley & Sons Ltd.

20. Lowry, D.H., Rosenbrough, N.J., Farr, A.L., and Randall, R.J. (1951): J. Biol. Chem., 193:265-275.

21. McGeer, E.G., Fibiger, H.C., and McGeer, P.L. (1971): Exp. Gerontol. 6:391-396.

22. McGeer, E.G., and McGeer, P.L. (1976): In: Neurobiology of Ageing, edited by R.D. Terry and S. Gershon, pp. 389-403. Raven Press, New York.

23. McGeer, P.L., and McGeer, E.G. (1976): J. Neurochem., 26:65-76.

24. McGeer, P.L., and McGeer, E.G. (1978): Adv. Exp. Med. Biol. 113: 41-57.

25. Meek, J.L., Bertilsson, L., Cheney, D.L., Zilla, G., and Costa, E. (1978): J. Gerontol. 12:129-131.

26. Meldrum, B., and Brierley, J.B. (1972): Brain Res., 48:361-365.

27. Mohan, C., and Radha, E. (1978): Exp. Gerontol., 13:349-308.

28. Morin, A.M., and Wasterlain, C.G. (1980): Neurochem. Res., 5:301-308.

29. Moudgil, V.K., and Kanungo, M.S. (1973): Biochem. Biophys. Acta, 329:211-220.

30. Mouritzen Dam, A. (1979): Neuropath. Applied Neurobiol., 5:249-264.

31. Nordberg, A., Adolfsson, R., Aquilonius, S.-M., Marklund, S., Oreland, L., and Winblad, B. (1980): In: Aging of the Brain and Dementia (Aging vol 13), edited by L. Amaducci, A.N. Davison and P. Antuono, pp. 169-171. Raven Press, New York.

32. Nordberg, A., and Larsson, C. (1981): In: Cholinergic Mechanisms: Phylogenetic Aspects, Central and Peripheral Synapses and Clinical Significance, edited by G. Pepen and H. Ladinsky, pp. 639-646. Plenum Press, New York.

33. Nordberg, A. and Wahlström, G. (1981): Abstracts Eighth International Congress of Pharmacology, Tokyo 1981, O-32 p. 827.

34. Nordberg, A., and Winblad, B. (1981): Life Sci. (in press).

35. Perry, E.K. (1980): Age and Ageing, 9:1-8.

36. Perry, E.K., Gibson, P.H., Blessed, G., Perry, R.H., and Tomlinson, B.E. (1977): J. Neurol Sci., 34:247-265.

37. Perry, E.K., and Perry, R.H. (1980): In: Biochemistry of Dementia, edited by P.J. Roberts, pp. 135-183. John Wiley & Sons Ltd.

38. Perry, E.K., Perry, R.H., Blessed, G., and Tomlinson, B.E. (1977): Lancet I, 189.

39. Perry, E.K., Perry, R.H., Blessed, G., and Tomlinson, B.E. (1978): Neuropath. Appl. Neurobiol. 4:273-277.

40. Perry, E.K., Perry, R.H., Gibson, P.H., Blessed, G., and Tomlinson, B.E. (1977): Neurosci. Lett., 6:85-89.

41. Perry, E.K., Tomlinson, B.E., Blessed, G., Bergmann, K., Gibson, P.H., and Perry, R.H. (1978): Br. Med. J., 2:1457-1459.

42. Pope, A., Hess, H.H., and Lewin, E. (1965): Trans Am. Neurol. Assoc., 89:15-16.

43. Reis, D.J., Ross, R.A., and Joh, T.H. (1977): Brain Res., 136: 465-474.

44. Reisine, T.D., Fields, J.Z., and Yamamura, H.I. (1977): Life Sci., 21:335-344.

45. Reisine, T.D., Yamamura, H.I., Bird, E.D., Spokes, E., and Enna, S.J. (1978): Brain Res., 159:477-480.

46. Rossor, M., Fahrenkrug, J., Emson, P., Mountjoy, C., Iversen, L., and Roth, M. (1980): Brain Res., 201:249-253.

47. Sims, N.R., Bowen, D.M., Smith, C.C.T., Flack, R.H.A., Davison, A.N., and Snowden, J.S. (1980): Lancet I:333-336.

48. Vijayan, V.K. (1977): Exp. Gerontol., 12:7-11.

49. White, P., Hiley, C.R., Goodhardt, M.J., Carrasco, L.H., Keet, J.P., Williams, I.E.I., and Bowen, D.M. (1977): Lancet I:668-670.

50. Winblad, B., Adolfsson, R., Carlsson, A., and Gottfries, C.-G. (1981): Proceedings from International Study Group on the Pharmacology of Memory Disorders Associated with Aging, Zürich, April 3-5.

The Aging Brain: Cellular and Molecular Mechanisms of Aging in the Nervous System, edited by E. Giacobini et al., Raven Press, New York © 1982.

Age-Associated Neurofibrillary Changes

Khalid Iqbal, Inge Grundke-Iqbal, Patricia A. Merz, and Henryk M. Wisniewski

New York State Institute for Developmental Disabilities, Staten Island, New York 10314

One of the cellular and molecular changes with aging the mechanism of which remains unknown is the formation of intra cellular neurofibrillary tangles in certain selected neurons of the aged human brain and to a much greater degree in several age-associated dementias especially the Alzheimer presenile and senile dementia. The number of these Alzheimer neurofibrillary tangles (ANT) correlates strongly with the degree of psychometric deficiency in the patients (36). It is this hallmark lesion of the aged human brain and dementias of the Alzheimer type which is discussed in this report.

I. FIBRILS OF A NORMAL NEURON

A normal mature neuron contains three types of fibers; neurotubules, neurofilaments and microfilaments. Neurotubules are the microtubules of the neuron and are apparently identical to microtubules in glial cells and all eukaryotic cells (29). Each microtubule measures 20-24 nm in diameter, has well defined lumen of about 15 nm and has short side arms. The protein subunit of microtubules is tubulin, a hetrodimeric protein. The apparent mol. wts. of human brain tubulin monomers are 56,000 for α and 53,000 for β. These tubulin monomers are acidic and differ slightly in amino acid composition and tryptic and cyanogen bromide peptide maps (6,17). About 80-85% of microtubule protein is tubulin, most of the remaining 15-20% protein is of two groups of high mol. wt. proteins, one group of about 250,000 to 350,000 mol. wt., called microtubule associated proteins or "MAPS" and the other of about 70,000 mol. wt., called "tau". In the absence of MAPS, microtubules assembled in vitro do not have side arms (4,28). Tau is believed to be required for the in vitro assembly of tubulin into microtubules (37). In vitro assembled brain microtubules also contain as contaminants small amounts of several other proteins including neurofilament proteins (see below) (17).

The neurofilaments are linear, 9-10 nm wide intermediate filaments of the neuron. They are found sparsely in the cell body, moderately in the dendrites and most abundantly in the axon (Fig. 1). Like microtubules, neurofilaments can be made to undergo in vitro disassembly-assembly cycles (22). However, the conditions for disassembly and assembly for neurofilaments are different from that for microtubules. Neurofilaments are biochemically different from intermediate filaments of other cell types and are made up of a triplet of about 70,000, 160,000 and 200,000

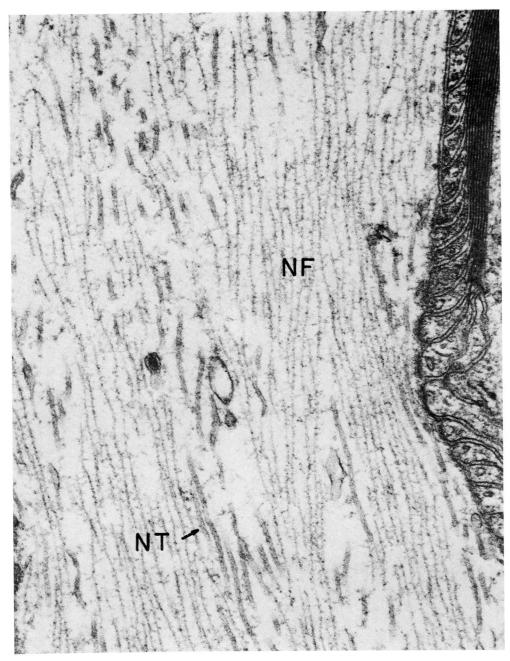

FIG. 1.   An electron micrograph showing normal neurofilaments (NF) and
neurotubules (NT) in an axon.   Magnification, X 62,500.

mol. wt. polypeptides, that are apparently unique to nerve cells (12,32, 34). Neurofilaments isolated from CNS contain varying amounts of a 50,000 mol. wt. polypeptide which is believed to be mostly the glial fibrillary acidic protein, the major protein of astroglial filaments (5).

Brain microfilaments, like those in muscle are 5 nm in diameter and are made up of actin (1), the 45,000 mol. wt. protein.

II. ALZHEIMER NEUROFIBRILLARY TANGLES (ANT)

a. Morphology

ANT produce green birefringence in polarized light after staining with Congo red. This optical property might be due to the β-pleated sheet nature of the fibrillar proteins making the ANT (38) in the same fashion as shown by Glenner, et.al., (9) in the case of amyloid. ANT are stained intensely with silver impregnation techniques. This is one of the most common histological methods used for detecting the presence of ANT in tissue. ANT are found mostly in the cerebral cortex, especially in the hippocampal pyramidal cells of Sommers sector, and small pyramidal neurons in the outer laminea of fronto-temporal cortex. They have not been seen in cerebellum, spinal cord, peripheral nervous system or extraneuronal tissues.

Ultrastructurally, ANT are composed of bundles of paired filaments (Fig. 2), each filament of the pair is 10-13 nm in diameter and helically wound around each other at regular intervals of 80 nm (26,39). These paired helical filaments (PHF), are also found in bundles in the degenerated neurites of the senile (neuritic) plaques and less frequently as individual fibers in myelinated axons. Senile (neuritic) plaque which is composed of degenerating neurites generally around a core of amyloid is the other leading lesion of Alzheimer dementia and the aged human brain. In neurons undergoing neurofibrillary changes, PHF appear to gradually become more densely packed and take over greater proportions of cell space displacing cytoplasmic organelles. It remains unclear whether accumulations of PHF lead to cell death. It is also unknown whether the affected cells can recover. Maintenance of synaptic contact has been observed in situations where pre and post synaptic processes are filled with PHF suggesting that a certain degree of function might persist in these affected synapses.

In addition to Alzheimer disease (AD) and senile dementia of the Alzheimer type (SDAT) which are believed to be the same disease with a different age of onset, PHF are also found in great abundance in Guam Parkinsonism dementia complex, dementia puglistica, postencephalitic Parkinsonism and adults with Down Syndrome. The ANT has also been reported in small numbers in several cases of subacute sclerosing panencephalitis (SSPE) and in rare cases of Hallerworden Spatz disease and juvenile neurovisceral lipid storage disease (for review see, 18, 41). Thus the accumulation of PHF is associated with normal aging, viral infection, chromosomal disorders and metabolic abnormalities. However, PHF of the Alzheimer type have never been observed in any aged animal species or have they been produced experimentally in animals.

The neurofibrillary changes in human disorders are not always of the Alzheimer type i.e. made up of PHF. For instance in progressive supranuclear palsy (PSP) some of the same neurons which contain tangles of PHF in Alzheimer brain have neurofibrillary tangles of 15 nm straight filaments (35). These tangles of 15 nm filaments in PSP are sometimes

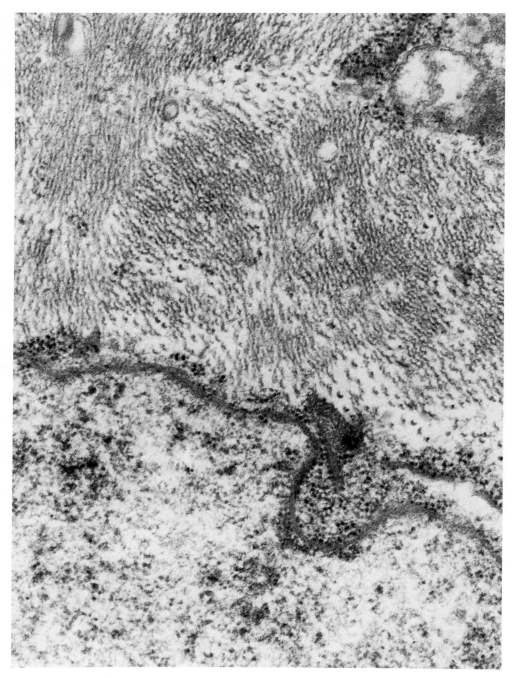

FIG. 2. An Alzheimer neurofibrillary tangle from a case of Alzheimer
dementia, showing bundles of PHF in the neuronal cytoplasm. The
neuronal nucleus is at the lower half. Magnification, X 56,000.

admixed with PHF (8). In sporadic motor neuron disease, vincristine neuropathy and infantile neuroaxonal dystrophy in humans the neuro-fibrillary changes are of 10 nm intermediate filament type. The 10 nm intermediate filament type neurofibrillary changes have been experi-mentally induced with aluminum, mitotic spindle inhibitors like colchicine, vinblastine and podophyllotoxin, various nitrates and acrylamide in animal (for review see, 18, 41). The aluminum-induced filamentous accumulation is apparently specific to the nervous system, while in the case of the mitotic spindle inhibitors similar changes occur in a wide range of cell types. In all of these intoxications, the fila-ments formed are morphologically identical to normal neurofilaments. These filaments induced with various agents have not yet been isolated and characterized. The neurofilamentous tangles induced with aluminum, colchicine, vinblastine and vincristine have been shown to immunostain with an antiserum to the 70 k neurofilament polypeptide but not with an antiserum to the 160 k neurofilament polypeptide (2,3). Whereas accord-ing to Selkoe, et.al., (33) the aluminum-induced neurofilamentous tangles are immunostained with an antiserum to the neurofilament 160 k polypep-tide and all the three polypeptides of the neurofilament triplet are enriched in neuronal perikarya isolated from spinal cord of rabbits with aluminum-induced neurofibrillary changes. Unlike PHF, both normal neuro-filaments and the aluminum induced filaments do not produce in polarized light the characteristic green birefringence after staining with Congo red (40). In contrast, according to a recent report by Linder, et.al., (27), the colchicine-induced filaments produce the Congo red green bire-fringence.

b. Bulk Isolation

Since PHF are unique to human brain, only this source of tissue can be used for the isolation of PHF. The PHF are structurally stable in both fresh and frozen autopsy tissue. Hippocampus, temporal and frontal cortices are the areas of the brain which are generally most affected by neurofibrillary changes. However, the number of ANT varies consider-ably from Alzheimer brain to brain and the amount of PHF for the purposes of biochemical isolation is generally extremely small even in the affected areas of the brain. Furthermore, any attempt to isolate PHF from whole tissue might be complicated by the presence of the astroglial filaments and neurofilaments which are present in large amounts. These difficul-ties have hampered progress in this important area of research on cerebral aging. Some of these difficulties were circumvented by the development of a technique for the bulk separation of neuronal perikarya and glial cells from fresh or frozen human autopsy tissue (13-15). Using this technique, a fraction modestly enriched in ANT was achieved by sub-cellular fractionation of the neuronal cell bodies isolated from affected areas of Alzheimer cerebral cortex (16). These preparations showed a consistant enrichment of a polypeptide, mol. wt. around 50,000 which was later partially characterized and shown to be localized to ANT (11,19). However, the PHF preparations were not highly purified and therefore of limited value for the purposes of further biochemical studies.

Taking advantage of the structural stability of PHF, a new method for the bulk isolation of highly purified preparations of PHF have now been developed (Iqbal, et.al., in preparation). The isolation of PHF is achieved by a combination of tissue disaggregation by sieving through

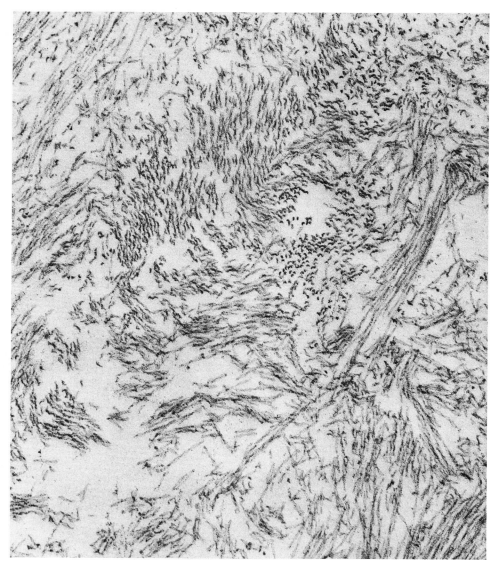

FIG. 3. An electron micrograph of isolated ANT showing
PHF. Magnification, X 64,500.

nylon bolting cloth, sucrose density gradient centrifugation and detergent treatment. ANT isolated by this procedure are highly purified as determined by light microscopy of Congo red stained preparations in polarized light, the isolated ANT produce green birefringence. The electron microscopic examination of the ANT preparations show highly purified PHF (Fig. 3). With these highly purified PHF, it is now possible to study the biochemistry of this lesion.

c.   Protein Profiles

SDS-polyacrylamide gel electrophoresis (SDS-PAGE) of isolated PHF have revealed three polypeptides, mol. wts. around 45,000, 50,000 and 55,000 and a very high mol. wt. (above 400,000) component which is seen near the top of the resolving gel (Iqbal, et.al., in preparation). As much as about 25% of the PHF protein sample does not enter the stacking gel during SDS-PAGE. However, reextractions and electrophoresis of this insoluble material has not revealed any polypeptides other than those observed in the first extraction of PHF. It thus appears that the material not entering the gel might be the insoluble pool of the same that is resolved on the SDS-PAGE. One or more of PHF polypeptides observed on SDS-PAGE might be the degradative product of a larger polypeptide, for instance, the one which migrated near the top of the resolving gel. Alternatively the possibility that one or two of these polypeptides represent contaminants in the isolated PHF fraction cannot be eliminated pending further characterization of these polypeptides. However, in either case the protein composition of PHF appears to be different from normal neurofilaments and microtubules. This biochemical evidence showing differences between PHF and normal neurofilaments and microtubules is supported by immunochemical studies showing lack of crossreactivity between PHF and neurofilaments and microtubules as described below.

III.   IMMUNOCHEMICAL RELATIONSHIP OF PHF WITH OTHER FIBRILS

a.   Plaque Amyloid

Antibodies to isolated PHF have been raised in rabbits (Grundke-Iqbal, et.al., in preparation). Staining of ANT and neurites of the neuritic (senile) plaques by the anti PHF serum was observed in all 14 cases of AD or ADAT studied. However, the plaque core amyloid was immunolabeled by the anti PHF serum in only one of these cases. The anti PHF serum did not label amyloid plaques in the brain of a mouse with scrapie. Different classes of immunoglobulin, neurofilament and albumin among other proteins have been detected in CNS amyloid (23,24,31). It is therefore likely that in rare cases of AD or SDAT antigens crossreacting with PHF might be present in plaque central core amyloid.

b.   ANT-crossreactive Antigens Present in Normal Young Brains

Alzheimer neurofibrillary tangle cross-reacting antigen/s (ANTCA) have been recently demonstrated in normal young human and animal brain by immunocytochemical labeling techniques (10,20). An antiserum raised against an in vitro assembled microtubule preparation labeled ANT immunocytochemically and the antibodies to ANTCA were absorbed with such microtubule preparations from several young human and calf brains. It was shown that this crossreactivity was not due to antibodies to tubulin or

other known microtubule proteins, but was due to some antigen/s
copurifying with microtubules in such preparations (20,21). Since then
additional anti brain microtubule sera have been raised and their
reaction with ANT extensively studied (Grundke-Iqbal, et.al. in preparation). Out of five anti microtubule sera, 2 stained tangles in Alzheimer
brains. A comparative study of these two antisera (anti ANTCA) with the
anti PHF serum showed that in the case of the anti ANTCA sera in some
brains the number of tangles immunostained was less than those labeled
with the anti PHF serum. Also, whereas the anti PHF serum labeled the
tangles in all AD and SDAT brains studied so far, staining of tangles
by an anti-ANTCA serum was only observed in about half of the cases.
Furthermore, while ANT staining with the anti ANTCA serum was easily
removed by absorption with small amounts of microtubule preparations,
in case of the anti PHF serum absorption with even 100-fold amounts of
microtubule preparations or brain homogenate did not completely remove
the ANT staining. These findings suggest that PHF contain some antigen/s
in addition to ANTCA discovered previously in normal brain (Grundke-Iqbal,
et.al., in preparation). It is possible that in normal brain tissue
homogenate, as well as in the microtubule preparations at the concentrations tested this additional PHF antigen/s might be present but not
in amounts large enough to completely absorb the antibodies to PHF. The
question of whether PHF contain any antigen/s absent in normal young/
adult brain will therefore have to be deferred until the availability of
isolated ANTCA'S for such studies. Isolation of ANTCA'S is currently
underway in Dr. Grundke-Iqbal's laboratory.

c. Neurofibrillary Changes of 15 nm and 10 nm Filaments

Immunocytochemical studies of two cases with PSP showed labeling of
the tangles with the anti PHF serum but not with antisera against neurofilament triplet. In contrast, anti PHF serum did not label tangles of
10 nm filaments induced with aluminum or colchicine, which are readily
labeled with antiserum to neurofilament P70 and P160. These results
suggest that Alzheimer PHF might be biochemically related to the 15 nm
filaments seen in PSP. Alternatively the reactivity of the anti PHF
serum with the PSP tangles might be due to PHF with which these tangles
are sometimes admixed (See above IIa). The neurofibrillary tangles of
10 nm filaments induced with aluminum or colchicine do not appear to be
biochemically related to the PHF (Grundke-Iqbal, et.al., in preparation).
Two groups have independently reported the presence of a 50,000 mol.
wt. polypeptide in calf (25) and chicken brain (7) crossreacting with
Alzheimer neurofibrillary tangles. Both groups believe these antigens
to be a neurofilament polypeptide. However, attempts to immunolabel ANT
with antisera to neurofilament triplet have been mostly unsuccessful (7).
Only in rare instances single neurons were observed containing some
immunolabeled material reminiscent of ANT. In general, increased staining was observed only at the periphery of the tangles which themselves
were standing out as unstained structures. A small percentage of ANT are
known to be composed of PHF admixed with a significant number of neurofilaments (30). This rare staining of ANT with antineurofilament sera
most probably is due to such neurofilament containing ANT. It thus
appears that the ANT crossreacting antigens observed by Ishii, et.al.
(25) and Gambetti, et.al. (7) in their neurofilament preparations are
other than the neurofilament triplet. The ANT crossreacting antigen/s
copurifying with microtubules and neurofilaments from normal brain are

probably the same.

IV. SUMMARY AND DISCUSSION

SDS-PAGE of highly purified PHF shows three polypeptides, mol. wt. 45,000, 50,000 and 55,000 and a very high mol. wt. component (greater than 400,000). This protein composition of isolated PHF is different from that of neurofilaments and microtubules. Immunochemically PHF do not crossreact with microtubules, neurofilaments, and 10 nm filaments induced with aluminum or colchicine, but some antigen/s (ANTCA) present in normal young brain crossreacts with PHF. However, antibodies to PHF appear to be only partially absorbed with ANTCA, suggesting that PHF might contain some antigenic sites in addition to those in ANTCA which copurifies with the in vitro assembled brain microtubule preparations. It is this modification of ANTCA or additional PHF antigen/s which is probably required for the formation of PHF. PHF might be the product of derepression of some previously repressed genes. Alternatively and most probably no new proteins are synthesized but post-transcriptional modifications take place in the affected neurons leading to the formation of PHF. These biochemical events might be initiated in the neuron by a variety of insults to the CNS including the interaction of some trans-missable agent on host cell protein/s. The nature of these biochemical changes which lead to the formation of PHF is not understood. One of these biochemical changes might be a shift towards the β-pleated con-formation of the proteins involved in the formation of PHF (38).

As stated earlier in this paper, though the evidence for biochemical relationship between plaque core amyloid and ANT is minimal, both are congophilic producing characteristic green birefringence in polarized light. Physicochemical studies of the amyloid fibrils from systemic amyloidosis have shown that they are made of proteins consisting of polypeptide chains arranged in β-pleated sheet conformation (9). Furthermore, it has been shown that the synthetic polypeptide, poly-l-lysine, and synthetic insulin and glucagon fibers, when converted to their β form, produce green birefringence in polarized light after Congo red staining identical to that of amyloid fibrils. The optical pro-perties of Congo-red stained fibrillar proteins thus appear to be dependent on the β-pleated sheet formation and this property is shared under appropriate conditions by a number of chemically unrelated proteins. Therefore PHF though chemically might be unrelated to amyloid are most likely made of β-pleated protein fibrils. Furthermore, PHF are insoluble under physiological conditions and are resistant to proteo-lytic digestion (Iqbal, et.al., in preparation) a characteristic of β-pleated sheet fibrils. This property should lead to the accumulation of fibrils made from such proteins which is indeed the case with ANT.

ACKNOWLEDGEMENTS

This work was supported in part by the National Institutes of Health grants NS 17487 and NS/HD 16971 and by an over-recovery Project Funds grant from the Research Foundation for Mental Hygiene.

Technical assistance was provided by Tanweer Zaidi, Christopher H. Thompson and Yunn-Chyn Tung, photographic work by Richard Weed and secretarial help by Adele Monaco. C. Rue helped in E.M.

Figure 1 was kindly supplied by Dr. Ricardo Madrid.

333

443

553

963

773

REFERENCES

1. Berl, S., Puszkin, S. and Nicklas, W.J. (1973): *Science*, 179: 441-433.
2. Dahl, D. and Bignami, A. (1978): *Exper. Neurol.* 58:74-80.
3. Dahl, D., Bignami, A., Bich, N.T. and Chi, N.H. (1980): *Acta Neuropathol. (Berl)*, 51:156-168.
4. Dentler, W.L., Garnett, S. and Rosenbaum, J.L. (1975): *J. Cell Biology,* 65:(1) 237-241.
5. Eng, L.F., Vanderhaegen, J.J., Bignami, A. and Gerstl, B. (1971): *Brain Res.*, 28:351-354.
6. Feit, H., Slusarek, L. and Shelanski, M.L. (1971): *Proc. Nat. Acad. Sci. USA,* 68:2028-2031.
7. Gambetti, P., Velasco, M.E., Dahl, D., Bignami, A., Roessmann, U. and Sindely, S.D. (1980): In: *Aging of the Brain and Dementia*, edited by L. Amaducci, A.N. Davison and P. Antuono, pp. 55-63 Raven Press, New York.
8. Ghatak, N.R., Nochlin, D. and Hadfield, M.G. (1980): *Acta Neuropathol. (Berl)*, 52:73-76.
9. Glenner, G.G., Eanes, E.D., Bladen, H.A., Linke, R.P. and Termine, J.D. (1974): *J. Histochem. Cytochem.*, 1141-1158.
10. Grundke-Iqbal, I., Johnson, A.B., Wisniewski, H.M., Terry, R.D. and Iqbal, K. (1979): *Lancet,* I:578-580.
11. Grundke-Iqbal, I., Johnson, A.B., Terry, R.D., Wisniewski, H.M. and Iqbal, K. (1979): *Ann. Neurol..* 6:532-537.
12. Hoffman, P.N. and Lasek, R.J. (1975): *J. Cell Biol.*, 66:351-356.
13. Iqbal, K. (1979): In: *Progress in Neuropathology,* edited by H.M. Zimmerman, pp. 125-140, Raven Press, New York.
14. Iqbal, K. and Tellez-Nagel, I. (1972): *Brain Res.*,45:296-301
15. Iqbal, K., Tellez-Nagel, I., and Grundke-Iqbal, I. (1974): *Brain Res.*, 76:178-184.
16. Iqbal, K., Wisniewski, H.M., Shelanski, M.L., Brostoff, S., Liwnicz, B.H. and Terry, R.D. (1974): *Brain Res.*, 77:337-343.
17. Iqbal, K., Grundke-Iqbal, I., Wisniewski, H.M. and Terry, R.D. (1977): *J. Neurochem.*, 29:417-424.
18. Iqbal, K., Wisniewski, H.M., Grundke-Iqbal, I. and Terry, R.D. (1977): In: *The Aging Brain and Senile Dementia*, edited by K. Nandy and I. Sherwin, pp. 209-277, Plenum Press, New York.
19. Iqbal, K., Grundke-Iqbal, I., Wisniewski, H.M. and Terry, R.D. (1978): *Brain Res.*, 142:321-332.
20. Iqbal, K., Johnson, A.B., Grundke-Iqbal, I. and Wisniewski, H.M. (1980): *J. Neuropath. Exp. Neurol.*, 39:363.
21. Iqbal, K., Grundke-Iqbal, I., Johnson, A.B. and Wisniewski, H.M. (1980): In: *Aging of the Brain and Dementia*, edited by L. Amaducci, A.N. Davison and P. Antuono, pp. 39-48, Raven Press, New York.
22. Iqbal, K., Merz, P., Grundke-Iqbal, I. and Wisniewski, H.M. (1981): *J. Neuropath. Exp. Neurol.*, 40:315.
23. Ishii, T., Haga, S. and Shimizu, F. (1975): *Acta Neuropathol. (Berl)*, 32:157-162.
24. Ishii, T., and Haga, S. (1976): *Acta Neuropathol. (Berl)*, 36:243-249.
25. Ishii, T., Haga, S. and Tobutake, S. (1979): *Acta Neuropathol. (Berl)* 48:105-112.
26. Kidd, M. (1963): *Nature (London)*, 197:192-193.
27. Linder, E., Lehto, V.P. and Virtanen, I. (1979): *Acta Path. Microbiol. Scand. Sect. A.*, 87:299-306.

28. Murphy, D.B. and Borisy, G.G. (1975): <u>Proc. Natl. Acad. Sci. USA</u> 72:2696-2700.
29. Olmsted, J.B. and Borisy, G.G. (1973): <u>Ann. Rev. Biochem.</u> 42:507-540.
30. Oyanagei, S. (1979): <u>Adv. Neurol. Sci.</u> (Japanese), 18:77-88.
31. Powers, J.M., Schlaepfer, W.W., Willingham, M.C. and Hall, J. (1981): <u>J. Neuropath. Exp. Neurol.</u>, 40:311.
32. Schlaepfer, W.W. (1977): <u>J. Cell Biol.</u>, 74:226-240.
33. Selkoe, D.J., Liem, K.H., Yen, S.H. and Shelanski, M.L. (1979): <u>Brain Res.</u>, 163:235-252.
34. Soifer, D., Iqbal, K., Czosnek, H., DeMartini, J., Sturman, J.A. and Wisniewski, H.M. (1981) <u>J. Neurosci.</u>, 1:461-470.
35. Tellez-Nagel, I. and Wisniewski, H.M. (1973): <u>Arch. Neurol.</u> 29:324-327.
36. Tomlinson, B.E., Blessed, G. and Roth, M. (1970): <u>J. Neuro. Sci.</u> 11:205-242.
37. Weingarten, M.D., Lockwood, A.H., Hwo, S.Y. and Kirschner, M.W. (1975): <u>Proc. Natl. Acad. Sci. USA,</u> 72(5):1858-1862.
38. Wisniewski, H.M. (1979): In: <u>Aging and Immunity</u>, edited by S.K. Singhal, N.R. Sinclair and C.R. Stiller, pp. 185-194, Elseiver North Holland, Inc., New York/Amsterdam.
39. Wisniewski, H.M., Narang, H.K. and Terry, R.D. (1976): <u>J. Neurol. Sci.</u>, 27:173-181.
40. Wisniewski, H.M., Sinatra, R.S., Iqbal, K. and Grundke-Iqbal, I. (In press) In: <u>Aging and Cell Structure</u>, Vol. 1 edited by J. Johnson, Plenum Press, New York.
41. Wisniewski, K., Jervis, G.A., Moretz, R.C. and Wisniewski, H.M. (1979): <u>Ann. Neurol.</u> 5:288-294.

The Aging Brain: Cellular and Molecular Mechanisms of Aging in the Nervous System, edited by E. Giacobini et al., Raven Press, New York © 1982.

Serum Prolactin Changes with Age, Senile Dementia, and Dihydroergotoxine Mesylate Treatment

T. Samorajski, Beng T. Ho, Patricia M. Kralik, and *James T. Hartford

*Departments of Neurobiology and Neurochemistry, Texas Research Institute of Mental Sciences, Houston, Texas 77030; *Department of Psychiatry, University of Cincinnati Medical Center, Cincinnati, Ohio 45267*

The progressive reduction of reproductive function and behavioral deficits which are associated with aging may be, in part, caused by disruption of the striatal and hypothalamic-hypophyseal control systems (9). Although the origin of these changes is uncertain, previous studies suggest that dopaminergic (DA) neurons are particularly susceptible to age- and disease-related decrements in number and function (review, 27).

Decreases in DA concentration and turnover have been reported in the striatum and other selected regions of aged rodent and human brains (1,6,12). In the hypothalamus, three DA neuronal systems have been identified: the incertohypothalamic, tuberohypophyseal, and tuberoinfundibular systems (5,21). Decreased function in the latter system may be particularly revelant to aging because changes in these neurons may influence the release of gonadotropic hormones (follicle-stimulating hormone, FSH; leuteinizing hormone, LH; and prolactin, PRL) from the anterior pituitary gland (20,30). Severe changes in hypothalamic neurons may result in senescence of endocrine glands and other target tissues (13,23).

Clinically, assays of PRL have proved useful in identifying infertility in young women who have high PRL levels; reduction of these levels by treatment with the ergot alkaloid 2-bromo-α-ergokryptine (bromocriptine, Sandoz) has helped them to conceive (25). High serum PRL levels are also associated with certain affective disorders (19). The ergot alkaloid derivative dihydroergotoxine mesylate (Hydergine, Sandoz) is useful in treating elderly patients suffering from a nonpsychotic organic brain syndrome (11,17). Hydergine has mixed agonist and antagonist effects on brain dopamine receptors and similarly mixed effects on phosphodiesterase and other neurochemical systems (4,8,10). Although its mechanism of action is not completely known, it is likely that Hydergine and other ergot alkaloid derivatives act as strong dopaminergic agonists at the level of the hypothalamus, inhibiting PRL secretion (2,8,14,18,31). There are, however, important quantitative differences when comparing different dopaminergic systems (22).

The present paper reports a study of PRL levels in a healthy population of men and women representing the reproductive and

postreproductive periods of the human lifespan. We also report the
results of a double-blind study on the effects of Hydergine on serum
prolactin levels, which was part of a larger investigation of cognitive
changes in elderly patients with chronic organic brain syndrome.
Changes in prolactin levels were correlated with duration of treatment
and clinical condition as determined by the <u>Sandoz Clinical Assessment
Geriatric</u> (SCAG) scale (29).

METHOD

Subjects

<u>Controls</u>.
Subjects were 61 employees of the Texas Research Institute of Mental
Sciences and volunteers from the Southwest YMCA in Houston, whose ages
ranged from 21 to 86 years. Of the 30 women and 31 men, 35 were
between ages 21 and 50 years, 11 between 51 and 70, and 15 were 71 years
old or older. None was chronically or acutely ill at the time of
testing. The participants were asked to abstain from food, smoking,
and drink except for water on the day blood samples were taken; they
were otherwise encouraged to follow normal daytime activities. Most
practiced some form of physical exercise; this included the older
subjects who were regular members in YMCA programs of calisthenics,
jogging, or swimming. Blood samples were collected between 10 and
12 a.m. in vacutainers coated with EDTA (ethylene diamine tetra acetic
acid).

<u>Patients</u>. The patient group included 26 persons whose ages ranged
from 60 to 95 years. There were 23 women and 3 men: one aged 60,
9 between ages 71 and 80, and 16 aged 81 or older. They were residents
of two nursing homes and had cognitive deficits (dementia) ranging from
mild to moderate.

Patients with a mild to moderate degree of dementia were selected
for a double-blind study using the SCAG rating scale (29), which
contains 18 items assessing interpersonal, cognitive, emotional (affect
and apathy) and physical (somatic) symptoms associated with mental
deterioration in the elderly. Severity of impairment was assessed with
a seven-point rating scale on which 1 indicates the absence of a
symptom and 7 indicates the presence of a severe symptom. Patients
with a mild to moderate degree of organic impairment (rating of 4 or 5)
were included in the study. All received a battery of medical and
laboratory tests and a physical examination.

Patients were assigned randomly to a drug or placebo group.
Nineteen of 26 patients completed the study. Nine patients received
Hydergine orally, 2 mg three times a day for 12 or 20 weeks; ten
patients received placebo orally, three times a day for 12 weeks.
Blood samples were drawn after a two-week, drug-free baseline period
and again at 6, 12, and 20 weeks during the treatment period. In
addition, five of the Hydergine-treated patients had blood drawn three
to six days after termination of Hydergine treatment.

<u>Procedure</u>. Serum was separated by centrifugation at 1.5 K rpm for
ten minutes from 6 to 8 ml of venous blood within 2 to 3 hours after
collection. Prolactin was determined by radioimmunoassay using the
human prolactin RIA kit from Calbiochem-Behring Corporation, with the
following modifications for increased sensitivity and liquid

scintillation spectrometry: Incubation time was increased from 5 to 24 hours after addition of the first antibody; following centrifugation, the supernatant was aspirated and the precipitate was suspended in 1 ml of distilled water, transferred to a glass counting vial and combined with a second 1-ml rinse; after the addition of 3 ml of methanol and 10 ml of Insta-Gel (Packard Instrument Co.), the samples were assayed by liquid scintillation spectrometry; a lower concentration of prolactin (2ng/ml) was included in the standard curves. Blood samples from five subjects were collected on five different days to measure daily variability. Individual variability ranged from 10 to 60 percent. The patient's physician recorded vital signs and his impression of the patient's psychological status on the SCAG form. Two-tailed tests were employed in the statistical comparisons.

RESULTS

The effects of age on serum prolactin levels of healthy men and women are summarized in Figure 1. Analysis of variance showed significant differences between women 21 to 50 years and those 51 to 70 and 71 to 90 years (p<0.025) thus, suggesting a significant decline with age. The difference between levels at middle (51 to 70 years) and old age (71 to 90 years) was not significant. A slight but insignificant serum prolactin decline with age was found in men. Differences between male and female levels were not significant.

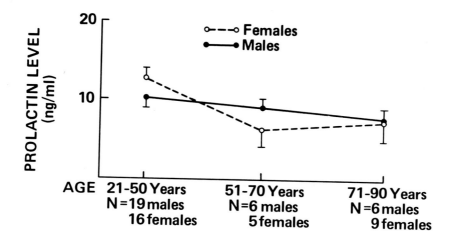

FIG. 1. Serum PRL levels in normal men and women of various age groups. Data are expressed as mean ± S.E.M. The difference between young (21-50) and old (51-70 and 71-90) women is significant at the P<0.025 level (ANOVA).

Serum prolactin values for the demented patients and age-matched controls are shown in Figure 2. In the 60- to 70-year-old groups there

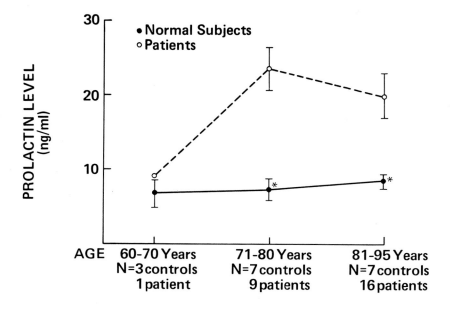

FIG. 2. Serum PRL levels in patients and age-matched controls. Each value is the mean ± S.E.M., *P<0.025.

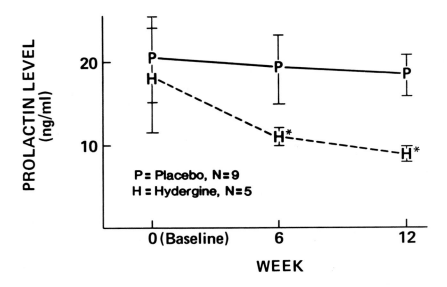

FIG. 3. Serum PRL values at baseline (Week 0) and after 6 and 12 weeks of placebo or Hydergine treatment (2 mg three times a day). Each value is the mean ± S.E.M., *P<0.05 (ANOVA).

was no apparent difference between the single patient and the three age-matched controls. A statistical comparison of the older groups (71 to 80 and 81 to 95), patients and age-matched controls, indicated that the patients had significantly higher prolactin levels ($p<0.025$). The difference between the serum prolactin levels of patients in the 71 to 80 and 81 to 95 age groups was not significant according to analysis of variance comparison.

A comparison of prolactin levels for Hydergine-treated patients with those observed in the placebo group at baseline (week 0) and at 6 and 12 weeks of treatment is illustrated in Figure 3. Both between- and within-group significance tests were performed. In the Hydergine-treated patients, prolactin levels decreased significantly at weeks 6 and 12 ($p<0.05$). The placebo group did not show a significant change in prolactin blood levels during the 12-week period.

The results shown in Figure 3 should be interpreted with caution because of the small sample size and the relatively large variability observed at baseline and in the placebo values. Nevertheless, it seems that, compared to baseline and placebo values, Hydergine (6 mg per day) lowers prolactin levels.

Examples of prolactin levels in patients at baseline, during Hydergine treatment, and three to six days after Hydergine was discontinued are shown in Table 1. Most of these show that prolactin levels were dramatically elevated when Hydergine was discontinued and returned rapidly to pretreatment levels. These results contrast with the gradual lowering of serum prolactin by Hydergine. One patient showed a lower value during the post-treatment phase, but this patient was switched to Deapril (dihydroergotoxine mesylate, Mead Johnson Pharm. Div.) at the end of 20 weeks of treatment with Hydergine.

TABLE 1. Serum prolactin levels in five subjects studied before, during and 3-6 days after termination of Hydergine treatment.

Patient number	Baseline values	Prolactin Levels at			Post-treatment (3-6 days)
		6 wks	12 wks	20 wks	
102	30.2	10.7			29.2
106	13.5	7.8	8.8	3.0	2.4 (a)
109	51.5	26.4			32.0
110	14.0	13.8	8.8	3.1	52.2
119	18.5	0.9			25.3
Mean ± SEM	25.5±7.2	11.9±4.2	8.8	3.1	28.2±8.0

(a)Patient received 3 mg Deapril (dihydroergotoxine mesylate, Mead Johnson Pharm. Div.).

Table 2 shows the relationship between changes in prolactin levels and composite scores on the SCAG, based on Pearson product-moment correlation coefficients. In this table, a positive correlation indicates that, as the prolactin level decreased, clinical response improved, supporting the hypothesis that decreasing prolactin levels

are positively correlated with clinical improvement. The correlation
coefficients are based on values observed for all patients, that is,
nine patients completing six weeks of treatment, and five from the same
group completing 12 weeks of treatment.

At week 6 the correlations were either negative or close to zero,
indicating little relationship between changes in prolactin levels and
changes recorded on the SCAG scale. At 12 weeks, however, the
correlation of all factors except affect and self-care tended to be more
positive. Values significantly different from zero include apathy,
overall impression and the total (average) of all items. Thus, at
least at 12 weeks, improvements in SCAG ratings are positively
correlated with decreasing prolactin levels although the magnitude of
the correlations are not large.

TABLE 2. Pearson product-moment correlation coefficients[a] for
change in prolactin vs. change in SCAG factor constructs

Item	Week 6 N= 9	Week 12 N= 5
1. Interpersonal relationships	.11	.14
2. Cognitive dysfunction	.07	.39
3. Affect	-.64	-.65
4. Apathy	.00	.51
5. Somatic functioning	-.03	.26
6. Self-care	-.10	-.33
7. Overall impression	-.22	.85
8. Average of 18 items	-.15	.54

[a] A positive correlation indicates that, as the prolactin level
decreases, the SCAG variable improves.

DISCUSSION

The normal PRL serum level in 16 premenopausal women was found to be
12.4 $\pm$ 1.5 ng/ml (Figure 1). Women between the ages of 51 and 70 years
and 71 to 90 years had values of 6.5 $\pm$ 0.8 and 7.9 $\pm$ 0.8, respectively;
these were significantly different from the premenopausal values
($p<0.025$ and $p<0.05$, respectively). These findings agree with those
of Pepperell et al. (25) and others (3,15,28). Normal PRL serum level
for men aged 21 to 50 years was 10.2 $\pm$ 1.2 ng/ml. The older males had
lower values (9.3 $\pm$ 1.7 and 8.0 $\pm$ 1.8) at 51 to 70 years and 71 to 90
years, respectively. An age-by-sex analysis failed to reveal
significant differences between genders.

PRL levels determined frequently in the same subject showed marked
fluctuations, and it is possible that serum PRL values of premenopausal
women fluctuate in accordance with different stages of the menstrual
cycle. Pepperell et al. (25), however, failed to find significant
differences between mean follicular and luteal phase values and did
not observe reproducible peaks in women with normal ovulation cycles.
Among men, fluctuations were as marked as those of the women. It is

unlikely, therefore, that ovulation cycles contribute to inter- and intrasubject variability. It is also possible that periodic variations of mood and such physiologic functions as sleep and physical activity alter prolactin levels.

Abnormalities in the 24-hour PRL profile in subtypes of depressed patients have been reported (24). While depression, decreased physical activity, and changes in sleep patterns are characteristic of some elderly individuals, we found that prolactin variability actually decreased with age in female subjects. These results suggest that prolactin variability, periodic variation of mood, and various physiological functions probably are not directly related. A thorough analysis of PRL fluctuations would require more frequent blood sampling and a detailed quantitative description of each secretory peak in relation to the physiological status of the subjects.

It has been postulated that serum PRL may be elevated in certain affective disorders (19). Our findings of significantly higher serum prolactin levels in demented patients compared to age-matched controls (Figure 2) agree with this suggestion. Our results indicate, further, that serum prolactin estimates should be part of the investigatory clinical profile of elderly patients impaired by chronic organic brain syndrome. Prolactin levels may provide additional information about symptom severity.

One problem in interpreting our data may be related to the comparison of healthy individuals and nursing home patients. Patients in nursing homes often have multiple disorders and chronic situational problems, leading to highly variable mood. Any or all of these situations could influence PRL independently, so that a correlation analysis of severity of cognitive dysfunction and prolactin levels might be misleading. The difference in PRL levels between the demented patients and age-matched controls shown in this study is strong enough, however, to warrant further investigation of the relation between serum PRL levels and severity of symptoms associated with chronic organic brain syndrome.

Serum prolactin has been shown to be decreased by dihydroergotoxine mesylate (Hydergine) at dosages of 1 mg three times a day, taken orally (18). In our study, a significant decline occurred with 2 mg three times daily (Figure 3). Gaitz et al. (17) have proposed that, because the ergot alkaloids are relatively slow-acting, patients may need to be treated several months at currently approved dosage levels before results will appear. It is of some interest, then, that prolactin levels in our Hydergine-treated group were significantly lower at 12 weeks of treatment than at 6 weeks. More surprising was the rapid return of prolactin to pretreatment levels within days after treatment was terminated (Table 1). The significance of this change in relation to behavioral influences, if any, is unknown.

Calculation of Pearson product-moment correlations at 6 and 12 weeks yielded some interesting differences (Table 2). At 6 weeks, the correlations were either negative or close to zero. At 12 weeks, however, the correlations tended to be more positive for all variables except affect and self-care. The values for overall impression and the total of all items are significantly different from zero. The correlation between apathy and lower prolactin approaches significance (0.51). This suggests that Hydergine may also have some positive affects on motor behavior and motivation concurrently with a lowering of prolactin levels.

It is possible that a longer course of therapy and the inclusion
of a larger number of patients would have produced more significant
results. It may also be true that Hydergine influences some behaviors
and prolactin indirectly, so that a correlation analysis would not
show significance. A problem in interpreting changes in affect
(mainly depression) and prolactin levels may relate to the possibility
that the SCAG test is not a suitable device for assessing mood in
depressed elderly patients. Some nursing home patients may remain
depressed because of severe and chronic problems (16 of the 26 patients
tested were 81 years of age or older).

Aging is associated with a progressive reduction of reproductive
function which may be caused, in part, by a disruption of the
hypothalamic-pituitary axis (9). Decreased function of the tuberoinfundibular system may be particularly pertinent to the study of aging
because of its influence on releasing the inhibitory factors associated
with endocrine function (Figure 4). The secretion of PRL by the
pituitary seems to be primarily controlled by dopaminergic inhibitory
neurons (7,16,20). Thus, a loss of tuberoinfundibular DA neurons may

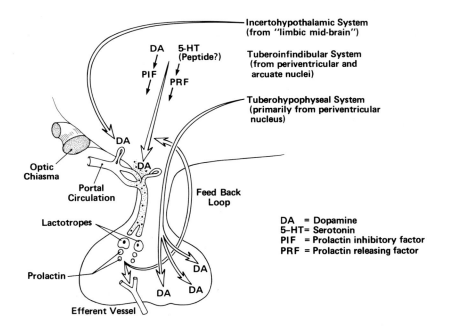

FIG. 4. Possible actions of dopamine on prolactin secretion.
Dopamine presumably reaches the lactotropes through the pituitary
portal system. Serum prolactin levels may reflect both the tone of the
tuberoinfundibular dopamine pathway and the sensitivity of the dopamine
receptor at the lactotrope. Three different fiber systems are
identified: incertohypothalamic, tuberoinfundibular, and tuberohypophyseal.

alter the balance between inhibitory and releasing factors produced by peptidergic neurons in the hypothalamus. A loss with aging, for example, may result in a decrease of prolactin-inhibitory activity or an increase in prolactin-releasing activity, with a concommitant increase in the production of PRL in the anterior pituitary. As schematically represented in Figure 4, the changes in the hypothalamic-pituitary axis may result, throughout the body, in further senescent changes associated with the mechanism of prolactin action on various biological systems (26). Hydergine, then, exerts its beneficial action by improving the function of hypothalamic DA neurons, possibly in the same way that L-dopa compensates for the loss of nigrostriatal DA neurons in patients suffering from Parkinsonism.

Hydergine was shown to be effective in suppressing serum PRL, and one might expect that other dopamine agonists which increase the amount of dopamine available to the receptor might provide alternative methods of treating symptoms associated with chronic organic brain syndrome. Further studies are needed to confirm the clinical utility of modulating dopaminergic neurotransmitter systems as a means of alleviating symptoms of senile dementia.

SUMMARY

Serum prolactin (PRL) levels were compared in 61 healthy subjects and 26 elderly nursing home patients suffering from a syndrome of dementia of light to moderate severity. Ages of normal subjects varied from 21 to 86 years. Women in this group showed a significant decline of PRL levels with age, while PRL levels of healthy men were slightly and insignificantly lower with age. In the demented patients, serum prolactin levels were significantly higher than those of age-matched controls. When a compound of ergot alkaloids (dihydroergotoxine mesylate; Hydergine, Sandoz) or placebo was given to the nursing home patients, those in the treatment group (6 and 12 weeks) experienced a significantly greater decline in serum PRL levels than did those in the placebo group. A significant correlation was found between PRL changes and changes in several behaviors measured by the Sandoz Clinical Assessment Geriatric (SCAG) scale. Cessation of Hydergine administration resulted in a rapid return of PRL to pretreatment levels. These results suggest that serum PRL estimates should form part of the investigatory clinical profile of elderly persons with symptoms of chronic organic brain syndrome. Prolactin values may also be useful in ascertaining possible effects of drugs in mediating behavioral changes associated with chronic organic brain syndrome.

ACKNOWLEDGMENTS

The authors are grateful to Lore Feldman, Lisa Hatfield, Diane Dunn, and Danielle Miller-Soule for their technical assistance and to the many volunteers whose participation made this study possible. We also thank John Patin and Dr. Dieter M. Loew, Sandoz, Inc., East Hanover, N.J., for statistical analysis, and review of the manuscript.

REFERENCES

1. Adolfsson: R., Gottfries, C.G., Oreland, L., Roos, B.E., and Winblad, B. (1978): In: Alzheimer's Disease: Senile Dementia and Related Disorders, edited by R. Katzman, R.D. Terry and K.L. Bick, pp. 441-451. Raven Press, New York.
2. Anlezark, G., Pycock, C., and Meldrum, B. (1976): European J. Pharmacol., 37:295-302.
3. Barberia, J.M., Abu-Fadil, S., Kletzky, O.A., Nakamura, R.M., and Mishell, Jr., D.R. (1975): Amer. J. Obstet. Gynec., 121:1107-1110.
4. Berde, B. and Schild, H.O., editors (1978): Ergot Alkaloids and Related Compounds. Springer-Verlag Berlin Heidelberg, New York.
5. Björklund, A., Moore, R.Y., Nobin, A., and Stenevi, U. (1973): Brain Res., 51:171-191.
6. Carlsson, A., and Winblad, B. (1976): J. Neural. Trans., 38:271-276.
7. Clemens: J.A. (1980): In: Advances in Biochemical Psychopharmacology, Vol. 23; Ergot Compounds and Brain Function: Neuroendocrine and Neuropsychiatric Aspects, edited by M. Goldstein, D.B. Calne, A. Lieberman, and M.O. Thorner, pp. 315-321. Raven Press, New York.
8. Cvejić, V., and Mršulja, B.B. (1981): Gerontology, 27:7-12.
9. Demarest, K.T., Riegle, G.D., and Moore, K.E. (1980): Neuroendocrinology, 31:222-227.
10. Djuričić, B.M., and Mršulja, B.B. (1980): Gerontology, 26:99-103.
11. Fanchamps: A. (1979): In: Geriatric Psychopharmacology, edited by K. Nandy, pp. 195-212. Elsevier North Holland, Inc., New York.
12. Finch, C.E. (1973): Brain Res., 52:261-276.
13. Finch: C.E. (1977): In: Handbook of the Biology of Aging, edited by C.E. Finch and L. Hayflick, pp. 262-280. Van Nostrand Reinhold, New York.
14. Flückiger, E., Markó, M., Doepfner, W., and Niederer, W. (1976): Post-graduate Medical J., 52(suppl. 1):57-61.
15. Fournier, P.J.R., Desjardins, P.D., and Friesen, H.G. (1974): Amer. J. Obstet. Gynec., 118:337-343.
16. Frantz: A.G. (1979): In: Endocrine Rhythms, edited by D.T. Krieger, pp. 175-186. Raven Press, New York.
17. Gaitz: C.M., and Hartford, J.T. (1979): In: Geriatric Psychopharmacology, edited by K. Nandy, pp. 213-224. Elsevier North Holland, Inc., New York.
18. Gross, R.J., Eisdorfer, C.E., Schiller, H.S., and Cox, G. (1979): Experimental Aging Res., 5:293-302.
19. Horrobin, D.F. (1973): Prolactin: physiology and clinical significance, pp. 158-169. Medical and Technical Publishing Co. Ltd., Lancaster, Great Britain.
20. Lawton, N.F., Evans, A.J., and Weller, R.O. (1981): J. Neurological Sciences, 49:229-239.
21. Lindvall: O., and Björklund, A.C. (1978): In: Handbook of Psychopharmacology, Vol. 9, edited by L.L. Iversen, S.D. Iversen, and S.H. Snyder, pp. 139-231. Plenum Press, New York.
22. Loew: D.M., Vigouret, J.M., and Jaton, A. (1980): In: Ergot Compounds and Brain Function: Neuroendocrine and Neuropsychiatric Aspects, edited by M. Goldstein, D.B. Calne, A. Lieberman, and M.O. Thorner, pp. 63-74. Raven Press, New York.
23. Meites: J., Huang, H.H., and Simpkins, J.W. (1978): In: The Aging

Reproductive System (Aging, Volume 4), edited by E.L. Schneider, pp. 213-235. Raven Press, New York.

24. Mendlewicz, J., Van Cauter, E., Linkowski, P., L'Hermite, M., and Robyn, C. (1980): Life Sciences, 27:2015-2024.
25. Pepperell, R.J., Bright, M., and Smith, M.A. (1977): Med. J. Aust., 1:85-89.
26. Rillema, J.A. (1980): Federation Proc., 39:2593-2598.
27. Samorajski: T., and Hartford, J. (1980): In: Handbook of Geriatric Psychiatry, edited by E.W. Busse, and D.G. Blazer, pp. 46-82. Van Nostrand Reinhold, New York.
28. Seki, K., Seki, M., Okumura, T., and Huang, K. (1976): Amer. J. Obstet. Gynec., 124:125-128.
29. Shader, R.I., Harmatz, J.S., and Salzman, C. (1974): J. American Geriatric Society, 22:107-113.
30. Weiner, R.I., and Ganong, W.F. (1978): Physiol. Rev., 58:905-976.
31. Willoughby, J.O., and Day, T.A. (1981): Neuroendocrinology, 32:65-69.

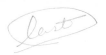

*The Aging Brain: Cellular and Molecular
Mechanisms of Aging in the Nervous System,*
edited by E. Giacobini et al., Raven Press, New
York © 1982.

Cellular and Molecular Mechanisms of Aging of the Nervous System: Toward a Unified Theory of Neuronal Aging

Ezio Giacobini

*Department of Biobehavioral Science, Laboratory of Neuropsychopharmacology,
University of Connecticut, Storrs, Connecticut 06268*

A. BASIC QUESTIONS RELATED TO A GENERAL THEORY OF CELLULAR AGING.

Numerous hypotheses have been put forward in an attempt to rationalize and unify the theories on cellular and molecular mechanisms of aging. Each of these hypotheses is concerned with the impairment of a particular subcellular mechanism implying most often the function of nucleic acids in aging cells. Some of these hypotheses have exerted an extraordinary stimulating effect on the whole field of experimental gerontology. A possible failure of nucleic acids function and metabolism has been stressed (40, 18). Many reasons for such a failure have been proposed, all resulting in an altered specificity of the translational step in protein synthesis. The reasons for a deficient function of nucleic acids and related enzymes can be multiple; quantitative changes in DNA or RNA content per cell, deficiency in DNA-repair capacity, free radicals pathology, etc. all leading to changes in content of information or in a disturbance of the mechanism of protein synthesis regulation. Some of these theories consider the possibility of errors leading to reduced specificity of information-handling enzymes thus causing increasing error frequency in protein synthesis. The effect of such errors may be cumulative, leading to "catastrophic" consequences for the function and survival of the cell. The weakness of such a theory is the present lack of demonstration of "wrong proteins" and of the subsequent steps as parts of a cascade of events which may be lethal to the cell. Other theories, in an attempt to explain increasing cell death during aging, try to rationalize the variation in the growth potential of individual cells within a culture (See section E. 2, 3, 4). These models may explain the variability in life-span of cultures grown under identical conditions, however, they fail to indicate specific molecular defects related to or causing aging processes. The inherent strength of these theories is the possibility of experimentally testing their predictions by making use of simpler models such as cell or tissue cultures (e.g. human fibroblasts), unicellular organisms, and tissues derived from invertebrates such as Drosophila. On the basis of the information collected through these studies it is presently difficult to conceive a single and universal mechanism of aging, rather we think of the phenomenon of aging as "a result from a combination of several, mutually independent mechanisms, both programmed and stochastic" (18). As methodologies of cellular and molecular biology become more refined it will become increasingly easier to test experimentally each of the present working hypotheses and make verifiable predictions on aging mechanisms.

B. <u>QUESTIONS SPECIFICALLY RELATED TO AGING OF THE NERVOUS SYSTEM</u>.

Human pathology of brain aging and decreased mental and physical performance, particularly motor activity, have been recognized and studied for many years. However, compared to other systems the amount of critical information related to the nervous system of experimental animals and humans is still relatively poor and does not allow the formulation of a general hypothesis of aging of the nervous tissue. A number of quantitative and descriptive data have been collected in cases of non-reversible senile dementia, mostly related to characteristic changes in the structure of the cytoskeleton or in the activities of neurotransmitter related enzymes (9, 7). Animal studies are still discontinuous and related only to a few and scattered ages. It is therefore difficult not only to formulate a general hypothesis on brain aging but to identify the precise period at which specific changes in structure and function may start to occur.

We feel that before attempting to formulate a working hypotheses on brain aging, some general questions should be asked:
1) Are there biochemical changes specifically related to aging, or can neurochemical decreases (e.g. decreased neurotransmitter synthesis and receptor binding) be explained by a selective decrease in the number of cells of synapses?

One of the most common interpretations of age related changes is a degeneration of nerve cells due to unknown factors acting on the aged neuron. However, in spite of the widely accepted belief that a progressive, large-scale neuronal loss occurs during aging, a survey of the literature (10, 16, 23, 24, 43) does not support the view of a generalized phenomenon of neuronal death.

Ponzio et al. (43) showed that in the rat the concentration of catecholamines is not significantly decreased in the striatum and hypothalamus. However, the NE content decreases in the brainstem. This is where the cell bodies of the neurons, which project to different parts of the brain, are located. Therefore, at least in some areas there is probably no loss of noradrenergic terminals due to aging. It may be that only selected populations of noradrenergic neurons projecting from the brainstem are lost or damaged as a consequence of aging. Presently, we ignore the mechanism which could produce such a selective loss of a specific neuronal population. In the peripheral nervous system there is so far no evidence for neuronal loss due to aging. In the ciliary ganglion the number of cells present at one month of age (approx. 2700) is the same as at 7 years (11), however profound changes have been described in the cholinergic innervation of the target organ (15, 29, 30, 31, 32, 33, 34, 35, 36, 37).

Similar changes have been described by Smith (this publ.) in the neuromuscular junction of the rat.

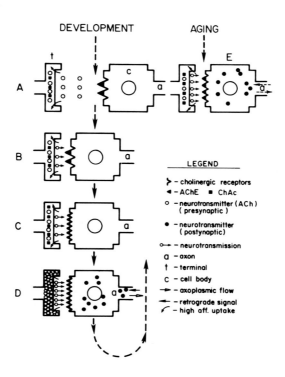

FIG. 1. Synaptogenesis and aging in the PNS of the chick.

A. Phase of innervation - low density of receptors, low level of
    neurotransmitter (NT) synthesis and release. Absence of synaptic
    structures. Appearance of uptake and inactivation.

B. Phase of neurotransmission - onset and maturation of synaptic
    activity in target organ. Rudimentary synaptic structures.

C. Phase of receptogenesis - sustained increase of receptors density.
    Primitive synaptic structures.

D. Phase of biochemical and structural maturation - accelerated syn-
    thesis, inactivation and transport of NT. Completion of synaptic
    stuctures (vesicles, membrane specialization, etc.).

E. Phase of regression and aging - decreased synthesis of NT, and of
    uptake of NT precursor.

2) Do age-dependent modifications involve all parts of the neuron (cell body, axon, terminals) or are some parts more vulnerable or more affected than others? The information accumulated so far in our studies (15, 30, 32, 33) on cholinergic mechanisms points to a selective vulnerability of the terminals during aging. (Fig. 1)

3) Are some biochemical mechanisms related to neurotransmission more affected than others? Our results indicate that uptake mechanisms may be more vulnerable in aging of cholinergic and adrenergic synapses (20, 21, 22, 30).

4) Are changes in neurotransmission due to a "cascade" phenomenon or to the sum of multiple and simultaneous defects taking place in the aging synapse? Our data (15, 29, 30, 31, 32, 33, 34, 35, 36, 37) do not support the hypothesis of a "cascade" phenomenon but favor the hypothesis of a sum of almost simultaneous events such as decreased enzyme activity, altered uptake mechanisms and modified turnover of the neurotransmitter. Although all the neurochemical parameters we have examined so far show some evidence of decline, some of them are more severely impaired than others. (Fig. 1)

5) Can biochemical damage explain a functional loss? We have seen that the levels of neurotransmitter synthesis in the iris during aging are as low as or lower than at embryonic ages. Could this phenomenon by itself lead to a great decrease in the function of the organ?

A final question is whether aging of the nervous system possesses any particular feature which makes it unique, or whether it is only part of the general process of cellular aging which involves the whole organism. In reviewing the literature we realized that most information is centered around the mechanism of neurotransmission and synaptic organization. By analyzing the results collected from published investigations and review articles we will attempt to suggest such a working hypothesis based on a general view of synaptic aging. This should not prevent us to consider alternative theories of brain aging taking into consideration other phenomena such as possible failure(s) in the cytoskeleton and transport system of the neuron. Both possibilities seem to be real in view of the findings of brain pathology in aging animals and humans.

C. CHANGES IN BRAIN CELLS WHICH HAVE BEEN DEMONSTRATED OR SUGGESTED TO BE AGE RELATED.

   1) Biochemical changes

   a) Decrease in neurotransmitter levels and in the capacity of synthesizing neurotransmitters.
      The decrease in NE (norepinephrine) levels seen in certain areas of human brain (45) may depend either on the increase seen in metabolizing enzymes (MAO) or in the decrease of enzyme activities related to synthesis (DDC, dopadecarboxylase); TH, tyrosine hydroxylase; (38). Declines in ChAc (cholineacetyltransferase) activities in the cortex have also been measured (38). By contrast, in the thelencephalon of the mouse ChAc activity was unaffected by aging (49).
   b) Decrease in receptor number or altered receptor sensitivity.
      These may depend on a loss of receptor due to a decreased rate of synthesis or to a decrease in radioligand binding. Other changes are: receptor desensitization, agonist induced down-regulation, and lower resistance to desensitization (28). A decreased capacity of synthesis

or mobility following denervation may cause a lower basal receptor number. Examples of these changes are decreases in DA (dopamine) HA (histamine), 5-HT and ACh receptor binding sites (28). In addition to a decreased density in β-adrenergic receptor binding, a decreased capacity for β-receptors to become supersensitive following denervation has been found (28). A decrease in DA receptor binding with ^{3}H-spiroperidol is accompanied by a decreased capacity for stimulation of adenylcyclase activity by DA and HA (28). Trabucchi et al. and Nomura et al. (this publ.) found significant decreases in both high and low affinity binding and in sensitivity to DA stimulation in various brain areas of rats. The decrease is not equal throughout the brain but region dependent (low in striatum, high in retina) and affects only one class of DA receptors. A decrease is also seen for DA stimulation of cAMP accumulation. This indicates that both neurotransmitter and receptor may be selectively modified and that the dopamine system is most vulnerable to aging. Some other receptor systems such as that for GABA seems to be resistant to aging (Enna, this publ.). It should be stressed that in general receptor modifications are different for various types of receptors and for different receptor areas. This selectivity in receptor modifications suggests differences in neuronally or non-neuronally located receptors. It should also be noted that a decrease in the number of receptors is functionally additive to any presynaptic loss. The pathological significance of a decreased number of receptors is important in interpreting the development and progression of Parkinsonism (e.g. DA receptors) or the deterioration of neuroendocrine functions (e.g. hypothalamus and amine receptors).

c) <u>Degeneration of cytoskeleton</u>.

This is represented by neurotubular changes such as twisted tubules or the production of neurofibrillary tangles (Alzheimer disease) and β-helical abnormal filament proteins. Such changes are discussed in detail in the chapters by Wisniewski, Iqbal, Bignami and Dahl (this publ.).

d) <u>Defects in ion transport capacity</u>.

This is associated to an age related decline in Na^+, K^+ ATPase activity which is common to myocardial, brain, spinal cord and renal tissue (27). Cell membranes are candidates for changes which may be responsible for impaired ion transport, activity and mobility of receptor proteins and accessibility of receptor binding sites. Table 1

The results of Porcellati et al. (this publ.) and of Calderini and Toffano (this publ.) suggest that ethanolamine and choline phosphotransferase as well as acetyltransferase activities are affected differently by aging. The biosynthetic ability decreases in some brain areas of aging rats (18 mo) indicating that incorporation of both glycerol and nitrogenous bases in brain membranes is affected by aging. On the contrary methylation of phospolipids increases, perhaps to compensate for the increased membrane viscosity observed during aging.

e) <u>Age associated decrease in local cerebral glucose utilization</u>.

The glucose utilization may be reduced by 25-30% in whole brain of rats. The loss is most pronounced in several CNS areas (but not cerebellum) of rats. An estimate of changes in glucose utilization which can affect ACh (acetylcholine) synthesis by limiting the supply of acetyl-CoA showed no significant variation in patients aged 15-68 years (Sims et al., this publ.). Synthesis of ACh, however, declined by 34-41% in the striatum of rats with no significant changes in glucose utilization. Gibson and Petersons (this publ.) findings in mice confirm the view that changes in $^{14}CO_2$ production from labelled carbohydrate precursors are insufficient to account for the decline in ACh synthesis. Alteration of ACh release and Ch uptake may be more important in this respect than changes in carbohydrate metabolism.

TABLE 1.   AGE RELATED CHANGES IN SYNAPTIC TRANSMISSION

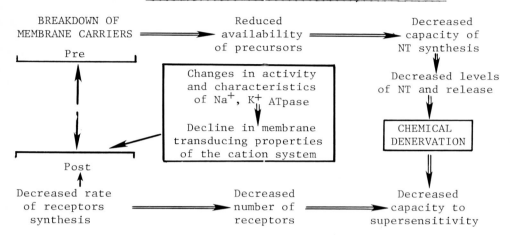

As indicated in Table 1 membrane related changes in neurotransmission could lead to a situation of chemical denervation.

D.   STRUCTURAL CHANGES.

1)   Neuronal loss and neuronal degeneration.

This phenomenon is strictly area-dependent: while in some brain areas no changes in the number of neurons has been observed, in other areas significant decreases have been reported. (See section B. 1.) Unfortunately, in most animal studies intermediate ages have not been examined (e.g. stages between 3 and 24 months in rats).

In human cerebral cortex, neuronal loss has been reported (1, 3) Purkinje cells and cells in the putamen of aging humans have been shown to decrease with age (19). However, no neuronal loss has been reported for nuclei of medulla, pons and hypothalamus of human brain. Only the locus coeruleus shows a significant age related loss of neurons (50). In this nucleus, Goldman and Coleman (16) showed no loss in neuron number with advancing age in Fisher 344 rats. This indicates that although some aging phenomena may correlate closely in rodent and man, the two species may not be completely equivalent with regard to brain aging.

2)   Loss of synapses and dendrites.

Changes in specific types of synapses have been reported. An example is the 27% decrease in axodendritic synapses seen in 24 months old rats (2). These changes are due to the presynaptic neuron and are not accompanied by neuronal loss. This phenomenon can be interpreted as either primary degeneration or as an excess of synapse destruction over synapse production. As pointed out by several authors (46) synapses may be continuously remodelled and reformed throughout adult life as part of an age-dependent process of synaptic reorganization. An example of considerable structural reorganization is the molecular

layer of the dentate gyrus during aging (2). In this layer an astrocytic hypertrophy is seen which may be compensatory for age-related
changes in synaptic transmission processes.

3) Decrease in synapse formation and plasticity in vitro.

Changes in synapse formation with age have been studied in cell
cultures. In cultures of rat striated muscles co-cultured with cholinergic cells, synapses are detected after 24 hrs (47). Similarly chick
embryo retina and muscle cells will produce synapses with a peak at
6-16 days of embryonic age. The period of maximal synaptic formation
is found in 8 day embryos. Although the results of these experiments
cannot be directly applied to the in situ situation (14), they indicate both an optimal age and a period of maximal activity for synaptic
formation in the embryo (44, 47).

4) Changes and errors in neuronal microenvironment.

It should be stressed that any error in the microenvironment of the
neuron produced by changes in number, distribution or structure of nonneuronal elements (capillaries, neuroglia) will also affect the neuronal metabolism. Most affected should be the energy metabolism of the
cell, ion transport mechanisms and synthesis, release, and reuptake of
neurotransmitters or precursors.

The chapters by Vernadakis and Cutler (this publ.) illustrate the
possible effect of epigenetic factors, associated with glia, involved
in regulation of neuronal plasticity. Vernadakis proposes that aging
in the CNS may be intimately related to changes in glial cells which
modulate the microenvironment of the aging neuron. This idea is developed into a theory by Cutler (this publ.), the epigenetic-dysdifferen-
tiation model of cellular aging, according to which both cellular environment and intrinsic production of toxic factors might slowly change
the cell from its proper state of differentiation.

5) Possible causes to cell- or synaptic loss.

Several possible causes of cell-or synaptic loss have been discussed, such as genetic factors in age-related programming. As listed
below (see section F.) other causes could be constituted by errors in
cell replication. These changes should affect mainly endothelial or
neuroglial cells since neurons do not usually replicate in adult life.
An error catastrophe in RNA composition, or a translational error,
could have similar consequences, particularly if this would be linked
to changes in specific brain proteins (e.g. S-100 or 14-3-2). Such
neuronal or non neuronal errors in protein synthesis are possible,
however, they have not been demonstrated in the nervous tissue so far
(see E.).

6) Pathological degeneration and neuronal loss.

An analogy between loss and degeneration of neurons under aging
conditions in humans and in cases of extrapyramidal syndromes such as
Parkinson (DA neurons), Guam-Parkinson dementia complex, and Huntington's Chorea (GABA neurons) represents an attractive hypothesis. It is
tempting to suggest that the process of synaptic and neuronal degeneration under these conditions may in fact have a common mechanism.

E. POSSIBLE CHANGES IN NUCLEIC ACIDS FUNCTION AND PROTEIN SYNTHESIS

The following changes have been postulated for other aging tissues but
have not been demonstrated in the nervous system.

1) Changes in thymidine metabolism and DNA synthesis.

Senescent cells (fibroblasts) which are not capable of replicating DNA still periodically activate the enzymes necessary for the synthesis of TTP (thymidine triphosphate) (39). The synthesis of TTP is temporally correlated with the replication of DNA. In this respect, senescent cells differ from quiescent cells and thus may be blocked at a different point of their reproductive cycle.

2) Loss of proliferative capacity.

An exponentially increasing number of cells is unable to respond to serum mitogens by initiating DNA synthesis. This condition which has been found to be true for human fibroblastlike cells (42) does not apply to adult neurons.

3) Metabolic (chronologic) tissue and/or number of replications as determinants of in vitro life span.

Life span of growing cultures is determined by the number of replications. In older cultures other factors such as serum deprivation appear to reduce the replicative potential (4).

4) Alterations of DNA-protein interactions.

A greater degree of DNA-protein interaction in post-mitotic tissues with advancing age has been demonstrated for several tissues including brain from Drosophila melanogaster (6). This may indicate and increase in binding strength of nuclear proteins to DNA.

5) Free radical pathology.

A number of investigators (5) have implicated free radical pathology in the aging process, particularly on the deleterious effect of free radicals on specific biological systems; i.e., membranes, protein and enzyme systems and DNA. A mutant of Drosophila melanogaster has been employed which is totally deficient in its DNA-repair capacity (5). The results indicated that mutations at loci affecting DNA repair capacity can alter species longevity.

F. CHANGES IN THE SYNTHESIS OF FACTORS NECESSARY FOR ADULT NEURONAL SURVIVAL.

Although in embryonic cells the presence of factors such as the NGF have been demonstrated to be indispensable for neuronal survival of dorsal root and sympathetic ganglion cells, no similar factors have yet been identified as necessary for adult neuron survival. Therefore it is still hypothetical to suppose their existence and to think of a possible reduced synthesis or availability during aging. (Table 2)

G. CHANGES IN NEUROENDOCRINE AND IMMUNE SYSTEMS.

Other possible changes may be related a) to the immune system producing immunodeficiency in old animals (e.g. decreased levels in immunoglobulin) or b) to the neuroendocrine system as changes in hormonal secretion (e.g. secretion of "antihormone agents" antagonizing the pituitary secretion). The impact of such changes to the function of the adult nervous system is presently difficult to assess. Various steroid receptors show differential patterns of age loss depending upon brain region and hormone (Roth, this publ.). Serum levels of certain hormones, such as prolactin were found to change significantly in elderly following drugs treatment. An example is the variation of serum prolactin

TABLE 2.

EFFECTS OF AGING ON NEURONAL SURVIVAL AND FUNCTION

EFFECT	SITE OF EFFECT	EFFECT OF AGING
NEURONAL SURVIVAL	NEURON	reduced synthesis of factor
MAINTENANCE OF SYNAPTIC CONTACTS	TARGET ORGAN	reduced synthesis of factor
SYNTHESIS AND REGULATION OF MEMBRANE COMPONENTS	TARGET ORGAN	reduced physiological activity
SYNTHESIS AND REGULATION OF NEUROTRANSMITTERS	NEURON	reduced availability of precursor

THIS SCHEME SHOWS THE POSSIBLE CAUSE AND EFFECT OF AGING PROCESSES ACTING ON VARIOUS BASIC NEURONAL MECHANISMS. THE PRESUMPTIVE SITE OR TARGET IS INCLUDED.

with treatment with ergot-alkaloids in non-psychotic brain-damaged elderly patients (Samorajski et al., this publ.). Serum levels of prolactin may be useful in ascertaining possible effects of drugs in mediating behavioral changes associated with chronic organic brain syndromes (Samorajski et al., this publ.). With regard to age related neuroendocrine modifications, it is of interest that manipulation of 5-HT levels by means of a tryptophan deficient diet induces alteration in neuroendocrine function as well as prolongation of physiologic competence in old rats (Timiras et al., this publ.).

H. CHANGES IN RESPONSE TO NERVE AND PHARMACOLOGICAL STIMULATION.

These changes may be related to either loss or decreases of synapses or to a change in number or in sensitivity of receptors. Most characteristic for the NE system is the decreased response to adrenergic agonists in the aging rat (25). With regard to the cholinergic system, one should recall the changes in negative chronotropic response to vagal stimulation showing an increased threshold to elicit bradycardia (13); the higher sensitivity to the hypotensive action of ACh (12) and the decreased effect of atropine on the heart rate in humans (8). The effect of vagotomy on heart rate is decreased in rats (26) and shows that the vagal control of the heart decreases with old age or, alternatively, that a decrease in sympathetic mediated increase in heart rate occurs.

These results indicate that both the vagus nerve and its cardiac muscarinic receptors show a diminished response with age. However, we are still unable to discriminate the sequence in time of this change.

I. BASIC CHANGES IN PERIPHERAL SYNAPSES AND NEUROMUSCULAR JUNCTIONS.

The following observations seem to be most relevant to the phenomenon of aging in striated muscle of the limbs of rodents:

a) a decrease in number of muscle fibers (17).
b) maintenance of the number of nerve fibers (17).
c) similarity between senile and postdenervation changes reminding of a functional denervation.
d) presence of dedifferentiation mechanism; i.e., fast-slow characteristics tends to be lost.
e) reduction in the level of ChAc activity in limb muscles of old rats which is greater than the fall in number of muscle fibers (48).
f) maintained size of muscle end-plate but more extensive arborization with increased number of terminals per end plate and synaptic vesicle per terminal (Smith, this publ.).
g) decreased levels of ACh per end-plate, smaller quantities of ACh released per action potential. Small alterations in ChAc and AChE activities. The lower levels in ACh are probably due to a limited precursor availability (Smith, this publ.).

The following observations have been reported in the avian ciliary ganglion-iris preparation (15, 30), which support the view that a) presynaptic components are relatively more affected by aging processes than postsynaptic components, b) the major defect in peripheral cholinergic function may be due to a failure in the uptake mechanism of the precursor molecule and in a decreased turnover rate of ACh in the aging synapse (Fig. 1E). The following results from our laboratory which support such a hypothesis are:

a) a significant decrease in ACh and Ch levels starting in the adult.
b) a moderate decrease in AChE and ChAc activity. The changes in AChE activity are not as pronounced as for ChAc.
c) a pronounced decrease in V_{max} values for Ch uptake with changes in its characteristics.
d) a moderate decrease in ABTX (alphabungarotoxin) binding.
e) a significant decrease in ACh turnover rate.

The scheme of Table 3 suggests a mechanism of age-related changes in neuronal mechanisms based on the findings reported above.

DEVELOPMENT OR AGING? A GENERAL DISCUSSION.

The largely descriptive character of our present knowledge of aging processes is emphasized by the abundant list of data and phenomena reported previously. Although the lack of complete and longitudinal studies makes it difficult to reach a conclusion, a continuum may exist between developmental and aging processes. This continuity seems to be more evident at the level of peripheral synapses (Fig. 1). Early changes in cholinergic binding properties as demonstrated by Nordberg et al. (this publ.) in the human hippocampus (period 3 days - 2 years) may indicate developmental features which may be part of a continuous process. A hypothesis of "progressive aging" or of "continuous development" could

TABLE 3.   AGE RELATED CHANGES IN NEURAL MECHANISMS

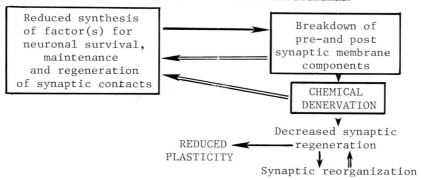

well be accommodated in the epigenetic – dysdifferentiation model of
Culver (this publ.). This theory implies that "developmentally related
changes in hormones and growth factors may slowly damage nerve cells over
a long period of exposure changing the cell from its proper state of differentiation." The question of cellular death as a major cause of aging
is still unsolved. However, it seems clear that a generalized phenomenon
of neuronal loss in all cerebral area does not represent a main feature
of the aging brain. While certain regions of the brain are thought to
lose neurons in the course of aging no neuronal loss has been demonstrated in other regions. In addition, there is a difference between species
(for example between the primate and the rodent brain locus coeruleus)
indicating that they may respond differently to aging. If certain
analogies between developmental and aging processes can be established,
some basic differences seem to emerge from the studies performed at the
level of peripheral synapses (ganglia, neuromuscular junctions and iris)
(Smith et al. and Marchi et al., this publ.). A process of constant regression and constant renewal seems to take place in the adult peripheral
synapse. A positive balance between degeneration and regeneration and a
process of constant "rejuvenation" and plasticity seems to be characteristic for the healthy adult synapse. Aged animals seem to lose the capacity of constant "rejuvenation." According to some authors (41) this
may be due to a decline in the process of terminal sprouting and axonal
regeneration which reverts neuromuscular junctions to structures of a
"smaller size and simpler branching pattern." As the ability of nerve
terminals and axons to sprout and regenerate becomes limited, plasticity
is also reduced. A different interpretation of the phenomenon is presented by others. According to Smith et al. (this publ.) in the aged
muscle the surface area of the end plate region does not change, but significantly more nerve terminals per end plates are present. This may indicate that the normal process of degeneration has slowed down producing
a net increase which is seen as a more extensive arborization. Also more
synaptic vesicles per terminal are seen in the aged terminal, which are
less functional as demonstrated in electrophysiological experiments. As
we have seen in the iris neuromuscular junction (30), the defect in the
cholinergic apparatus is probably not related to a decrease in enzyme
activities or in receptor numbers but rather to lower ACh levels due to
a limited precursor availability (Fig. 1). Given these two contrasting
interpretations of the same phenomenon (Smith, this publ.; (41)), more

studies will be necessary in order to establish which kind of imbalance is present between processes of degeneration and regeneration of aging synapses.

It is apparent from the conclusions of several authors that we are still far from a suggestion for a "rejuvenation" of old synapses. However, it is interesting to note that dietary manipulations of neurotransmitter levels, as proposed by Timiras et al. (this publ.) could lead to a prolongation of physiologic competence in rodents.

Some age associated changes seem to be universally valid for all species investigated so far, they are: neuronal atrophy, presence of lipofuscin, loss of dendritic arborization and astrocytic reactions. The only modifications which seem to be characteristic of the human brain are the so-called neurofibrillary tangles, however, these are seen both in cases of senile dementia and in normal subjects. Other structural changes of nerve terminals, such as poor preservation of synaptic vesicles, accumulation of mitochondria, etc., are now being described (Wisniewski, this publ.). The new findings may contribute to fill the gap between biochemical and pathological findings which has been so far particularly wide in studies of aging of the human brain.

ACKNOWLEDGEMENTS

The investigations carried out in the author's laboratory were supported by PHS grants NS-11496, NS-11430, NS-15086, and NSF grant GB-41475 to E.G. and by grants from the University of Connecticut Research Foundation.

REFERENCES

1.   Brody, H. (1955): J. Comp. Neurol., 102:511-556.
2.   Bondareff, W. (1980): In: Neural Regulatory Mechanisms During Aging, edited by R.C. Adelman, J. Roberts, G.T. Baker, S.I. Baskin, and V.J. Cristofalo, pp. 143-158. Alan R. Liss, Inc., New York.
3.   Colon, E.J. (1972): Psychiat. Neurol. Neurochir. 75:261-270.
4.   Cristofalo, V.J., Palazzo, R., and Charpentier, R.L. (1980): In: Neural Regulatory Mechanisms During Aging, edited by R.C. Adelman, J. Roberts, G.T. Baker, S.I. Baskin, and V.J. Cristofalo, pp. 203-206. Alan R. Liss, Inc., New York.
5.   Daly, R.N., Jacobson, M., Cunningham, E.T., Davis, F.A., and Baker, G.T. (1980): In: Neural Regulatory Mechanisms During Aging, edited by R.C. Adelman, J. Roberts, G.T. Baker, S.I. Baskin, and V.J. Cristofalo, pp. 209-210. Alan R. Liss, Inc. New York.
6.   Darocha, I.B., and Baker, G.T. (1980): In: Neural Regulatory Mechanisms During Aging, edited by R.C. Adelman, J. Roberts, G.T. Baker, S.I. Baskin, and V.J. Cristofalo, pp. 207-208. Alan R. Liss, Inc., New York.
7.   Domino, E.F., Dren, A.T., and Giardina, W.J. (1978): In: Psychopharmacology: A Generation of Progress, edited by M.A. Lipton, A. Di Mascio, and K.F. Killam, pp. 1507-1515. Raven Press, New York.
8.   Dauchot, P., and Gravenstein, J.S. (1971): Clin. Pharmacol. Therap., 12:274.

9. Eisdorfer, C. (1980): In: <u>Neural Regulatory Mechanisms During Aging</u>, edited by R.C. Adelman, J. Roberts, G.T. Baker, S.I. Baskin, and V.J. Cristofalo, pp. 53-69. Alan R. Liss, Inc., New York.
10. Finch, C.E. (1973): <u>Brain Res.</u>, 52:261-276.
11. Fiori, M.G., and Mugnaini, E. (1979): <u>9th Ann. Meet. Soc. Neurosci.</u> Abst. 10, p. 5.
12. Frolkis, V.V. (1968): <u>Triangle</u>, 8:322.
13. Frolkis, V.V., Bezrukov, V.V., Duplenko, Y.K., Shchegoleva, I.V., Shevtchuk, V.G., and Verkhratsky, N.S.(1973): <u>Gerontologia</u>, 19:45.
14. Giacobini, E. (1980): In: <u>Tissue Culture in Neurobiology</u>, edited by E. Giacobini, A. Shahar, and A. Vernadakis, pp. 187-204, Raven Press, New York.
15. Giacobini, E. (1982): In: <u>Advances in Cellular Neurobiology</u>, 3, edited by S. Fedoroff and L. Hertz, Academic Press, New York. (In press).
16. Goldman, G., and Coleman, P.D.(1981): <u>Neurobiol. Aging</u>, 2:33-36.
17. Gutmann, E., and Hanzlikova, V. (1972/73): <u>Mech. Age. Dev.</u> 1:327-329.
18. Hahn, H.P., von (1973): <u>Triangle</u>, 12:149-152.
19. Hinds, J.W., and McNelly, N.A. (1977): <u>J. Comp. Neurol.</u> 171:345-368.
20. Hoffman, D.W., and Giacobini, E. (1980): <u>Brain Res.</u> 201:57-70.
21. Hoffman, D.W., Marchi, M., and Giacobini, E. (1980): In: <u>Neurobiol. of Aging</u>, 1:65-68.
22. Hoffman, D.W., Salzman, S.K., Marchi, M., and Giacobini, E. (1980): <u>J. Neurochem.</u>, 34(6):1785-1787.
23. Jacobson, M. (1978): In: <u>Developmental Neurobiology</u>, 2nd ed. pp. 111-112. Plenum Press, New York.
24. Kanowski, S. (1977): <u>Prog. Neuro-Psychopharmacol.</u> 1:249-256.
25. Kelliher, G.J., and Stoner, S.A. (1978): <u>Gerontology</u>, 18-88.
26. Kelliher, G.J., and Conahan, S.T. (1980): In: <u>Neural Regulatory Mechanisms During Aging</u>, edited by R.C. Adelman, J. Roberts, G.T. Baker, S.I. Baskin, and V.J. Cristofalo, pp. 187-189. Alan R. Liss, Inc., New York
27. Kendrick, Z.V., Goldfarb, A.H., Roberts, J., and Baskin, S.I. (1980): In: <u>Neural Regulatory Mechanisms During Aging</u>, edited by R.C. Adelman, J. Roberts, G.T. Baker, S.I. Baskin, and V.J. Cristofalo, pp. 223-225, Alan R. Liss, Inc., New York.
28. Makman, M.H., Gardner, E.L., Thal, L.J., Hirschhorn, I.D., Seeger, T.F., and Bhargava, G. (1980): In: <u>Neural Regulatory Mechanisms During Aging</u>, edited by R.C. Adelman, J. Roberts, G.T. Baker, S.I. Baskin, and V.J. Cristofalo, pp. 91-127. Alan R. Liss, Inc., New York.
29. Marchi, M., and Giacobini, E. (1980): <u>Dev. Neurosci.</u> 3:39-48.
30. Marchi, M., and Giacobini, E. (1981): In: <u>Proc. Meet. on Cholinergic Mechanisms</u>, edited by G. Pepeu, Plenum Press, New York. (In press).
31. Marchi, M., Giacobini, E., and Hruschak, K. (1979): <u>Dev. Neurosci.</u>, 2:201-212.

32. Marchi, M., Hoffman, D.W., and Giacobini, E. (1980): In: Aging of the Brain and Dementia, edited by L. Amaducci et al., pp. 159–166, Raven Press, New York.

33. Marchi, M., Hoffman, D.W., and Giacobini, E. (1980): In: Neural Regulatory Mechanisms During Aging, edited by R.C. Adelman, J. Roberts, G.T. Baker, S.I. Baskin, and V.J. Cristofalo, pp. 215–219. Alan R. Liss, Inc., New York.

34. Marchi, M., Hoffman, D.W., Giacobini, E., and Fredrickson, T. (1980): Brain Res. 195:423–431.

35. Marchi, M., Hoffman, D.W., Giacobini, E., and Fredrickson, T. (1980): Dev. Neurosci., 3:235–247.

36. Marchi, M., Hoffman, D.W., Mussini, I., and Giacobini, E. (1980): Dev. Neurosci., 3:185–198.

37. Marchi, M., Yurkewicz, L., Giacobini, E., and Fredrickson, T. (1981): Dev. Neurosci., 4:258–266.

38. McGeer, E.G. (1978): In: Alzheimer's Disease: Senile Dementia and Related Disorders, edited by R. Katzman, R. Terry, and K. Bick, Raven Press, New York.

39. Olashaw, N., Kress, E.D., and Cristofalo, V.J. (1980): In: Neural Regulatory Mechanisms During Aging, edited by R.C. Adelman, J. Roberts, G.T. Baker, S.I. Baskin, and V.J. Cristofalo, pp. 195–197, Alan R. Liss, Inc., New York.

40. Orgel, L.E. (1963): Proc. Nat. Acad. Sci. (Wash.) 49, 517.

41. Pestronk, A., Drachman, D.B., and Griffin, J.W. (1980): Exptl. Neurol. 70:65–82.

42. Phillips, P.D., and Cristofalo, V.J. (1980): In: Neural Regulatory Mechanisms During Aging, edited by R.C. Adelman, J. Roberts, G.T. Baker, S.I. Baskin, and V.J. Cristofalo, pp. 199–202. Alan R. Liss, Inc., New York.

43. Ponzio, F., Brunello, N., and Algeri, S. (1978): J. Neurochem. 30:1617–1620.

44. Ruffolo, R., Eisenbarth, G., Thompson, J., and Nirenberg, M. (1978): Proc. Natl. Acad. Sci. USA, 75:2281–2285.

45. Samorajski, T., (1975): In: Aging, 1, edited by H. Brody, D. Herman, and J.M. Ordy, p. 199. Raven Press, New York.

46. Sotelo, C., and Palay, S.L. (1971): Lab. Invest. 25:653–671.

47. Thompson, J.M. (1980): In: Neural Regulatory Mechanisms During Aging, edited by R.C. Adelman, J. Roberts, G.T. Baker, S.I. Baskin, and V.J. Cristofalo, pp. 221–222. Alan R. Liss, Inc., New York.

48. Tucek, S., and Gutman, E. (1973): Expl. Neurol. 38:349–360.

49. Unsworth, B.R., Fleming, L.H., and Caron, P.C. (1980): Mech. Age. Dev. 13:205–217.

50. Vijayashankar, N., and Brody, H. (1979): J. Neuropath. exp. Neurol. 38:490–497.

Subject Index

DATE DUE